Health Informatics

WILLIAM HARVEY LIBRARY

This book is due for return on or before the last date shown below
28 DAY LOAN

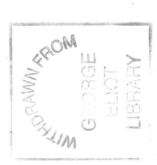

Christoph U. Lehmann • George R. Kim
Kevin B. Johnson
Editors

Pediatric Informatics

Computer Applications in Child Health

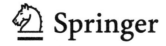 Springer

Editors
Christoph U. Lehmann
The Johns Hopkins School of Medicine
Baltimore, MD
USA

George R. Kim
The Johns Hopkins School of Medicine
Baltimore, MD
USA

Kevin B. Johnson
Vanderbilt University School of Medicine
Nashville, TN
USA

ISBN: 978-1-4419-9294-9 (PB)
ISBN: 978-0-387-76445-0 (HB)   e-ISBN: 978-0-387-76446-7
DOI: 10.1007/978-0-387-76446-7
Springer Dordrecht Heidelberg London New York

Library of Congress Control Number: 2009926513

Series Preface

This series is directed to Health care professionals who are leading the transformation of health care by using information and knowledge. Historically the series was launched in 1988 as Computers in Health Care, to offer a broad range of titles: some addressed to specific professions such as nursing, medicine, and health administration; others to special areas of practice such as trauma and radiology; still other books in the series focused on interdisciplinary issues, such as the computer based patient record, electronic health records, and networked Health care systems. Renamed Health Informatics in 1998 to reflect the rapid evolution in the discipline known as health Informatics, the series continued to add titles that contribute to the evolution of the field. In the series, eminent experts, serving as editors or authors, offer their accounts of innovations in health Informatics. Increasingly, these accounts go beyond hardware and software to address the role of information in influencing the transformation of Health care delivery systems around the world. The series also increasingly focused on the users of the information and systems: the organizational, behavioral, and societal changes that accompany the diffusion of information technology in health services environments.

Developments in health care delivery are constant; most recently developments in proteomics and genomics are increasingly becoming relevant to clinical decision making and emerging standards of care. The data resources emerging from molecular biology are beyond the capacity of the human brain to integrate and beyond the scope of paper based decision trees. Thus, bioinformatics has emerged as a new field in health informatics to support emerging and ongoing developments in molecular biology. Translational informatics supports acceleration, from bench to bedside, i.e. the appropriate use of molecular biology research findings and bioinformatics in clinical care of patients.

At the same time, further continual evolution of the field of Health informatics is reflected in the introduction of concepts at the macro or health systems delivery level with major national initiatives related to electronic health records (EHR), data standards and public health informatics such as the Health care Information Technology Standards Panel (HITSP) in the United States, Canada Health Infoway, NHS Connecting for Health in the UK.

We have consciously retained the series title Health Informatics as the single umbrella term that encompasses both the microscopic elements of bioinformatics and the macroscopic aspects of large national health information systems. Ongoing changes to both the micro and macro perspectives on health informatics will continue to shape health services in the twenty-first century. By making full and creative use of the technology to tame data and to transform information, health Informatics will foster the development and use of new knowledge in health care. As coeditors, we pledge to support our professional colleagues and the series readers as they share advances in the emerging and exciting field of Health Informatics.

Kathryn J. Hannah
Marion J. Ball

Foreword

Clinical informatics by its very nature is flexible, interdisciplinary, and dynamic. Ever changing, ever adjusting to novel clinical needs and emerging information technologies, it focuses upon a constantly moving target. If the field is so dynamic, why is a text still useful in a Web 2.0 era? Two major reasons come to mind.

First, pediatric informatics is a new and emerging field and it is crucial that learners have access to a definitive source that lays out the boundaries of the discipline. This book does just that for the first time and does it well. It will be very apparent to the reader that the discipline is growing exponentially, supporting routine clinical care, offering more timely communications with parents and patients via personal health records, transforming practice through dynamic decision support, linking data to population and public health objectives, and supporting clinical and informatics research.

Second, clinical informatics can enhance equity, safety, efficiency, timeliness, and effectiveness and can make the patient, the child or adolescent along with his or her loved ones much more the center of action. While the book contains chapters on informatics topics that are not unique to pediatrics, its authors focus on the direct linkage of informatics and information technology to pediatric clinical work. They illustrate through many examples the transformative potential of informatics to impact positively on pediatric practice by addressing longstanding weaknesses of solely memory-based clinical care and strengthening connections among families and caregivers through communications technology.

Clinical informatics will play a vital role in defining new standards for clinical excellence. The American Medical Informatics Association (AMIA) believes the pool of health professionals who bring informatics knowledge, attitudes, and skills to clinical domains such as pediatrics must expand and deepen. For the last several years, AMIA has worked (with support from the Robert Wood Johnson Foundation) to create a medical sub-specialty of clinical informatics for all 24 boards recognized by the American Board of Medical Specialties. In 2008, it began active work to strengthening training and establishing informatics certification for other doctorally-prepared clinicians (e.g., nurses, pharmacists, and dentists among others).

I am confident that pediatricians will constitute a solid part of this expanded pool of clinical informaticians. Indeed, until such properly trained pediatric informaticians working in interdisciplinary teams can integrate informatics and communications technology into practice, children and their families will be the lesser for it.

This text will prove useful to a wide set of readers interested in clinical informatics and serve as an anchoring text for the emergence of a new full member of the health care team, the well-trained clinical pediatric informatician.

Don E. Detmer, MD, MA, FACMI, FACS
President and CEO, American Medical Informatics Association, Bethesda, MD
Professor of Medical Education, University of Virginia, Charlottesville, VA

Preface

This book is the product of over 2 years of collaboration by colleagues who have been involved in pediatric informatics. The evolution of this community has been driven by common interests of pediatricians that have coalesced because of increasing concerns about patient safety, the desire to improve and measure the quality of patient care and the growing realization that health information technology has much to offer to improve child health, but that it must be tailored to meet those needs. The growth of the community has been facilitated by the increasing availability and use of e-mail and other communication tools by pediatricians, which has kindled interest.

Many pediatricians became acquainted with pediatric health information technology (health IT) and informatics through a special interest group (SIG), the Section on Computers and Other Technologies (SCOT) in the American Academy of Pediatrics (AAP). This informal group of pediatricians, assembled by pediatrician Byron Oberst, MD FAAP, met once or twice yearly, sharing explorations and experiments with "new" computing technologies (remember the Newton?) in practice. Through the 1990s, the AAP moved from being primarily a paper-based information organization to a "wired" one, moving publications, member notifications (of events such as changes in immunization schedules) and child advocacy to the electronic superhighway. SCOT and the affiliated Task Force on Medical Informatics (TFOMI) became the Steering Committee (SCOCIT) and currently is the Council on Clinical Information Technology (COCIT). Membership grew and COCIT is now a source of educational programs, policy statements, and technical expertise on health IT as it applies to child health and pediatric management.

The community has been buoyed by connections to other communities, ranging from university informatics training programs (supported by the National Library of Medicine), health information exchanges (HIEs), government agencies, patient safety groups and other domains, including pediatric nursing, pediatric pharmacy, and medical education. In all these arenas, there have been pediatric leaders who have helped shape the agenda of pediatric informatics.

We live in an "interesting time" as the US faces many challenges. Pediatric practices face new and growing pressures for accountability and reporting of quality measures as well as the need to improve practice and demonstrate value. Health IT can provide solutions but currently has low adoption in practice and requires financial investment and risk that practices that operate at low margins including safety net clinics may not be able to afford, given the current economic climate and the increasing costs and complexities of care (such as interruptions in vaccine availability). In addition, for pediatric practices, some aspects of health IT and standards is still in development. These factors, among others, have been the driving force for the creation of this text.

The intent of this book is twofold. One is to introduce pediatricians to current concepts in health IT relevant to child health and to provide linkages to available literature, resources and expertise and experience on the various topics covered. The second is to introduce informaticians and other health IT professionals to the needs and nuances of child health with regard to technology and information standards development. It does not replace authoritative texts in pediatrics or medical informatics, but creates necessary connections in this area of clinical informatics.

Christoph U. Lehmann, MD, FAAP
George R. Kim, MD, FAAP
Kevin B. Johnson, MD FAAP

Acknowledgments

The editors would like to acknowledge persons and groups who have contributed directly and indirectly to the completion of this text:

- Marion J. Ball EdD, for creating the opportunity for us to put this together
- The individual chapter authors, for their time and expertise
- Don E. Detmer MD MA, from the American Medical Informatics Association
- Beki Marshall, Jen Mansour and Errol R. Alden MD FAAP from the American Academy of Pediatrics (AAP) and its Council on Clinical Information Technology (COCIT)
- The Johns Hopkins University School of Medicine Divisions of Health Sciences Informatics and Neonatology
- S. Andrew Spooner MD MS FAAP from the Cincinnati Children's Hospital Medical Center for feedback and discussion
- Teresa Gillespie from Vanderbilt University, for editorial assistance and support
- Susan and Jerry Aronson (both MD FAAP), friends, colleagues, mentors, pediatricians, and leaders in advocacy and the use of technology in child health
- The staff at Springer: Cate Rogers Padmaja Sudhaker and Grant Weston for publication support

Christoph U. Lehmann, MD, FAAP
George R. Kim, MD, FAAP
Kevin B. Johnson, MD FAAP

How to Use This book

This book is the first attempt at a comprehensive text on Pediatric Informatics. Compiling the information took over two years and fifty authors. Pediatrics is an ever changing science and research in Pediatric Informatics continues to generate new knowledge. While this book represents the compiled knowledge of the editors and authors of the field, readers are advised to use the information as a basis for further research. This book will serve as a starting point for health IT implementation endeavors, but it does not absolve readers from conducting further due diligence efforts. The editors and the authors are not endorsing any of the products mentioned in this book.

Contents

Part VII   A Vision and Current Landscape of Pediatrics

Contributors

William G. Adams, MD FAAP
Associate Professor of Pediatrics
Director, Child Health Informatics
Department of Pediatrics
Boston University School of Medicine, Boston MA

Michael Apkon, MD PhD FAAP
Associate Clinical Professor of Pediatrics
Yale University School of Medicine
Vice President, Executive Director
Yale-New Haven Children's Hospital, New Haven CT

John M. A. Bohnen, MD FRCSC FACS
Professor of Surgery and Health Policy, Management and Evaluation
Vice-Dean, Clinical Affairs
University of Toronto, Toronto ON Canada

John S. Clark, PharmD MS BCPS
Associate Director of Pharmacy,
Pharmacy Residency Program Director,
University of Michigan Hospitals and Health Centers
Assistant Clinical Professor
University of Michigan College of Pharmacy, Ann Arbor MI

Bernard A. Cohen, MD FAAP
Professor of Dermatology and Pediatrics
The Johns Hopkins University School of Medicine
Director of Pediatric Dermatology
The Johns Hopkins Children's Center, Baltimore MD

Prudence W. Dalrymple, PhD AHIP MS (Informatics)
Director, Institute for Healthcare Informatics
The iSchool at Drexel, College of Information Science & Technology
Drexel University, Philadephia PA

Donna M. D'Alessandro, MD FAAP
Professor of Pediatrics
University of Iowa, Iowa City IA
Communications Director, Academic Pediatric Association
Member, Executive Committee of the Council on Clinical Information
Technology
American Academy of Pediatrics

Mark A. Del Beccaro, MD FAAP
Professor of Pediatrics
Pediatrician-in-Chief, Chief Medical Information Officer
Seattle Children's Hospital, Seattle WA
Policy Committee Chair, Council on Clinical Information Technology
American Academy of Pediatrics

Larry W Desch, MD FAAP
Clinical Associate Professor
Department of Pediatrics
University of Illinois-Chicago School of Medicine, Chicago IL
Developmental Pediatrician
Advocate Health Care, Oak Lawn, IL

Don E. Detmer, MD, MA
President and Chief Executive Officer
American Medical Informatics Association, Bethesda, MD

Willa H. Drummond, MD MS (Informatics)
Professor of Pediatrics, Physiology, and Large Animal Clinical Sciences
Division on Neonatology
University of Florida Colleges of Medicine & Veterinary Medicine,
Gainesville FL
Member, Executive Committee of the Council on Clinical Information
Technology
American Academy of Pediatrics

Mitchell J. Feldman, MD FAAP
Assistant Clinical Professor of Pediatrics
Harvard Medical School
Assistant in Computer Science, Department of Medicine and in Pediatrics
Massachusetts General Hospital, Boston MA

Jeffrey M. Ferranti, MD MS
Associate Chief Information Officer
Enterprise Analytics and Patient Safety
Duke University Health System, Durham NC

Catherine Garger, RN BSN
Nursing Project Analyst
The Johns Hopkins Children's Center, Baltimore, MD

Robert S. Gerstle, MD FAAP
Assistant Professor of Pediatrics
Tufts University School of Medicine, Boston MA
Pediatric Faculty, Division of Academic General Pediatrics
Baystate Medical Center, Springfield MA

Peter S. Greene, MD
Executive Director
MedBiquitous Consortium, Baltimore MD
Chief Medical Information Officer
The Johns Hopkins Medical Institutions, Baltimore MD

Peter R. Holbrook, MD FAAP
Chief Medical Officer
Children's National Medical Center
Professor of Anesthesiology and Critical Care Medicine
George Washington University School of Medicine, Washington DC

Howard E. Jeffries, MD FAAP
Clinical Associate Professor of Pediatrics
Medical Director, Continuous Performance Improvement
Seattle Children's Hospital, Seattle WA

Kevin B. Johnson, MD MS FAAP
Associate Professor & Vice Chair of Biomedical Informatics
Associate Professor of Pediatrics
Vanderbilt University School of Medicine, Nashville TN

George R. Kim, MD FAAP
Research Associate in Pediatrics and Health Sciences Informatics
The Johns Hopkins School of Medicine, Baltimore, Maryland
Member, Executive Committee of the Council on Clinical Information
Technology
American Academy of Pediatrics

Joy Kuhl
Director, Health Information Technology
Alliance for Pediatric Quality
(American Academy of Pediatrics, American Board of Pediatrics,
Child Health Corporation of America and the
National Association of Childrens Hospitals and Related Institutions)
Administrative Co Chair, HL7 Child Health Work Group
Member, CCHIT Child Health Work Group

Paul A. Law, MD MPH FAAP
Director, Medical Informatics
Kennedy Krieger Institute
Assistant Professor of Pediatrics
The Johns Hopkins School of Medicine, Baltimore MD

Christoph U. Lehmann, MD FAAP
Director of Clinical Information Technology
The Johns Hopkins Children's Center
Associate Professor of Pediatrics and Health Sciences Informatics
The Johns Hopkins School of Medicine, Baltimore MD
Member, Board of Directors, American Medical Informatics Association

Harold P. Lehmann, MD PhD FAAP
Associate Professor of Pediatrics and Health Sciences Informatics
The Johns Hopkins University School of Medicine, Baltimore MD

Michael G. Leu, MD MS MHS FAAP
Medical Director, Clinical Effectiveness
Pediatric Hospitalist/Informatician
Seattle Children's Hospital, Seattle WA
Applications Committee Chair, Council on Clinical Information Technology
American Academy of Pediatrics

Donald E. Lighter, MD MBA FAAP FACHE
Director, The Institute for Healthcare Quality Research and Education
Knoxville TN
Professor, College of Business Administration
University of Tennessee, Knoxville TN

Paul H. Lipkin, MD FAAP
Associate Professor of Pediatrics
The Kennedy Krieger Institute
The Johns Hopkins Children's Center, Baltimore, MD

Carol Matlin, RN MS
Pediatric Nurse Educator
The Johns Hopkins Children's Center, Baltimore MD

Anne Matlow, MD FRCPC
Professor of Pediatrics, Laboratory Medicine and Pathobiology
University of Toronto, Toronto ON Canada
Director of the Infection Prevention & Control Programme
Medical Director, Patient Safety
Sick Kids Hospital, Toronto ON Canada

Robert E. Miller, MD
Associate Professor of Pathology, Biomedical Engineering and Health Sciences
Informatics
Director of Pathology Informatics
Johns Hopkins University School of Medicine, Baltimore MD

Sandra H. Mitchell, RPh MSIS
Senior Consultant
maxIT Healthcare, Westfield IN

Declan O'Riordan, DO FAAP
Pediatrician, Neonatal-Perinatal Medicine
St Luke's Children's Hospital, Boise ID

David Mark N. Paperny, MD FSAM FAAP
Adolescent Medicine Specialist
Kaiser Permanente Hawaii, Honolulu HI

Ari H Pollack, MD FAAP
Clinical Instructor of Pediatrics
University of Washington School of Medicine
Informatics Physician
Seattle Children's Hospital, Seattle WA

Peter J. Porcelli Jr., MD MS FAAP
Associate Professor of Pediatrics
Wake Forest University School of Medicine, Winston-Salem, NC

Molly Reyna, BA
Senior Program Manager
Pediatric Telemedicine Program
Children's National Medical Center, Washington, DC

Samuel Trent Rosenbloom, MD MPH FAAP
Assistant Professor, Departments of Biomedical Informatics, Internal Medicine
and Pediatrics
Assistant Professor, School of Nursing
Vanderbilt University School of Medicine, Nashville TN

Craig Sable, MD FAAP FACC
Director, Echocardiography and Pediatric Cardiology Fellowship Training
Medical Director, Telemedicine
Children's National Medical Center
Associate Professor of Pediatrics
George Washington University School of Medicine, Washington DC

Joseph H. Schneider, MD MBA FAAP
Chief Medical Information Officer & Medical Director of Clinical Informatics
Baylor Health Care System, Dallas TX
Chair, Council on Clinical Information Technology
American Academy of Pediatrics

Richard N. Shiffman, MD MCIS FAAP
Professor of Pediatrics
Yale Center for Medical Informatics
Yale University, New Haven CT

Mark M. Simonian, MD FAAP
General solo pediatrician, Clovis CA
Immediate past chair, Council on Clinical Information Technology
American Academy of Pediatrics

Anthony D. Slonim, MD DrPH
Vice President of Medical Affairs
Carilion Medical Center, Roanoke, Virginia
Professor of Internal Medicine, Pediatrics and Public Health
University of Virginia School of Medicine, Charlottesville VA

Valerie Smothers, MA
Deputy Director
MedBiquitous Consortium, Baltimore MD

David C. Stockwell, MD FAAP
Medical Director of Patient Safety
Assistant Professor of Pediatrics
Children's National Medical Center, Washington DC

Allen Y. Tien, MD
Adjunct Associate Professor of Health Sciences Informatics
The Johns Hopkins University School of Medicine, Baltimore MD
Founder, President and Research Director
Medical Decision Logic Inc, Baltimore MD

Toby Vandemark, BA
Consultant in Information Technology, Winter Park FL

Michael A. Veltri, PharmD
Director, Pediatric Pharmacy
The Johns Hopkins Children's Center, Baltimore MD

Carl G. M. Weigle, MD FAAP
Professor of Pediatrics, Medical College of Wisconsin
Chief Medical Information Officer, Children's Hospital of Wisconsin
Member, Children's Specialty Group
Children's Hospital of Wisconsin, Milwaukee WI

Stuart T. Weinberg, MD FAAP
Assistant Professor of Biomedical Informatics and Pediatrics
Vanderbilt University School of Medicine, Nashville TN

Alan E. Zuckerman, MD FAAP
Assistant Professor of Family Medicine
Director of Primary Care Informatics
Georgetown University, Washington DC
Member, Executive Committee of the Council on Clinical Information
Technology
American Academy of Pediatrics

Part I
Introduction to Pediatric Informatics

Chapter 1
Snapshots of Child Health and Information Technology

George R. Kim

> *"In a time of turbulence and change, it is more true than ever that knowledge is power"*
>
> – John F. Kennedy

Health care is in "a time of turbulence and change." One characteristic of this time is the growing awareness by the public, government and health care industry that the safety, cost-effectiveness and outcomes of US medical care can and must improve. Another is the overwhelming belief by policy-makers, health experts and patients that technology will help bring about improvements and savings through better control and accounting of health care processes and information.

For pediatricians and the families for whom they provide care, this time creates new challenges. Children, especially those with special health care needs, encounter barriers to timely appropriate care and are at high risk for harms from medical errors, and there is growing concern among pediatric providers that current health information technologies (health IT), designed for adults, do not meet pediatric needs and may in fact create new vulnerabilities and risks to child health and safety.

For pediatricians, these challenges present opportunities to:

- Bring expertise in child health to technology developers to create information tools and standards that will make pediatric practice safer, more efficient and that will optimize and strengthen the value of pediatric care.
- Share evidence and experience on successful strategies for adopting health IT into pediatric workflows that minimize risk to patients and maximize benefits to all.

1.1 Organization of the Book

This book presents medical, technical, organizational, and economic perspectives on information technology in child health, drawing on shared expertise from general and specialty pediatrics, health care leadership, pediatric nursing, pharmacy, medical education, quality and safety, and information technology. In many chapters, contributors have provided Case Studies that illustrate or expand on some aspect of their topics, through discussion of literature references and/or specific or hypothetical examples.

- **Part I** begins the book with a general introduction to pediatric informatics.
- **Part II** covers the distinct information needs of pediatric care, in general and for specific populations: neonates, adolescents, children with special health care needs and in emergency and critical care situations.
- **Part III** covers the pediatric data-knowledge-care continuum, starting with a discussion of the complexities of health care processes and how standardization seeks to reduce their inherent risks. This is followed by an introduction to the use of evidence-based medicine tools, guidelines and online knowledge resources for pediatric practice, and concludes with a description of how IT standards are and will be used to track continuous professional development of pediatricians.
- **Part IV** covers informatics in pediatric ambulatory care, beginning with a business case for the Medical Home and discussions of prioritization and alignment of health IT in small and large practices. This is followed by discussions about specific health IT tools: electronic health records, electronic prescribing, telemedicine, personal health records, privacy issues, electronic mail, and online practice portal tools.
- **Part V** covers informatics and pediatric inpatient practice, beginning with an overview and discussions on different steps of the medication delivery: prescribing/ordering (computerized provider order entry/CPOE), dispensing (pharmacy information systems) and administration (bar-coding, radio-frequency identification, smart pumps, electronic medication administration records). The section concludes with two chapters on preventing and reporting errors.
- **Part VI** covers "frontier" or development areas in pediatric informatics: health information exchanges, pediatric data and terminologies and informatics in pediatric research.
- **Part VII** concludes the book with an example of a vision of pediatric care using tools discussed in previous sections and a listing of organizations that form a community of practice for pediatric informatics.

The aim of this text is to promote knowledge sharing within the pediatric community on the opportunities and challenges that health IT presents to improving child health. With no pretense to being comprehensive, it serves as an introduction to pediatric informatics concepts for ongoing discussion among child health professionals as health IT adoption progresses.

Chapter 2
Informatics and Pediatric Health Care

Kevin B. Johnson and George R. Kim

Objectives

- To introduce basic concepts of clinical informatics in pediatrics
- To outline the roles of pediatricians in clinical informatics
- To provide pointers in current thinking about informatics training for clinicians

2.1 Introduction

The incorporation of information technology (IT) to improve the quality, safety, and efficiency of medical care has gained popularity among the public, policy-makers, and clinicians. The application of IT tools to address the special vulnerabilities of children, to meet the data needs of their care and to avert medical errors and their consequences, is natural if not compelling. However, the successful and safe adoption of IT into pediatric care requires participation of professionals who understand both child health and clinical informatics.

2.2 The Special Needs of Children

The pediatric mantra that children "are not just little adults" reflects their special needs and vulnerabilities that must be considered when planning health interventions that are safe and effective. The distinctions and special needs (physiologic, psychosocial, and demographic) of children, apart from adults, create data management challenges that must be addressed in a systematic and comprehensive fashion to provide the best care within a technology-driven health care environment.

Children (as a population) are diverse and complex, across dimensions of growth (premature infants to young adults), development (precocious and age-appropriate to significant delay), health (well children to those with special health care needs) and socio-economic status. Pediatric care affects a diverse and complex population within a health care system that is itself complex and largely designed for adults. As child advocates, pediatricians must assure that all health systems and clinical environments

C.U. Lehmann et al. (eds.), *Pediatric Informatics: Computer Applications in Child Health,* Health Informatics,
© Springer Science+Business Media, LLC 2011

Infant Mortality, 2005

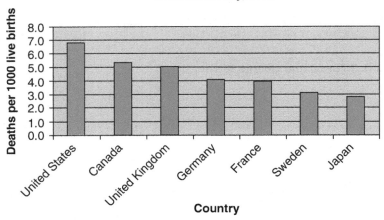

Fig. 2.1 Infant mortality by country, 2005[1]

that provide medical care for children do so with the highest quality and safety. As partners in child health, pediatricians must lead and educate others about the special needs of children in different age/developmental stages[1,2] and health categories.[3]

Despite efforts to assure equitable care for all children, including outreach to poor and disenfranchised populations (federally qualified health care centers,[4] mobile vans to provide vaccines and care in urban areas,[5] free vaccine programs[6]), the US health care system, while state-of-the-art, has largely failed to achieve clinical outcomes commensurate with its national financial investment in comparison with other industrialized nations. Infant mortality rates continue to be high (Fig. 2.1) in comparison to other countries, disparities in immunization rates persist[7] and patient safety statistics show a need for improvement.[8,9]

2.3 Clinical Informatics in Meeting Pediatric Health Needs

Pediatrics is concerned with the health of infants, children, and adolescents; their growth and development; and their opportunity to achieve full potential as adults. Pediatricians must be concerned not only with particular organ systems and biologic processes, but also with environmental and social influences, which have a major impact on the physical, emotional, and mental health and social well-being of children and their families.[10] Pediatricians have diagnostic tools, medications, and vaccines to promote well-being, but most importantly, pediatricians possess knowledge of children and their illnesses and data derived from their care. Informatics and information technology have great potential to leverage clinical data to improve health outcomes.

Biomedical informatics is the science and technology of understanding and managing data and knowledge to solve health problems. This rapidly evolving field can be broadly divided into two domains: *bioinformatics* (genetic and genomic data and knowledge as they relate subcellular processes to health) and *clinical informatics* (the management of medical data and knowledge as they relate to the health of individuals, families, communities, and populations).

Clinical informatics, the focus of this book, has been in existence for over 30 years. In the past decade, it has received increasing interest as the adoption of health IT tools have been promoted as a solution to improve patient safety, efficiency, and cost effectiveness. Pediatric informatics, a subset, can be defined as "clinical informatics that advances child health," and as such, is a translational field, in that it transforms results from information science and technology into new methods and tools for diagnosis, therapy, and prevention and into general pediatric practice.[11] The increasing availability of IT environments that allow rapid development of operational tools and the progressive adoption of computational tools into health care infrastructures have facilitated the translation of pilot projects into successful production-level applications without extensive technical expertise by clinical innovators.

IT functions that can improve quality and safety in health care include: speeding and organizing access to longitudinal personal health data and related information, standardizing and streamlining communication and transactions, automating tracking and auditing, providing decision support and clinician guidance, translating evidence into practice, and reusing clinical data for practice and public health planning. IT functions that can improve the efficiency and cost-effectiveness of care include: standardizing and automating documentation, reducing clerical and transcription errors, coordinating care services, and improving the accuracy of charge capture. To take advantage of these IT functionalities, health care systems must have a common infrastructure that spans and connects many health institutions and entities (hospitals, physician offices, pharmacies, laboratories, etc.) to enable real-time data sharing, as advocated by the IOM[12] and other leaders in health care.

However, as there is great promise, there are also caveats to disseminating information technology in health care. First, technology must solve the problems for which it was intended. Although there may be evidence that a particular technology will improve safety, its inappropriate implementation may have unintended and/or hazardous consequences. Second, sufficient planning and resources must be allocated to assure a viable and sustainable deployment. The business plan for a technical solution must include pragmatic considerations for its continuation and growth. Third, clinician and cultural resistance to adopting new technologies can be strong, especially if applications unproven in practice are associated with high financial investments and require major organizational and behavior change. Past bad experiences with specific applications may cause practitioners to question and oppose the adoption of health IT. Thus, clinical informatics goes beyond the realm of IT alone and into its interactions with people, organizations, and processes as they affect health outcomes.

2.4 Pediatricians' Role in Health Information Technology Adoption

As advocates for children, pediatricians should be very interested in health information technology and its adoption into practice for several reasons.

2.4.1   Improving the Quality and Safety of Pediatric Care Requires Detailed Medical Knowledge of Children's Needs and of the Problems in Health Care Processes

In addition to the previously described statistics, other findings include the Institute of Medicine (IOM) report *To Err is Human*[99] finding that 44,000–98,000 people die in hospitals each year as a result of preventable medical errors. A recent study from the New England Journal of Medicine revealed that (similar to adults) children receive approximately half of indicated care in acute and preventive care.[13] The Joint Commission has reported that children may be at three times the risk that adults have for medication errors.[14] Efforts to improve safety have started at pediatric hospitals, such as collaborations through the Child Health Corporation of America (CHCA)[15] with the Institute for Health Care Improvement (IHI, led by pediatrician Donald Berwick), including the development of data-driven "trigger" tools to identify proactively adverse drug events in neonatology[16] and pediatric inpatients.[17] To achieve the ideal of "Do no harm," pediatricians must take the lead in reducing harm that is inherent in the health system.

In addition to being able to provide clinical insights for tools such as weight-based drug dosing algorithms for electronic prescribing and age-based decision support, pediatricians have insights weaknesses in the information infrastructure. In day-to-day care, practitioners routinely make clinical decisions with incomplete and fragmented patient data: lost immunization records, missing specialist reports for the child with special health care needs, unavailable medical histories of children in foster care are common problems for pediatricians. In addition, practitioners have firsthand experience with the time demands of practice and information overload and other barriers to providing effective preventive care.[18–21] Historically, pediatricians have collective experience with efforts and difficulties in creating and sustaining registries and information systems to track and assure immunizations, blood lead and newborn metabolic screening. For these reasons, pediatricians are essential to the incorporation of health IT into pediatric practice.

2.4.2   Improving the Quality and Safety of Information Tools for Pediatrics Requires Pediatrician Advocacy in Technology Development

A primary function that a pediatrician trained in informatics serves in health IT adoption is to understand which questions must be asked about information systems, their possibilities, their application, their use by clinicians, and their limitations. These questions are the subject of active research in informatics as they are informed by pediatric and child health agendas. A sample of these questions is outlined in Table 2.1.

The purpose of questions is to stimulate dialogue with information technology developers and to educate them on the needs of pediatrics. In turn, developers can guide pediatricians in focusing their clinical knowledge and representing them explicitly as data, in the perspectives, interpretations, and granularity required to assure correct execution by applications. Thus, pediatricians also serve as child advocates at the developers' table.

As with many fields, the bulk of published evidence supporting the value of clinical informatics has been derived from data involving (nonpregnant, nongeriatric) adults. This limits generalization of findings to other populations, neglecting important distinctions between general adult medicine and pediatrics (for example) that may affect the design, implementation, and outcomes of interventions that use clinical informatics applications. Examples of distinctions between pediatric and adult medicine data needs are listed in Table 2.2.

Health IT advocacy may go beyond the institutions in which pediatricians practice. Much of pediatric informatics data and research has been derived from academic pediatric centers, and often in inpatient settings. However, much of pediatric care occurs in ambulatory settings and in community hospitals, in which children and infants receive care but where there may be no certified pediatricians.[22]

Table 2.1 Sample questions for pediatric informatics

Pediatric area of concern	Special clinical informatics issues
Premature infants and their associated medical problems	How can clinical systems automatically adjust to expected developmental ages and needs of premature infants?
Injury prevention	How can injuries be prevented in inpatient settings?
	How can parent knowledge about injury risks be assessed and improved by primary care practitioners?
	How can physician/parent adherence to injury prevention guidelines be improved?
Well child care	What are the advantages of well-child care documentation by computer?
Congenital issues (anomalies AND disease)	How should pediatricians be trained in the age of genomic medicine?
Drug prescribing	How can errors and miscommunications in weight-based prescriptions for children be reduced or eliminated?
Office of the future	How might pediatric office visits better utilize telemedicine/teleconferencing to better inform caregivers?
	How might aggregate public health data improve home management and triage? How should the privacy considerations for adolescents be managed in the electronic age?
Parent engagement (systems approach to care)	How can personal health records improve parent activation?
	What is the impact of improved school information systems on medication adherence?

2.4.3 Regulation and Legislation of Health Information Tools and Their Use in Child Health Requires Active Input from Pediatric Clinicians

Another area of health IT advocacy in which pediatricians need to serve is in legislative and regulatory issues regarding pediatric-specific IT. The organizational and political drive to improve patient safety through the adoption of HIT has many stakeholders including patient groups, physicians, nurses, health care administrators, and regulators. In addition, the business case to improve efficiency and decrease costs, and the increasing availability of tools and techniques that facilitate application development and evaluation have created a marketplace with vendors

Table 2.2 Distinctions between adult and pediatric data

Clinical data	Adult nuances	Pediatric nuances
Age	Unit granularity (years, months)	Unit granularity (years, months, weeks, days, hours) Correction for prematurity
Body measures	Weight (not required)	Weight (required)
	Height	Height
		Head circumference
		Age-specific normal percentiles
Blood pressure	Arm side (left, right)	Extremity (arm, leg)
	Position (standing, sitting, supine)	Extremity side (left, right)
		Cuff size used (neonatal, pediatric, adult)
		Age/gender specific norms
HR, RR	Normal ranges	Age-specific normals
Temperature	Route (oral, otic)	Route (oral, otic, rectal, axillary)
		Route-specific normal values
Laboratory values	Normal range of values	Age-adjusted values
Drug doses	Usually single dose amount (occasionally wt/BSA based)	Usually weight/BSA based (up to adult dose amount)
Immunizations	Infrequent (except influenza vaccination)	Frequent during years 1, 2
		Age-based sequence and timing to achieve adequate protection
Basal Fluid requirements	1,000–1,500 cc/day	Usually higher relative need due to increased BSA/ weight ratio and metabolic expenditures
X-Ray radiation dose	Standard dose?	Much less for infants

and entrepreneurs eager to partner with health care providers. The pediatric portion of the market place is small, but important, which is driven by advocacy for pediatric-specific applications. As applications and their use become standard, legislation and regulation of health IT adoption and use (as a sign of quality) is becoming more prevalent, in the forms of increased reporting requirements by practices and pay-for-performance[23] driven by sentinel events and pressures from stakeholders. This is met by resistance to change without incentives, since the burden and risk of health IT adoption belongs to practices while the go not only to patients, but to health insurance payors, information technology vendors and regulatory commissions (who benefit from increased knowledge from reporting). Therefore, it is in pediatricians' interest to lead in the technical, organizational, political, and the economic aspects of pediatric health IT adoption.

2.5 Pediatricians' Training in Informatics

The training required by pediatricians to perform these functions varies, depending on the location and nature of practice (inpatient setting, pediatric hospital, academic medical center, ambulatory practice of varying sizes, rural or urban, etc.). To remain competitive, practitioners will need to understand how to leverage information technology as a part of business. In addition to using electronic health records (Chapters 15, 18), and electronic prescribing (Chapter 19) for health maintenance and disease management,[22-26] practices will integrate pediatric disease-based clinical practice guidelines into standard workflows. In addition, adoption of new information tools such as the Internet by families as an adjunct source of health information stimulates health discussions with their providers.[27]

Health IT has been embraced by new pediatric graduates within their training (as a part of systems-based practice[28] and patient safety[29]), with appreciation of the functionality that health IT plays in reporting quality metrics to governmental and regulatory agencies. Beyond general knowledge and awareness of health IT use, practitioners will likely participate in additional learning of information technology and informatics for advanced learning. Programs vary in length of time, financial investment and the depth of knowledge. Short programs are offered by the American Medical Informatics Association (AMIA 10 × 10 program[30]), Stanford University[31] and the National Library of Medicine,[32] with longer programs offered by universities funded by the National Library of Medicine,[33] up to and including doctoral and postdoctoral programs.

Curricula vary according to local expertize. Beyond the United States, the International Medical Informatics Association (IMIA) supports a "world-wide systems approach to health care...that is supported by informatics-based information and communication systems and technologies." A scientific map of the breadth and the depth of informatics knowledge in the context of clinical science is shown in Table 2.3 serves to guide the development of formal training programs.

Table 2.3 IMIA scientific knowledge map[34,35]

Applied technology	Infrastructure	Data related	Applications and products	Human – organizational	Education and knowledge
Algorithms	Archival repository systems for medical records- EPR-CPR-EMR	Classification	Biostatistics	Assessment	Bibliographic
Bioinformatics	Authentication	Coding systems	Clinical trials	Compliance	Cognitive learning
Bio-signal processing	Chip cards in health care	Concept representation-preservation	Computer-supported surgery	Cognitive tasks	Computer aided instruction
Boolean logic	Distributed systems	Data acquisition-data capture	Decision support	Collaboration	Computer-supported Training
Cryptology	Health professional workstation	Data analysis-extraction tools	Diagnosis related	Communication	Consumer education
Human genome related	Interfaces	Data entry	Disease mgt.-EPR-CPR-EMR	Economics of IT	Continuing education
Human interfaces	Knowledge based systems	Data policies	Epidemiological research	Ethics	Digital libraries
Image processing	Networks	Data protection	Hospital IS	Implementation-deployment	E-business
Mathematical models in medicine	Neural networks	Database design	Event-based systems	Diffusion of IT	Health/medical informatics education
Pattern recognition	Pen based	Indexing	Evidence based guidelines	Evaluation	Information management-dissemination
	Security	Syntax	Expert systems	Human factors	Knowledge bases
	Speech recognition	Language representation	Health services research	Legal issues, implementing national laws	Knowledge
		Lexicons	HIS management	Management	
				Managing change	
				Needs assessment	

Standards
Systems architecture
Telehealth
User interfaces

Linguistics
Modeling
Nomenclatures
Standards
Terminology-vocabulary
Thesaurus tools

Knowledge-based systems
Laboratory data
Image processing
Operations/resource management
Outcomes research and measurement
Quality management
Patient identification
Patient monitoring
Minimum data sets
Supply chain
Telematics
Telemedicine

Organizational redesign processes
Organizational transformation
Planning
Policy issues
Privacy
Project Management
Security
Strategic plans
Unique Identifiers
User-computer management
Learning models
Online/distance education

Clinical Disciplines: Anesthesia, Behavioral, Cardio/Thoracic, Cardiovascular, Dentistry, Dermatology, Emergency Medicine, Environmental health, Gastroenterology, Human genetics, Internal Medicine, Neurosurgery, Nursing, Obstetrics & Gynecology, Ophthalmology, Orthopedics, Pathology, Pediatrics, Pharmacy, Primary care, Psychiatry, Radiology, Surgery, Urology

2.6 Conclusion

As the adoption of health information technology into clinical infrastructures becomes more of a reality, pediatricians will need to advocate for the needs of children and pediatrics in technical development, in incentive alignment, in resource allocation and in regulatory issues. The contents of this book describe current informatics work in many of the different sub-domains of pediatrics. As clinical informatics disciplines from pediatrics, nursing, pharmacy, and others mature and converge, it may one day be unnecessary to maintain the distinctions of pediatric informatics as health systems meet the goals of providing the best in quality and safe care for all children.

References

1. American Academy of Pediatrics, Maternal Child Health Bureau. Bright Futures; 2008. Available at: http://brightfutures.aap.org. Accessed April 22, 2008.
2. Brazelton TB. *To Listen to a Child: Understanding the Normal Problems of Growing Up*. New York: Da Capo Press; 1992.
3. American Academy of Pediatrics, Council on Children with Disabilities. Care coordination in the medical home: integrating health and related systems of care for children with special health care needs. *Pediatrics*. 2005;116:1238–1244.
4. Hoag SD, Norton SA, Rajan S. Fderally qualified health centers: surviving Medicaid managed care, but not thriving. *Health Care Financ Rev*. 2000;22(2):103–117.
5. The Children's Health Fund. National Network. Available at: http://www.childrenshealthfund.org/programs/index.php. Accessed April 22, 2008.
6. Rosenthal J, Rodewald L, McCauley M, et al. Immunization coverage levels among 19- to 35-month-old children in 4 diverse, medically underserved areas of the United States. *Pediatrics*. 2004 April;113(4):e296–302.
7. Smith PJ, Stevenson J. Racial/ethnic disparities in vaccination coverage by 19 months of age: an evaluation of the impact of missing data resulting from record scattering. *Stat Med*. 2008; 27(20):4107–18.
8. Smith RB, Cheung R, Owens P, Wilson RM, Simpson L. Medicaid markets and pediatric patient safety in hospitals. *Health Serv Res*. 2007 October;42(5):1981–1998.
9. Kohn KT, Corrigan JM, Donaldson MS. *To Err Is Human: Building a Safer Health System*. Washington, DC: National Academy Press; 1999.
10. Organisation for Economic Co-operation and Development. OECD Health Data; 2007. Available at: http://www.ecosante.org/index2.php?base=OCDE&langs=ENG&langh=ENG&ref=YES&sessionid=17e0465732f39d116056695b6334ca93. Accessed April 22, 2008.
11. Stanton B, Behrman RE. Overview of pediatrics. In: Kliegman RM, Behrman RE, Jensen HB, Stanton BF, eds. *Nelson Textbook of Pediatrics*. 18th ed. Philadelphia, PA: Saunders; 2007.
12. Woolf SH. The meaning of translational research and why it matters. *JAMA*. 2008 Jan 9;299(2):211–213.
13. Aspden P, Corrigan JM, Wolcott J, Erickson SM. *Patient safety: Achieving a new standard for care*. Washington, DC: National Academy Press; 2003.
14. Mangione-Smith R, DeCristofaro AH, Setodji CM et al. The quality of ambulatory care delivered to children in the United States. *N Engl J Med*. 2007 October 11;357(15):1515–1523.
15. The Joint Commission. Sentinel Event Alert: Preventing Pediatric Medication Errors. Issue 39; 2008. Available at: http://www.jointcommission.org/SentinelEvents/SentinelEventAlert/sea_39.htm. Accessed April 22, 2008.

16. Child Health Corporation of America. CHCA Website; 2008. Available at: http://www.chca.com/index_flash.html. Accessed April 22, 2008.
17. Sharek PJ, Horbar JG, Mason W, et al. Adverse events in the neonatal intensive care unit: development, testing, and findings of a NICU-focused Trigger Tool to identify harm in North American NICUs. *Pediatrics*. 2006;118(4):1332–1340.
18. Takata GS, Mason W, Taketomo C, Logsdon T, Sharek PJ. Development, testing, and findings of a pediatric-focused trigger tool to identify medication-related harm in US children's hospitals. *Pediatrics*. April 2008;121(4):e927–e935.
19. Reisinger KS, Bires JA. Anticipatory guidance in pediatric practice. *Pediatrics*. 1980; 66(6):889–892.
20. LeBaron CW, Rodewald L, Humiston S. How much time is spent on well-child care and vaccinations? *Arch Pediatr Adolesc Med*. 1999:153(11):1154–1159.
21. Frame PS. Health maintenance in clinical practice: strategies and barriers. *Am Fam Physician*. 1992;45(3):1192–1200.
22. Kuo AA, Inkelas M, Lotstein DS, Samson KM, Schor EL, Halfon N. Rethinking well-child care in the United States: an international comparison. *Pediatrics*. 2006;118(4):1692–1702.
23. Freed GL, Uren RL, Hudson EJ, Lakhani I, Wheeler JR, Stockman JA 3rd. Research Advisory Committee of the American Board of Pediatrics. Policies and practices related to the role of board certification and recertification of pediatricians in hospital privileging. *JAMA*. 2006;295(8):905–912.
24. Cusack CM. Electronic health records and electronic prescribing: promise and pitfalls. *Obstet Gynecol Clin North Am*. 2008;35(1):63–79, ix.
25. Cooley KA, Frame PS, Eberly SW. After the grant runs out. Long-term provider health maintenance compliance using a computer-based tracking system. *Arch Fam Med*. 1999;8(1):13–17.
26. Frame PS. Automated health maintenance reminders: tools do not make a system. *J Am Board Fam Pract*. 2003;16(4):350–351.
27. Frame PS, Zimmer JG, Werth PL, Hall WJ, Eberly SW. Computer-based vs manual health maintenance tracking. A controlled trial. *Arch Fam Med*. 1994;3(7):581–588.
28. Christakis DA, Zimmerman FJ, Rivara FP, Ebel B. Improving pediatric prevention via the internet: a randomized, controlled trial. *Pediatrics*. 2006;118(3):1157–1166.
29. Accreditation Council for Graduate Medical Education. (2007) Common Program Requirements: General Competencies; 2007. Available at: http://www.acgme.org/outcome/comp/GeneralCompetenciesStandards21307.pdf. Accessed April 23, 2008.
30. Singh R, Naughton B, Taylor JS, et al. Comprehensive collaborative patient safety residency curriculum to address the ACGME core competencies. *Med Educ*. 2005;39(12):1195–1204.
31. American Medical Informatics Association. AMIA 10×10 Website; 2008. Available at: http://www.amia.org/10×10/. Accessed April 23, 2008.
32. Stanford University. Medical Informatics Introductory Short Crse (Online); 2008. Available at: http://bmir.stanford.edu/pages/view.php/education. Accessed April 23, 2008.
33. Marine Biology Laboratory, National Library of Medicine. BioMedical Informatics Course; 2008. Available at: http://courses.mbl.edu/mi/. Accessed April 23, 2008.
34. National Library of Medicine. NLM's University-based Biomedical Informatics Research Training Programs; 2008. Available at: http://www.nlm.nih.gov/ep/GrantTrainInstitute.html. Accessed April 23, 2008.
35. International Medical Informatics Association. Towards IMIA 2015 - the IMIA Strategic Plan; 2007. Available at: http://www.imia.org/images/imia_strategic_plan.pdf. Accessed April 23, 2008.
36. International Medical Informatics Association, Working Group 1. Health and Medical Informatics Education. Recommendations of the International Medical Informatics Association (IMIA) on Education in Health and Medical Informatics. *Meth Inf Med*. 2000;39:267–277.

Part II
Special Considerations in Pediatric Care

Chapter 3
Core Pediatric Data

Kevin B. Johnson, Stuart T. Weinberg and George R. Kim

Objectives

- To distinguish pediatrics from other medical domains in terms of clinical data
- To outline a framework of core pediatric data, knowledge, and functionality to articulate information needs for different tasks

3.1 Introduction

The distinguishing characteristic of pediatrics as a unique medical domain is the breadth and depth of human growth and development that it covers. The range and variation in these parameters create many contexts in which clinical and administrative data is collected, interpreted, and used to provide appropriate care: to diagnose, plan, and manage therapy of an individual child's illness, to create relevant and effective care on group and population levels, and to study the needs of child health.

Consider the following vignettes:

- *You are in the newborn nursery evaluating a 1-day-old baby who has begun to grunting and is showing evidence of jaundice.*
- *You are in office seeing a toddler whose mother states that this morning the child has begun to have difficulty breathing, has had a yellowing of his eyes and has been urinating dark brown.*
- *You are in the emergency department of your local hospital seeing a teenager who has complained of chest pain on deep breathing, feels tired and has noted a yellowing of her skin and eyes.*

With only the above pieces of information being presented, the clinical thought process is guided by the pediatrician's knowledge of relevant issues in the each age category, which demands specific clinical data:

C.U. Lehmann et al. (eds.), *Pediatric Informatics: Computer Applications in Child Health,* Health Informatics,
© Springer Science+Business Media, LLC 2011

- For the infant, initial clinical questions surround the maternal and perinatal history: the gestational age of the infant, the results of prenatal screening tests (including those for bacterial and viral infections and blood types), the medical condition and treatment of the mother prior to delivery.
- For the toddler, questions will revolve around the child's recent illnesses, activities, and exposures, presence of fever, to be confirmed by examination and laboratory testing.
- For the adolescent, the questions will include medical and family history, medications, exposures to sexual contacts and substance use, in addition to reports of similar illnesses from the patient's family and community.

The different lists of questions (plus others that are not included), their appropriate choice and use to create differential diagnoses to guide further testing, treatment, and outreach and follow-up are second nature to most practicing pediatricians, based on clinical training and experience.

3.2   Core Data, Knowledge, and Functionality

The organization and codification of clinical questions, their answers and their contexts for communication with other practitioners and for use in computerized systems begins with three levels of abstraction of the information needs of pediatricians for specific tasks (such as patient care, administration, and research).

Core clinical data is a basic set of defined medical, historical, and demographic information about a patient or set of patients necessary for specified clinical tasks. Core clinical data is typically in text, numerical, or categorical forms, although it may also consist of multimedia (imaging, audio) or complex (genomic, physiologic (ECG, EEG)) forms in the future. Example of core clinical data include: patient identifiers, examination findings, and laboratory results for a patient or set of patients at a given date and time.

Core clinical knowledge is a synthesis of core clinical data from a patient or set of patients that provides medical meaning or significance in the context of clinical tasks. One example of core clinical knowledge is a list of reference values for normal blood pressures and weights of children over different age ranges based upon a statistical inference of measurements from a large population of healthy children at different ages.

Core clinical functionality is the application of clinical knowledge and patient data within the context of a clinical task. Examples include: the generation of an appropriate dose (from a pediatric formulary) of a specific medication according to a patient's weight (from a patient record) for an outpatient prescription and the automated calculation of a patient's body mass index according to a patient's height, weight, and population normal values for a pre-participation sports physical examination.

3.3 Pediatric Information Tasks Across the Age Spectrum

Tasks that use clinical data, knowledge, and functionalities include the collection, storage, retrieval, and use of longitudinal patient information for clinical decision-making and health maintenance. These tasks include:

- **Coordinating maternal and newborn health information**
  - Collecting, recording, interpreting, and sharing genetic histories for prenatal counseling and family planning
  - Linking prenatal care data with infant birth information for timely and emergent care and health maintenance (newborn metabolic and hearing screening)
  - Aggregating maternal and neonatal outcomes data for research and quality improvement

- **Tracking and reporting of immunization information**
  - Collecting and recording immunization administration dates from clinic encounters
  - Providing decision support and reminders for timely completion of immunization series according to periodic schedules
  - Generating vaccination reports for individuals, practices, and populations

- **Monitoring and documentation of growth and development**
  - Recording and presenting changes in weight, height, head circumference over sequential visits
  - Calculating body mass index values over time, in health maintenance and as part of weight management
  - Tracking growth over time within the context of medication therapy (such as for attention deficit/hyperactivity disorder (AD/HD))

- **Providing age-appropriate medication dosing and laboratory test result interpretation**
  - Recommending weight-based dosing of specific drugs
  - Alerting prescribers to known adverse reactions
  - Checking dose-range limits
  - Rounding to safe and convenient doses (such as school day dosing)
  - Incorporating age-based normal values based on published values

- **Protecting patient privacy appropriately**
  - Restricting record access to guardians
  - Including patient access for emancipated minors
  - Assuring adolescent privacy for substance abuse and sexuality issues
  - Providing appropriate emergency access to records

- **Identifying patient data accurately and precisely**
  - Tracking patient name changes (such as for newborns)
  - Handling information on patients with ambiguous gender

- Presenting numerical data to the appropriate precision (weight in grams and age in hours for newborns and in kilograms, years, and months for older children)

3.4 Pediatric Core Data for Practice Administration

A common use of data is for practice administration functions, such as billing. Core data includes patients' demographic and insurance information, dates of encounters, assigned diagnoses, and services used (including pharmacy prescriptions).

Claims data can be used to study service utilization and to improve health outcomes. One example is the use of immunization information systems to identify children with asthma for influenza vaccination reminders[1] for Medicaid populations. The biases of claims data such as incompleteness (in identifying all patients at risk) can limit generalization of use of such data. However, administrative medication claims data may show adverse health trends, such as one study which showed an association of high pharmacy cost-sharing with lower use of bronchodilators, inhaled corticosteroids, and leukotriene receptor antagonists in for children in private drug plans.[2]

Claims data may be used to assess quality in ambulatory care, however, it frequently underestimates measures. Although this is the most readily available data in most practices, its current use is limited in clinical tasks related to quality and safety.[3]

3.5 Pediatric Core Data for Clinical Care

In addition to the framework of data/knowledge/functionality and general clinical information tasks, core data can be specified on the basis of age groups (premature and term newborns, infants, toddlers, school-aged children, preteens, adolescents, and young adults) and populations with specific needs and conditions (well children, children with special health care needs, precocious children, foster children, children with chronic and acute disease). Each group and condition range has specific core data:

- Infants: Chapter 4
- Adolescents: Chapter 5

Forms and templates, as organizing devices for structured communication and recording of core clinical data are well known to practitioners. The adaptation and conversion of structured (and unstructured) data for use in electronic records, practice management systems, health registries, and other tools that share pediatric personal health information require consensus and planning:

- Structured data for electronic health records: Chapter 18
- Pediatric data standards and terminologies: Chapters 32 and 33
- Structured data for research: Chapter 34

3.6 Pediatric Core Data for Quality Improvement and Clinical Research

The potential of pediatric data to provide insights for improvements in quality and safety for patient care and population health outcomes has been well appreciated.

The federal government periodically collects population data for understanding trends and setting norms for national health measures. The Centers for Disease Control and Prevention,[4] the National Center for Health Statistics (NCVHS)[5] and the Agency for Health Quality Research (AHRQ)[6,7] among others have created large reference data sets (and tools to use them) for child health quality improvement and research, including the National Health and Nutrition Examination Survey (NHANES),[8] the National Immunization Survey (NIS)[9] and the National Vital Statistics System (NVSS).[10] One large prospective study sponsored by the US Department of Health and Human Services and the Environmental Protection agency, the National Children's Study[11] is collecting core pediatric data on exposures to environmental hazards on a national sample over several decades. Similar efforts are occurring in other countries.

Professional collaborative projects to collect clinical data for research, quality measurement and for evaluating the impact of interventions on health outcomes that define core data elements for reporting have been growing as electronic communications and computing power grow. Examples of such projects include the Vermont Oxford Network for neonatology,[12] the Interactive Autism Network (described in Chapter 34) and the National Pediatric Trauma Database.[13] New data types, including genomic information, have been added to core data sets used in disease registries to help identify patients at risk and who may benefit from new therapies and clinical trials.

Interest in reusing de-identified clinical data for research has grown as the capability for collecting, storing, and retrieving it for analytic processes[14] has increased. New uses, such as adverse drug event alerting systems[15] and clinical dashboards[16] that provide real-time measures of key performance indicators for clinical and practice decisions as well as research insights.

3.7 Conclusion

Core pediatric data has many uses that vary according the age, the health needs and the purpose for which it is needed. Advances in information technology provide new opportunities and challenges[17] for leveraging the power of these data in unprecedented ways to improve health care on individual, practice and population levels.

References

1. Dombkowski KJ, Leung SW, Clark SJ. Provider attitudes regarding use of an immunization information system to identify children with asthma for influenza vaccination. *J Public Health Manage Pract.* 2007;13(6):567–571.
2. Ungar WJ, Kozyrskyj A, Paterson M, Ahmad F. Effect of cost-sharing on use of asthma medication in children. *Arch Pediatr Adolesc Med.* 2008;162(2):104–110.
3. Naessens JM, Ruud KL, Tulledge-Scheitel SM, Stroebel RJ, Cabanela RL. Comparison of provider claims data versus medical records review for assessing provision of adult preventive services. *J Ambul Care Manage.* 2008;31(2):178–186.
4. Centers for Disease Control and Prevention. CDC Website; 2008. Available at: http://www.cdc.gov. Accessed April 22, 2008.
5. National Center for Health Statistics. NCHS Website; 2008. Available at: http://www.cdc.gov/nchs/Default.htm. Accessed April 22, 2008.
6. Agency for Healthcare Research and Quality. Medical Expenditure Panel Survey; 2006. Available at: http://www.meps.ahrq.gov/mepsweb/. Accessed April 22, 2008.
7. Agency for Healthcare Research and Quality. Hospital Cost and Utilization Project (H-CUP); 2008. Available at: http://www.ahrq.gov/data/hcup/. Accessed April 22, 2008.
8. National Center for Health Statistics. National Health and Nutrition Examination Survey (NHANES); 2008. Available at: http://www.cdc.gov/nchs/nhanes.htm. Accessed April 22, 2008.
9. National Center for Health Statistics. National Immunization Survey; 2008. Available at: http://www.cdc.gov/nis/. Accessed April 22, 2008.
10. Centers for Disease Control and Prevention. National Vital Statistics System; 2008. Available at: http://www.cdc.gov/nchs/nvss.htm. Accessed April 22, 2008.
11. US Department of Health and Human Services, US Environmental Protection Agency. The National Children's Study; 2008. Available at: http://www.nationalchildrensstudy.gov/. Accessed April 22, 2008.
12. Vermont Oxford Network. VON Website; 2008. Available at: http://www.vtoxford.org/. Accessed April 2008.
13. Tepas JJ 3rd. The national pediatric trauma registry: a legacy of commitment to control of childhood injury. *Semin Pediatr Surg.* 2004;13(2):126–132.
14. Hammarstedt R, Bulger D. Performance improvement: a "left brain meets right brain" approach. *Healthc Financ Manage.* 2006;60(12):100–104, 106.
15. Almenoff JS, Pattishall EN, Gibbs TG, DuMouchel W, Evans SJ, Yuen N. Novel statistical tools for monitoring the safety of marketed drugs. *Clin Pharmacol Ther.* 2007;82(2):157–166.
16. Barrett JS, Mondick JT, Narayan M, Vijayakumar K, Vijayakumar S. Integration of modeling and simulation into hospital-based decision support systems guiding pediatric pharmacotherapy. *BMC Med Inform Decis Mak.* 2008;28;8:6.
17. Berner ES, Moss J. Informatics challenges for the impending patient information explosion. *J Am Med Inform Assoc.* 2005;12(6):614–617.

Chapter 4
Neonatal Care and Data

Declan O'Riordan and Peter J. Porcelli Jr.

Objectives

- To characterize baseline information about pregnancy, labor, and delivery needed by neonatal practitioners during birth and transition from obstetrical to pediatric care
- To outline medical concerns of premature infants, the levels and environments of neonatal care and the information needs in the transition from neonatal to primary care
- To describe information challenges in neonatal care

4.1 Introduction

Neonatology encompasses the care of all infants: from term newborns to extremely premature infants, from healthy infants to those suffering from severe infections or genetic disorders. While the management of infants can vary greatly, there are essential core data and knowledge that is needed to care for them.

4.2 The Mother–Infant Dyad

In neonatal care, the medical history covers two patients: the mother and the infant. Thorough knowledge of the maternal history (medical, obstetrical, medication, and social) is crucial for evaluating any newborn. The efficient and accurate transfer of this information from the obstetrical to neonatal providers is a great challenge, but can benefit care tremendously.

C.U. Lehmann et al. (eds.), *Pediatric Informatics: Computer Applications in Child Health,* Health Informatics,
© Springer Science + Business Media, LLC 2011

4.2.1 Maternal Medical and Obstetrical History

Essential maternal medical and obstetrical information includes:

Maternal Age—Pregnancies in women who are young (teenage) or older than 35 years of age are at risk for complications. Risks that younger pregnant women face include preeclampsia, sexually transmitted diseases, lack of family and financial resources and others.[1-3] Problems faced by older pregnant women include increased risks for eclampsia, needs for caesarean delivery, diabetes, and abruption, as well as increased probabilities of genetic abnormalities in offspring.[4]

Maternal Past Medical History—The developing fetus is an integral part of the mother, and systemic maternal conditions, such as diabetes, hypertension, and diseases such as systemic lupus erythematosis or hyperthyroidism can have profound effects on its growth. Knowledge of the severity and etiology of maternal conditions and relevant maternal data near delivery is important for newborn care. For example, mild maternal gestational diabetes mellitus can evoke fetal secretion of insulin leading to macrosomia and neonatal hypoglycemia shortly postdelivery, while severe diabetes of long standing may compromise fetal growth due the negative effects on the placenta from vascular disease.[5] Some neonatal conditions influenced by maternal medical conditions may not be evident until well after hospital discharge. Continuity between the maternal record and the ongoing infant record is important to the primary care pediatrician.

Prior Pregnancies and Neonatal Illnesses—Conditions from prior pregnancies also often present in subsequent pregnancies. For example, Group B Streptococcal (GBS) disease in one newborn also places subsequent newborns at risk for this infection.[6] Examples abound and any obstetrical/neonatal information tracking system must allow for flexible and thorough documentation of prior pregnancies.

Family History—The family history is an important component of any medical evaluation. While adult diseases (coronary artery disease, adult onset cancer, etc.) often contribute little to newborn care, extended families may have histories of unexplained childhood deaths or illnesses that can raise suspicion for potential illness (metabolic, structural, respiratory, etc.) in the newborn.

4.2.2 History of the Current Pregnancy

Detailed knowledge of the current pregnancy is vital, but may be difficult to obtain, particularly when complications prompt emergency delivery. Prenatal obstetrical care is largely delivered in outpatient centers that are associated to labor and delivery wards of delivering hospitals. A major impediment to the development of complete electronic patient records has been the inherent difficulty of integrating timely outpatient data into inpatient records, particularly during nonbusiness hours (nights, weekends, and holidays).

Essential prenatal information includes:

Gestational Age—An infant may be term (between 37 and 42 weeks gestation), preterm (<37 weeks) or postterm (>42 weeks),[7] where weeks are counted from the date of the last menstrual period (LMP), sometimes called post-menstrual age (PMA). The date of (term) delivery (also called the "estimated date of confinement" or EDC) can be calculated from the gestational age, when known or estimated from physical exam. Obstetricians may modify the estimated due date based on ultrasound, if the mother's LMP is unknown. The gestational age (in days) of fetuses conceived via assisted reproduction (ART) is determined by adding 14 to the number of days since implantation of the fertilized egg.[8]

Number of Expected Fetuses—Until recently, higher ordered multiple gestations (triplets, quadruplets, etc.) were rare. Assisted reproduction has made twins and triplets commonplace. Between 1980 and 1997, the number of twin live births rose 52% and the number of triplets and higher order deliveries rose 404%.[9] Higher-order pregnancies are at higher risk for complications and prematurity is commonplace.

Prenatal Studies—Prenatal care usually includes a standard battery of prenatal laboratory tests at various points during pregnancy. Some tests (screens for maternal HIV, group B streptococcal and drugs of abuse) may prompt treatment protocols for mother and infant. These test results are a vital part of the prenatal and infant record and must be easily available as they can influence care shortly after birth.

Prenatal laboratory test results include:

- Maternal blood type and Rh (Rhesus antigen)
- Maternal antibodies against known blood antigens
- Group B Streptococcal (GBS) screen
- Maternal antibodies for syphilis—VDRL or RPR
- Presence of Hepatitis B surface antigen and antibody
- Maternal immunity to toxoplasma, rubella, cytomegalovirus, and herpes
- Maternal tests for HIV, gonorrhea, and chlamydia (often sent at obstetrician's discretion)
- Maternal toxicology screen

Each of these results has implications for evaluation and treatment of the newborn, such as the administration of Hepatitis B immune globulin in addition to Hepatitis B vaccine.[10]

A major challenge of neonatal care is collection and processing of maternal data from obstetric records when outpatient offices are closed. In some cases, this may leads to duplication of maternal testing and possible unnecessary treatments of the infant. Linkage of information between hospitals and obstetric offices could decrease this problem. In some cases, maternal prenatal lab tests processed at the intended delivery hospital can facilitate data availability at delivery.

Pregnancy Complications—The evolution of a pregnancy greatly impacts neonatal conditions. Potential complications include premature labor, fetal growth restriction, pregnancy-induced hypertension, pre-eclampsia, and others. These complications can extend maternal hospitalization, sometimes for weeks, well before delivery.

Fetal Ultrasounds/Echocardiograms—Prenatal ultrasound provides an opportunity to estimate gestational age and identify problems in the developing fetus. A suspected heart malformation prompts a fetal echocardiogram and cardiology evaluation. An ultrasound-detected heart or other malformation may critically determine the location of delivery, the resuscitation protocol and treatment plan shortly after birth.

Maternal Infections During Pregnancy—Infections by viruses, bacteria, and fungi may affect the developing fetus and newborn. Some infections, particularly viral infections, may cross the placenta and have severe, sometimes fatal effects. Other maternal infections, such as urinary tract infections, place the infant at higher risk for bacterial infections after birth. Others, such as TORCH infections, may place the infant at risk for life-long complications. The prenatal course and treatment of maternal infection may help determine the extent of evaluation and need for treatment of the newborn.

Pregnancy Interventions—Perinatologists and surgeons are increasingly able to directly intervene in the course of fetal development. Some of these interventions have been well accepted (amniotic fluid sampling, fetal transfusions), while others (fetal surgery) are experimental. Nevertheless, fetal interventions will likely become more frequent in the future and their incorporation into a maternal–fetal record electronic record should be standard.

Consulting Physicians—Pediatric subspecialists (geneticists, nephrologists, cardiologist, neonatologists, and others) may meet with expecting parents prior to delivery and may participate in postnatal care. Easy access to information about specialists' involvement and their contact information may help to streamline infant care after delivery.

4.2.3   Labor and Delivery

Delivery records must document the onset of labor, time of rupture of membranes, presence of maternal fever, type and timing of medications/anesthesia administered to mother and method of delivery (vaginal, Caesarean, forceps, or vacuum). Obstetricians often note the presence of fetal heart rate decelerations prior to delivery that comprise four varieties: early, late, variable, and prolonged. While documentation may indicate only the presence of "decels," the type, frequency, duration, and severity of fetal heart rate deceleration may indicate placental insufficiency.[7] Meconium may be passed in utero and its presence in amniotic fluid place the infant at risk for fetal meconium aspiration and respiratory distress after birth. Additionally, infection of the amniotic fluid, chorioamnionitis, may produce malodorous, cloudy amniotic fluid and place the newborn at high risk for bacterial infection.

4.3   The Infant

4.3.1   Neonatal Resuscitation

As a part of delivery, the newborn's condition is immediately assessed. Many infants are initially cyanotic with rapid improvement as breathing begins. Some infants require resuscitation, which may be complex and prolonged, for a variety of reasons, including persistent apnea, prolonged cyanosis, bradycardia, or poor tone. The APGAR score is assigned to describe the infant's initial condition and response to resuscitation (Table 4.1).[11] Good documentation of resuscitation describes an infant's condition, resuscitation steps instituted and response to resuscitation. Because resuscitation may be prolonged and time is often short, thorough documentation may be difficult and may follow resuscitation and stabilization of the infant. While real-time documentation of resuscitation would be ideal, manpower and space for a human scribe are often limited in the delivery or operating room.

4.3.2   Is It a Boy or a Girl?—The Special Cases of Ambiguous Genitalia

While many parents learn the gender of the newborn during an antenatal ultrasound, some prefer wait to know until delivery. In most cases, the gender is readily apparent, but in a small percentage of newborns, the gender is not immediately evident in the delivery room and assignment must be deferred. Ambiguous genitalia require careful discussions between all members of the treatment team and parents.[12] As such, premature assignment of gender is inappropriate.

4.3.3   How Big Is the Baby?

The birthweight, length, and head circumference determine whether an infant is appropriately sized for the estimated gestational age based on normative values readily available on growth charts. Infants who are smaller than expected (<10%) are *small for gestational age* (SGA) while infants who are larger than

Table 4.1 The APGAR score

Score parameter	0	1	2
Color	Cyanotic or pale	Acrocyanosis	Pink
Pulse	0 (Asystolic)	<100/min	>100/min
Reflex irritability	None	Grimace	Cries
Tone	Flaccid	Decreased	Active motion
Respirations	Apneic/gasping	Irregular	Good
Total			

expected (>90%) are *large for gestational age* (LGA).[13] Those infants whose weight, head circumference, and length are between the 10th to 19th percentiles are *appropriate for gestational age* (AGA). While parents in United States almost exclusively use the English system (pounds, ounces, inches) when referring to the weight and length of the newborn, medical care of newborns, particularly medication dosing, requires these measurements in metric.

4.4 Well Baby Care

4.4.1 The Newborn Nursery

In many cases, term newborns stay in the mother's room to facilitate bonding and feeding or are admitted to a well baby nursery, with anticipated discharge in 48–72 h. Routine newborn care is often high-volume and information systems that link obstetrical care to newborn nursery to primary pediatric care may bring benefits in multidisciplinary care and patient satisfaction.[14]

4.4.1.1 Challenges of the Newborn Nursery

In a typical community nursery, primary care practitioners (pediatricians and family practitioners) examine infants and review their records in the morning prior to seeing patients in the outpatient setting. Challenges include:

Identifying Subtle Signs of Illness—Early signs of illness in the newborn may be subtle. Some, such as difficulty in establishing feedings after delivery or heart murmurs may not manifest until after discharge, yet can be life-threatening if not detected early.

High Patient Volume—Newborn nurseries vary greatly in size. Larger nurseries may employ hospitalists in addition to private pediatricians and family physicians to examine newborns prior to discharge. A challenge to planning newborn nursery information systems is the collection of examination data for documentation and conveyance to primary care practices efficiently, particularly when patient loads are high.

Critical Laboratory Values—Efficient and coordinated notification of abnormal laboratory test results, such as direct antibody tests (DAT), complete blood counts (CBCs), electrolytes, blood glucoses, and blood gas determinations may alert nursery physicians to potentials for problems that may delay discharge or require further workup or referral to a neonatal intensive care unit.

Identification of Infants Who Will Require Close Follow-Up—Most infants are discharged from the nursery by 48 h of age with office follow-up at 1 week, but some may be eligible to go home with closer follow-up. Issues such as resolving jaundice, early discharge from the hospital and first-time breast feeding mothers may require a coordinated follow-up visit sooner than 1–2 weeks. Continuity of care from the nursery to primary care can be enhanced by phone calls to follow-up physicians, in addition to hospital documentation. The typical summary for term newborns contains:

- Maternal medical and obstetrical history, including maternal medications
- Labor and delivery history, including prenatal test results (Group B Strep status, RPR, Rubella, HIV, maternal blood type, maternal gonorrhea, and chlamydia results)
- A summary of the neonate's course, including resuscitation and Apgar scores, physical exam, birth and discharge weights, laboratory values (bilirubin levels, infant/mother blood types, DAT, CBC), stooling/voiding patterns, administration of hepatitis B vaccine, and infant feeding.

Newborn Screening—Newborn screening test results are usually unavailable at the time an infant is discharge, and require follow-up with the primary care practitioner. These screens include:

- Metabolic testing (which varies from state to state)[15]
- Newborn hearing screen[16]
- Specific tests for infants at risk (genetic testing, intrauterine infection screens (TORCH[17]))

4.4.1.2 Ill Term Infants at a Community Hospital

Although many hospitals provide low level neonatal intensive care, very ill term infants requiring mechanical ventilation and advance life support must be stabilized and transported to the closest neonatal intensive care unit (NICU)[18]. Term nursery planning includes standardized procedures for the management and transfer of such infants, including:

- Medical stabilization protocols for infants (including appropriate equipment and trained physicians)
- Coordination and transport of infants to known NICUs
- Information transfer and documentation of care

Well-designed information systems within a regional network can facilitate the gathering of needed information. Transfer documentation for neonatal transport includes: a summary by the clinician of the infant's course and copies of the nursing flow sheets, medication records, laboratory results, and radiographic studies. Design of computerized systems, in addition to collecting and making necessary information available, should facilitate its summarization and organization for optimal care.

4.5   Neonatal Intensive Care

Premature births currently account for 10–12.5% of all births in the United States.[19,20] Advances have extended survival of infants as early as 23 weeks gestation, with standard treatments for previously fatal diseases such as respiratory distress syndrome (RDS).

4.5.1   NICU Environments

Neonatal nurseries comprise a range of facilities of different sizes and capabilities. The March of Dimes reports "Toward Improving the Outcome of Pregnancy" (TIOP I and TIOP II) described criteria stratifying nurseries according to the complexity of care.[18, 21,22] Level I nurseries offer basic resuscitation and care for uncomplicated deliveries. Level II (specialty) nurseries offer care for limited conditions that are expected to resolve quickly and that do not require extensive care. Level III (subspecialty) nurseries offer complex care, including surgical interventions, for critically ill term and preterm infants. Further classification, that addresses the need for regionalization of specialized critical care, such as extracorporeal membrane oxygenation (ECMO) and neonatal cardiac surgery, has been proposed.[23] Higher level NICUs employ high-risk obstetricians, perinatologists, neonatalogists, pediatric subspecialists, and neonatal nurses, dieticians, pharmacists, and respiratory therapists.

4.5.2   Crucial Issues of Prematurity

Prematurity is defined as birth occurring at less than 37 completed weeks since the onset of the LMP. The range of gestational ages of premature infants conveys a range of birth weights (that may extend to as low as 400–500 g) and risks for both morbidity and mortality. Viability indicates the possibility, but not the probability of long term survival. The limit of viability varies but may be estimated to be 23–25 weeks. Because of their premature systems, these infants are at risk for a number of problems.

4.5.2.1   Pulmonary Immaturity

Respiratory insufficiency or failure is a frequent consequence of prematurity and may be multifactorial in nature. Premature infants are at risk for *respiratory distress syndrome* (RDS), due to surfactant deficiency and structural lung immaturity. Therapies to support infants with immature lungs include endotracheal administration of surfactant and ventilatory support. Premature infants with RDS are at risk for subsequent chronic lung disease (*bronchopulmonary dysplasia*).[24]

Measures of respiratory distress include: vital signs (respiratory rate, heart rate, and oxygen saturation), the physical exam and arterial blood gas results (pH, PaO_2, $PaCO_2$) and physiologic measures such as mean airway pressure (MAP) and inspired oxygen (FiO_2), with the Oxygenation Index (OI)[25] as a calculated measure whose trends can be tracked over time.

$$OI = (MAP \times FiO_2 \times 100)/PaO_2$$

Infants with relatively mild respiratory insufficiency may be placed on one of several varieties of continuous positive airway pressure (CPAP, a device that blows air into the nose at a controlled pressure): bubble CPAP, mask CPAP, and prong CPAP. CPAP pressure must be tracked as it follows potential improvement or worsening of respiratory status. Infants who experience failure with CPAP require mechanical ventilation.

Mechanical ventilation of the premature neonate is a complex and controversial topic. Two general varieties of mechanical ventilation are available: *conventional ventilation* and *high frequency ventilation*. Conventional ventilation provides a standard breath (pressure or volume) into the lungs at a given minimum rate per minute, dependent on the ventilator settings. Available neonatal systems incorporate these varieties and offer the user the ability to adjust variables (tidal volume, peak pressure, rate, PEEP, and others). The second major classification of ventilators is the high-frequency ventilator. Several types of these ventilators are available.[26] High frequency ventilation provides small gas volumes at rapid rates to decrease the pulmonary trauma. The most common type is *high-frequency oscillatory ventilator* (HFOV or oscillator) which cycles air in and out of the lungs rapidly. The oscillator has relatively few variables to track: mean airway pressure (MAP), displacement (delta P), frequency, and FIO_2. While the individual level of these variables is very important, the trends of the variables and blood gas results provide a highly useful picture of an infant's respiratory status. Two other types of high frequency ventilators are in general use include the *jet ventilator*, which is similar to the oscillator, but cumulatively provides for oxygenation and removal of waste gases and *high frequency flow interrupters (HFFI)*. The jet ventilator is used in combination with a conventional ventilator to provide positive end-expiratory pressure (PEEP) and intermittent breaths. It is more complex than a conventional ventilator, with different variables: jet peak pressure (JPIP), inspiratory time, back up PEEP (baseline pressure), back up rate (0 to several breaths per minute) and back up peak pressure. HFFI is similar to jet ventilation but uses slower rates.[27]

Airway pressure release ventilators (APRV) have also been used on neonates, but on a more limited basis.[28]

4.5.2.2   Cardiovascular Instability

The tremendous cardiovascular changes occur during the transition from intrauterine to extrauterine life place premature infants are at high risk for two particular cardiovascular problems: patent ductus arteriosus (PDA) and hypotension. PDA is a persistence of an essential fetal connection (the ductus arteriosus) between the pulmonary artery and aorta that normally closes within 12–24 h in term neonates. In premature infants, the PDA can worsen respiratory distress and lower systemic blood pressure. Various medical and surgical therapies are used to close the duct.[29]

Hypotension, another complication of prematurity, is a poorly defined entity in extremely preterm infants. At this time, neonatalogists commonly attempt to keep the mean blood pressure at least the gestational age during the first several days after birth.[30]

$$\text{Mean blood pressure} = DBP + 1/3 * (SBP - DBP)^{31}$$

The medical management of hypotension includes:

Continuous intravenous infusions of vasopressors (dopamine, dobutamine, epinephrine) are administered on a *microgram per kilogram per minute* rate (unlike narcotics, which are infused on *a microgram per kilogram per hour* rate). Manual calculation of infusion rates and doses is error-prone. Errors can be reduced through the design and mandated use of calculators[32] that can be used in stressful situations. In addition to calculators, the mandated use of standard concentrations for continuous infusion medications[33] by the Joint Commission, which limits available concentrations of medications, thus reducing pharmacy preparation errors. The large variations in neonatal weights may create fluid overload for premature infants, but this may be offset by the use of computerized "smart" pumps (See Chapter 28).

Steroids (in particular hydrocortisone), dosed by weight (mg/kg/day) or by body surface area (BSA) may help stabilize blood pressure (using calculator support):

$$\text{Neonatal Estimated BSA } (m^2) = 0.05 \times Wt \ (Kg) + 0.05$$

4.5.2.3 Neurologic Immaturity and Vulnerability

Extremely premature infants are at risk for brain damage due to hypoxic and ischemic insults to the developing brain and nervous system. Infants less than 34 weeks gestational age (at birth) are at significant risk for *intraventricular hemorrhage* (IVH).[23] Hemorrhages, detected using cranial ultrasonography, can range from very small to catastrophic, lethal hemorrhagic infarctions,[34] which may create *posthemorrhagic hydrocephalus*, requiring neurosurgical intervention. *Periventricular leukomalacia* (PVL), resulting from blood flow instability and exposure to infection among extremely premature infants, may be detected by cranial ultrasound and places an infant at significant risk for long term developmental problems. The presence of intraventricular hemorrhages, periventricular leukomalacia, or hydrocephalus is vitally important for future medical and developmental care and this information must be clearly conveyed to future physicians and allied developmental professionals.

4.5.2.4 Susceptibility to Infection

Premature infants are immunologically naïve and vulnerable to a number of serious systemic infections, not only from maternal sources, but also those associated with hospitalization: vascular catheters, ventilator associated pneumonias, and necrotizing enterocolitis.[35]

4.5.2.5 Nutrition and Growth

In extremely premature neonates, use of the gut is limited initially, and therefore they must be supported at first with intravenous nutrition (*total parenteral nutrition, TPN*). As enteral nutrition is increased, the TPN is decreased accordingly. The management of premature infant nutrition is complex, requiring calculation of daily caloric, protein, fat, minerals, vitamins, and fluid needs as well as monitoring of growth and biochemical parameters. Computer applications can reduce the time spent in performing these calculations and the errors inherent in detailed information tracking. Applications that support TPN formulations have been described in the literature,[36] with demonstrated reductions in both time spent and errors.[37–40] In addition, systems have been deployed over several hospitals to extend standardization of TPN formulation.

We are entering a new era for growth and nutrition monitoring that individualizes postnatal growth by integrating perinatal, family, and postnatal data. A multitude of peri- and postnatal factors influence infants' postnatal growth to determine what is "best," according to gestational age and pathology. Determining adequacy of postnatal growth is more difficult than anticipated. An important distinction should be made between an *intrauterine growth curves* and a *postnatal growth curves*. Intrauterine growth curves describe the distribution of fetal weights based on gestational age. They can be used to determine whether a newborn is small or large for gestational age. A postnatal growth curve describes the growth in weight, head circumference, and length after birth. Superimposing the curves for premature infants reveals a striking deviation of the postnatal curve below the intrauterine curve, indicating a period of growth failure, particularly among those infants born most prematurely.[41] While the intrauterine growth curve may represent ideal postnatal growth, with the current state of neonatal care, intrauterine growth curves cannot be used to assess the adequacy of postnatal growth of premature infants.

In evaluating any standardized growth curve for use, several questions must be considered:

- From which population (ethnicity, gestational ages, socioeconomic status, etc.) was the reference standard generated?
- Does this population accurately reflect the infants whose growth will be assessed with the chart in question? For example, standard intrauterine growth curves include only Caucasian infant's from 26 to 42 weeks gestation in Denver from 1948 to 1961.[42] A more recent study using a more diverse population with larger numbers of infants at each gestational age describes birth weight percentages for

infants between 24 to 37 weeks (including a small number of infants between 22 to 23 weeks gestation).[43]
- When was the population (from which the growth curve was derived) studied? As advances in obstetrics, neonatology, and neonatal nutrition improve the care of premature neonates, recent studies may better reflect current care. For example, one of the earliest postnatal growth curves for premature infants demonstrated that 1 kg infants regained birthweight by 17 days, while a more recent curve reveals birth weight is regained much sooner (12.8 days).[41,44]

4.6   From Neonatal Care to Follow-Up Care

Ongoing care of infants requires accurate and efficient transfer of care plans and results of studies to the primary care pediatrician. The tremendous volume of information and documentation generated during a prolonged neonatal hospitalization is compounded by the fragmented nature of NICU care. An extremely premature infant may have many attending neonatologists, consultants, and trainees prior to discharge from the hospital. A major benefit of an effective information system in the NICU is the ability to locate and organize crucial information for follow-up of neonatal problems.

4.6.1   Metabolic Screening

States vary in the number of diseases included in the newborn screening panel and the number of newborn screens administered to each infant. The first sample is usually sent shortly after birth (after the first feeding) and the second sample between day 10 and 14. Samples are sent to state laboratories and results return in 1–2 weeks. Accurate and timely collection and tracking of metabolic screens is vitally important and failure may result in preventable or treatable disease with devastating complications. Regional registries, in conjunction with dedicated support personnel, can facilitate sharing of information and completion of follow-up with primary care physicians and specialists.[45]

4.6.2   Hearing Screening

Newborn hearing screens are performed prior to infant hospital discharge. NICU infants are at particular risk for hearing loss (up to 6% in one series of infants born between 500 to 750 g.[46]) Information about the necessity and timing of additional hearing tests for all infants should be transparent to parents and follow-up physicians.

4.6.3 Immunizations

Premature infants currently are covered by the same immunization schedule as term infants. A 24 week gestational age premature infant receives 2 month immunizations at a post-menstrual age of 32 weeks. It is not uncommon for very premature infants to be hospitalized for months, with multiple immunizations given in the hospital.

Palivizumab, a monoclonal antibody against respiratory syncytial virus (RSV), is recommended to prevent RSV infection in many premature infants or those with chronic lung or congenital heart disease. Eligible infants should be given as monthly injections during the RSV season, for up to the first 2 years of life.[47]

Communication of administered immunization, dates, and adverse reactions, must be communicated to the primary care physician to avoid lapses and unnecessary duplication of immunization doses.

4.6.4 Retinopathy of Prematurity

Retinopathy of prematurity (ROP) refers to the disordered growth of blood vessels supplying the developing retina. Very premature infants are at greatest risk for ROP and its sequelae because of the underdevelopment of retinal vessels. Regular eye exams by a pediatric ophthalmologist are necessary to monitor the growth of retinal blood vessels and for the development and progression of ROP. Frequency of ophthalmologic examinations is scheduled according to disease progression, the risk of complications (permanent blindness) and the need for intervention (retinal ablative surgery) to lessen the risk for retinal detachment.[48, 49] Neonatal follow-up tracking systems for premature infants should include the ability to track scheduling, completion, and reports of ophthalmology exams to the primary care physician and to parents to ensure appropriate future care.[49]

4.7 Specific Issues for Neonatal Information Systems

4.7.1 Handling Infant Name Changes

Although many infants assume the shared surname of parents, particularly if they are married, a significant portion of infants will not retain the surname initially assigned by the birth hospital. Changes in parental marital and legal status, as well as adoption, may result in infant name changes. These issues (and potential for errors) are increased with multiple gestations and infants with the same name in the same nursery, and when the infant is discharged to follow-up with the primary care physician. NICUs and neonatal identification systems must be able to disambiguate infants, even when names are changed, in the NICU and after discharge.

4.7.2 Improving NICU Medication Delivery

The 1999 Institute of Medicine report stating that tens of thousands of patients die yearly in the US from medical errors.[50] Infants in the NICU are particularly vulnerable to errors and their impacts.

4.7.2.1 Neonatal Drug Dosing

Pediatric medications dosing is based on patient weight. The small weights of premature infants, with rapid weight and body surface area changes and variable physiologies place sick neonates at high risk for medication errors. In the NICU, preterm neonates may receive multiple medications, which increase the likelihood of errors and drug interactions. The task of prescribing in the NICU is made even more difficult by the lack of accepted dosing guidelines for medications and the high rate of "off label" medication use due to overall paucity of studies specifically looking at medication use in neonates.

NICU medication errors commonly occur at the ordering stage. Extremely premature (low weight) infants are at risk for decimal place errors in dosing, that can be exacerbated with poor handwriting. In addition, many neonatal drugs are dispensed in vials from which very small amounts of drug must be withdrawn, which enable order of magnitude errors in ordering and administration.[51] Medication ordering error frequencies appear to be inversely proportional to body weight,[52] with 71% of errors occurred at the prescribing and 29% of errors at administration.[51] The two most common types of errors were incorrect dose and dosing interval, with increased rates of dosing errors occurring when new housestaff rotated through the NICU.

Additional risks for errors are incurred with complex calculations, such as discussed previously for continuous infusion ("drips") and total parenteral nutrition.[33] In addition to calculators, standard concentrations for continuous infusions,[53] with smart-pump technology and improved medication labeling have been associated with marked decreases in continuous infusion errors.[54]

Quality improvement in medication delivery demands consideration of the entire delivery process rather than independent events. *Failure mode and effects analysis* (FMEA), a quality improvement technique developed in industry to improve safety, has identified general lack of awareness of medication safety, problems with administration and ordering of medications to be the most significant issues in NICU medication delivery.[55]

Integration of information technology into ordering, dispensing, and administration of medications in inpatient environments is examined in Chapter 26.

4.7.2.2 Delivering Drugs in Emergencies: The Code Card

Code Cards detail specific emergency medications and their doses according to weight in both milligrams and milliliters to be given during resuscitations. During neonatal resuscitation, drug doses are ordered, drawn from stock vials and administered emergently, and errors may easily occur. A preterm infant's weight may change markedly over a short period of time, and therefore, code cards must be updated frequently. One benefit of computer-generated code cards (that can be created using commercially available software, such as a spreadsheet) is automated updating, especially if the dosing is linked to the current weight (from an electronic record), or as part of the regular care routine.

4.8 Conclusion

Though medicine has been late to incorporate computers into daily routines, use of computers in neonatology is growing. Linkage with obstetrical information systems can streamline entry of information into the neonate's record. Growth may be more easily monitored. Crucial information for follow-up physicians can be easily tracked and synthesized into discharge summaries. Patient safety can be enhanced by decreasing errors in medication and TPN orders. As obstetricians, neonatologists, nurses, and pharmacists increasingly incorporate computer systems, a major challenge will be to synthesize these systems into a cohesive outpatient and inpatient network.

References

1. Conde-Agudelo A, Belizan JM, Lammers C. Maternal-perinatal morbidity and mortality associated with adolescent pregnancy in Latin America: cross-sectional study. *Am J Obstet Gynecol*. 2005;192(2):342–349.
2. Quinlivan JA, Luehr B, Evans SF. Teenage mother's predictions of their support levels before and actual support levels after having a child. *J Pediatr Adolesc Gynecol*. 2004;17:273–278.
3. Orvos J, Nyirati I, Hajdu J, Pal A, Nyari T, Kovacs L. Is adolescent pregnancy associated with adverse perinatal outcome? *J Perinat Med*. 1999;27(3):199–203.
4. Braveman FR. Pregnancy in patients of advanced maternal age. *Anesthiol Clin*. 2006; 24:637–646.
5. Galerneau F, Inzucchi SE. Diabetes mellitus in pregnancy. *Obstet Gynecol Clin N Am*. 2004;31:907–933.
6. Adair CE, Kowalsky L, Quon H, Ma D, Stoffman, J, McGeer A, Robertson S, Mucenski M, Davies HD. Risk factors for early-onset group B streptococcal disease in neonates: A population-based case-control study. *CMAJ*. 2003;169(3):198–203.
7. Gabbe SG, Niebyl JH, Simpson JL. *Obstetrics - Normal and Problem Pregnancies*. 4th ed. New York: Churchill Livingstone; 2007.
8. Kalish RB, Thaler HT, Chasen ST, Gupta M, Berman SJ, Rosenwaks Z, Chervenak FA. First- and second-trimester ultrasound assessment of gestational age. *Am J Ostet Gynecol*. 2004;191:975–978.

9. Endres L, Wilkins I. Epidemiology and biology of multiple gestations. *Clin Perinatol.* 2005;32:301–314.
10. Pickering LK, Baker CJ, Overturf GD, Prober CG. Committee on Infectious Diseases. *2003 Report of the Committee on Infectious Diseases.* 26th ed. American Academy of Pediatrics. Elk Grove village, Illinoin; 2003.
11. Finster M, Wood M. The Apgar score has survived the test of time. *Anesthesiology.* 2005;102:855–857.
12. Hyun G, Kolon TF. A practical approach to intersex in the newborn period. *Urol Clin N Am.* 2004;31:435–443.
13. Watterberg K, Gallaher KJ. Signs and symptoms of neonatal illness. In: *Primary Pediatric Care.* 3rd ed. St. Louis, MO: Mosby; 1997:533.
14. Hayward-Rowse L, Whittle T. A pilot project to design, implement and evaluate an electronic integrated care pathway. *J Nurs Manage.* 2006;14(7):564–571.
15. Ananth CV, Vintzileos AM. Epidemiology of preterm birth and its clinical subtypes. *J Matern Fetal Neonatal Med.* 2006;19(12):773–782.
16. American Academy of Pediatrics, Joint Committee on Infant Hearing. Year 2007 position statement: Principles and guidelines for early hearing detection and intervention programs. *Pediatrics.* 2007;120(4):898–921.
17. Mets MB, Chhabra MS. Eye manifestations of intrauterine infections and their impact on childhood blindness. *Surv Ophthalmol.* 2008;53(2):95–111.
18. Stark AR. American Academy of Pediatrics Committee on Fetus and Newborn. Levels of neonatal care. *Pediatrics.* 2004;114(5):1341–1347.
19. Ananth CV, Joseph KS, Oyelse Y, Kemissie K, Vintzileos AM. Trends in preterm birth and perinatal mortality among singletons: United States, 1989 through 2000. *Obstet Gynecol.* 2005;105(5 Pt 1):1084–1091.
20. March of Dimes Committee on Perinatal Health. *Toward improving the Outcome of Pregnancy: Recommendations for the Regional Development of Matrnal and Perinatal Health Services.* White Plains, NY: March of Dimes National Foundation; 1976.
21. March of Dimes Committee on Perinatal Health. *Toward Improving the Outcome of Pregnancy: The 90s and Beyond.* White Plains, NY: March of Dimes Birth Defects Foundation; 1993.
22. American Academy of Pediatrics Committee on Fetus and Newborn. Levels of neonatal care (policy statement). *Pediatrics.* 2004;114(5):1341–1347.
23. Adams-Chapman I. Neurodevelopmental outcome of the late preterm infant. *Clin Perinat.* 2006;33:947–964.
24. Eichenwald EC, Stark AR. Management and outcomes of very low birth weight. *N Engl J Med.* 2008;358(16):1700–1711.
25. Bollen CW, van Vught AJ, Uiterwaal CS. High-frequency ventilation is/is not the optimal physiological approach to ventilate ARDS patients. *J Appl Physiol.* 2008;104(4):1238.
26. Donn SM, Sinha SK. Invasive and noninvasive neonatal mechanical ventilation. *Respir Care.* 2003;48(4):426–439.
27. Craft AP, Bhandari V, Finer NN. The sy-fi study: a randomized prospective trial of synchronized intermittent mandatory ventilation versus a high-frequency flow interrupter in infants less than 1000 g. *J Perinatol.* 2003;23(1):14–19.
28. Habashi NM. Other approaches to open-lung ventilation: airway pressure release ventilation. *Crit Care Med.* 2005;33(3 suppl):S228–S240.
29. Giroud JM, Jacobs JP. Evolution of strategies for management of the patent arterial duct. *Cardiol Young.* 2005;17(2 suppl):68–74.
30. Barrington KJ, Dempsey EM. Cardiovascular support in the preterm: treatments in search of indications. *J Pediatr.* 2006;148(3):289–291.
31. Mohrman DE, Heller LJ. *Cardiovascular Physiology.* New York: McGraw-Hill; 1991.
32. Lehmann CU, Kim GR, Gujral R, et al. Decreasing errors in pediatric continuous intravenous infusions. *Pediatr Crit Care Med.* 2006;7(3):1–6.
33. Joint Commision on Accreditation of Healthcare Organizations. Requirement 3B of Joint Commission 2006 National Patient Safety Goals Implementation Expectations; 2006.

Available at: http://www.jointcommission.org/PatientSafety/NationalPatientSafetyGoals/06_
npsgs.htm. Accessed December 14, 2008.

34. Bassan H, Feldman HA, Limperopoulos C, et al. Periventricular hemorrhagic infarction: risk factors and neonatal outcome. *Pediatr Neurol.* 2006;35(2):85–92.

35. Geffers C, Baerwolff S, Schwab F, Gastmeier P. Incidence of healthcare-associated infections in high-risk neonates: results from the German surveillance system for very-low-birthweight infants. *J Hosp Infect.* 2008;68(3):214–221.

36. Horn W, Popow C, Miksch S, et al. Development and evaluation of VIE-PNN, a knowledge-based system for calculating the parenteral nutrition of newborn infants. *Artif Intell Med.* 2002;24:217–228.

37. Costakos DT. Of lobsters, electronic medical records and neonatal total parenteral nutrition. *Pediatrics.* 2006;117:328–332.

38. Lehmann CU, Kim GR. Using information technology to reduce pediatric medication errors. *J Clin Outcomes Manage.* 2005;12(10):511–518.

39. Lehmann CU, Conner KG, Cox JM. Preventing provider errors: online total parenteral nutrition calculator. *Pediatrics.* 2004;113:748–753.

40. Riskin A, Shiff Y, Shamir R. Parenteral nutrition in neonatology–to standardize or individualize. *Isr Med Assoc J.* 2006;8(9):641–645.

41. Ehrenkranz RA, Younes N, Lemons JA, et al. Longitudinal growth of hospitalized very low birth weight infants. *Pediatrics.* 1999;104(2):280–289.

42. Lubchenco LO, Hansman C, Boyd E. Intrauterine growth in length and head circumference as estimated from live births at gestational ages from 26 to 42 weeks. *Pediatrics.* 1966:37(3):403–408.

43. Riddle WR, DonLevy SC, LaFleur BJ, Rosenbloom ST, Shenai JP. Equations describing percentiles for birthweight, head circumference, and length of preterm infants. *J Perinatol.* 2006;26:556–561.

44. Dancis J, O'Connell JR, Holt LE. A grid for recording the weight of premature infants. *J Pediatr.* 1948;33:570–572.

45. American Academy of Pediatrics Newborn Screening Authoring Committee. Newborn screening expands: recommendations for pediatricians and medical homes–implications for the system. *Pediatrics.* 2008;121(1):192–217.

46. Hack M, Friedman H, Fanaroff AA. Outcomes of extremely low birth weight infants. *Pediatrics.* 1966;98(5):931–937.

47. American Academy of Pediatrics Committee on Infectious Diseases and Committee on Fetus and Newborn. Policy statement. *Pediatrics.* 2003;112(6):1442–1446.

48. Marshall DD. Primary care follow-up of the neonatal intensive care unit graduate. *Clin Fam Pract.* 2003;5(2):243–263.

49. Demorest BH. Retinopathy of prematurity requires diligent follow-up care. *Surv Ophth.* 1996;41(2):175–178.

50. Institute of Medicine. *To Err Is Human: Building a Safer Health System.* Washington, DC. National Academy Press; 1999.

51. Chappell K, Newman C. Potential tenfold drug overdoses on a neonatal unit. *Arch Dis Child Fetal Neonatal Ed.* 2004;89:483–484.

52. Kaushal R, Bates DW, Landrigan C, et al. Medication errors and incidents in pediatric inpatients. *JAMA.* 2001;285(16):2114–2120.

53. Simpson JH, Ahmed I, McLaren J, Skeoch CH. Use of nasal continuous positive airway pressure during neonatal transfer. *Arch Dis Child Fetal Neonatal Ed.* 2004;89(4):F374–F375.

54. Larsen GY, Parker HB, Cash J, et al. Standard drug concentrations and smart-pump technology reduce continuous-medication-infusion errors in pediatric patients. *Pediatrics.* 2005;116:21–25.

55. Kunac DL, Reith DM. Identification of priorities for medication safety in neonatal intensive care. *Drug Safety.* 2005;28(3):251–261.

Chapter 5
Special Health Information Needs of Adolescent Care

David M.N. Paperny

Objectives

- To outline the unique confidentiality requirements for adolescent health information systems
- To define parameters and techniques for adolescent health screening and education
- To describe issues involved in protecting teens from online health risks

5.1 Introduction

Adolescent medicine concerns the biological, psychological, and social changes in the transition from childhood to adulthood, and its core clinical data and knowledge comprise a mixture of both pediatric and adult concerns. Adolescent morbidity is predominately the consequence of preventable risk behaviors.[1] The importance of preventive services and interventions to adolescents at-risk demands that practitioners address a broad range of concerns during encounters, including physical and mental health screening, detection of and response to hidden agendas, assurance of patient privacy, and guaranteeing access to care for this vulnerable population.[2]

5.2 Information Tasks for Adolescent Health Care

Tasks related to medical (and practice) management

- Create and retrieve records securely from office, hospital, emergency departments, consultants
- Access laboratory and imaging test results securely
- Communicate with the adolescent patients privately
- Collect and analyze practice population data
- Submit mandated reporting data

C.U. Lehmann et al. (eds.), *Pediatric Informatics: Computer Applications in Child Health,* Health Informatics,
© Springer Science+Business Media, LLC 2011

Tasks related to health care and anticipatory guidance
- Screen for and manage health problems (acute and chronic illnesses, acne, obesity, eating disorders)
- Schedule sexual health care (family planning, Depo-Provera, STIs, Pap smears, pregnancy)
- Detect latent and active illnesses (HIV, substance abuse, maltreatment, domestic violence)
- Provide age, race, gender, and literacy-appropriate anticipatory guidance
- Monitor patient health in the context of family history (blood pressure, obesity, cardiac disease)

Tasks related to practice operation

- Communicate (telephone, fax, e-mail, secure messaging)
- Schedule appointments with practitioners
- Prescribe safely, securely and accurately (e-prescribing)
- Provide population-appropriate patient educational materials and resources
- Assure confidentiality, integrity, and availability of medical records

Tasks related to financial management

- Bill appropriately
- Preserve confidentiality

Adolescents are not simply large children. In addition to the complex physical growth and maturational changes they undergo, teens also have four major developmental tasks to accomplish from age 11–24 years old. They must establish:

- Personal identity
- Independence
- Adult sexuality
- Vocational choice

These involve intellectual, psychological, and emotional growth and maturity as well as social, cultural, and legal changes, which may have profound impacts on the relationships between the patient and the physician, the physician and the family, and the patient and the family. These changes may also expose the growing youth to risks from self-injurious or harmful behaviors.

For the clinician, obtaining information on these issues may be challenging. Identification of high-risk behaviors in adolescents may be difficult because of physical, legal, cultural, and/or economic barriers to seeking care, because of confidentiality and trust issues in discussing hidden agendas and because of health literacy and physician cultural competence issues. The sensitive nature of health and non-health issues, especially in a population that is discussing them for the first time in a medical setting, may create patient or clinician discomfort and confidentiality issues. As a result, clinician "forgetfulness" may contribute to low rates of sensitive issues addressed. In addition, the health system may pit patient privacy against adequate care and/or public health reporting mandates. Clinicians treating teens may often be faced with these conflicts when handling patient data. Computerized prompting systems,[3] screening questionnaires,[4] and automated health assessments[5] address some of these barriers and have been shown to improve services for adolescents.

5.3 Core Clinical Data

In addition to knowledge of transitional developmental issues into adulthood and general health issues of teens and developing adults, providers of primary and specialty adolescent health care must collect, record, and communicate:

Biological data

- Vital signs, growth parameters, and physiologic measures in contrast to normal adult values (blood pressure, heart rate, weight, body-mass index, electrocardiogram)
- Anatomic, physiologic and physical maturity (sometimes including: bone age), parental heights, musculoskeletal strength, endurance and performance
  - Sexual maturity rating (Tanner scores, both genders), gonadal endocrine functions (including laboratory parameters, both genders), physical examination normal findings
  - Obstetric/gynecologic data (gravidity, parity, menstrual parameters)
- Medical history (including hospitalizations, surgeries, medications, allergies)
- Physical findings suggesting risky behavior (constitutional, skin, oral/dental)
- Disease-specific findings, diagnoses, and therapies
- Genetics and family history (hypertension, asthma, hyperlipidemia, diabetes)

Psychological data

- Cognitive and intellectual functions, including intelligence, language, and literacy/numeracy
- Affective functions, including depression, suicidal ideation

Social data

- School achievement and job readiness/performance
- Legal and economic status, including emancipation, homelessness, marital, and insurance status

Cultural data

- Religion and effects on health care preferences
- Customs and culture-specific health practices

Sexuality data

- Gender, orientation
- Practices (including contraception and high risk sexual experiences)

Behavioral risk data

- Harm exposures
  - Abuse (physical, sexual)
  - Bullying
  - Firearms
  - Suicide attempts, self mutilation
  - Bike helmet use
- Automotive
  - Seat belt
  - Driving while intoxicated, driving with someone who is intoxicated
  - Mobile and cellular communication use while driving
  - Speeding and racing
- Substance use and abuse

Nutrition and eating behaviors

- Diet (caloric and fat intake, in conjunction with physical activity)
- Eating disorders

Physical activity

- Caloric expenditure (in conjunction with diet)
- Sports activities and performance enhancement

Media use and abuse

- Displacement time from other activities
- Exposure to sexual, violent, or harmful media content
- Online exposure to predators, and access to alcohol, tobacco, and drugs

The clinical paradigm shift from pediatric disease/intervention to adolescent prevention/health-promotion places a greater emphasis on targeted social/behavioral morbidities and on risky behaviors. Technology must be able to focus on both preventive and interventional aspects of care and to assess and document the severity of morbidities.

5.4   Opportunities, Barriers and Threats

5.4.1   Maintaining Confidentiality

Assurance of confidentiality concerning sexuality, alcohol and substance abuse and mental health with parents, teachers, and authorities is a major issue and barrier in adolescent health care. Analyses of costs that result when teens don't seek care because a health care program does not *provide* appropriate confidential health services estimate annual costs $611 per teen.[6] Although access to care may be available, their concern about loss of confidentiality may be too high for teens to seek timely care.

Other aspects of the health system that may contribute to this include:

- Adolescents may not be able to articulate or know how to ask about confidentiality.
- Medical office and school-based clinical information on specific diseases (such as sexually transmitted infections) may have public health reporting requirements (with subsequent outreach to patients by government agencies). However, free clinic information is often held anonymously or by alias.
- Services for adolescents may be on parents' health plans, which may not automatically provide needed confidentiality, therefore the *default arrangement* must necessarily provide confidentiality.
  - For clinician services, this may require waiving advance payment for visits.
  - For laboratory services, arrangements are needed (for private offices) to handle "confidential" services for teens who cannot afford to pay for tests (at all or for a specific visit). Requests for drug testing for *substances of abuse* by parents or schools requires documented *consent by the teen* for testing (sometimes implied by giving a urine sample), as well as informed consent by both parent and teen that results may have future consequences (positive drug test result in medical chart may effect future health insurance & life insurance applications, security clearances, government job applications, etc.).

5.4.1.1   Case Study 1

A 15 year old girl seeing her private pediatrician for STD screening and contraception is given a pelvic exam, has a pregnancy screening test (sent to the lab) and receives a prescription for birth control pills. The patient could not pay much for the confidential visit, so the physician charged her $20 cash and suppressed the office visit bill to her parent's insurance. The girl went to a pharmacy where she paid $10 cash for her first month of oral contraceptives. The nurse logged the STD test into the office information system and sent it to the usual commercial lab, which automatically generated a bill sent to the girl's parents' insurance. The parents were furious that she had gone for testing because of sexual activity.

5.4.1.2   Opportunities

To help optimize care while assuring confidentiality, information technology and workflow approaches in this scenario include:

- Clinical decision support (e.g., informing the practitioner of the need for a Pap test 3 years after first intercourse).
- Creation of special comprehensive billing processes and procedures for confidential services that include consideration of all necessary (including laboratory) services, or alerts that patients need to be referred to free clinics.
- Manage a temporary alternate confidential address for bills associated to a particular VISIT (for which a teen patient *can* pay, but not on day of service) and

for outside ancillary services (laboratory, pharmacy) to be sent instead of the parents' address. Additional management functions should allow confidentiality to be assigned to portions of a visit (such as the family planning portion of a health maintenance encounter). This may require the creation of two visits on the same day/encounter, resulting in two separate bills (Chapter 22).

5.4.2   Screening Teens Who Are at Risk for Health Problems

Adolescent risk behaviors may surface in various ways:

- Chart review by a clinician at the beginning of a visit
- Screening questionnaires that trigger further investigation
    - CAGE questions for alcohol abuse
    - Perceived Benefit of Drinking Scale (PBDS) for alcohol abuse[7]
    - Various generic health screening instruments[8] including HEADSS
    - AMA Guidelines for Adolescent Preventive Services (GAPS) questionnaires[9]
    - Youth Health Program(YHP) computerized screening[10]
- Discovery of hidden agendas during the interview and examination
- Laboratory testing requests or results, either routine, voluntary, or mandated
- Follow up visits and communications with patients
- Review of practice performance for quality assurance

5.4.2.1   Case Study 2

Dr Jones evaluates his panel of high risk adolescents by selecting ages 14–17, and all those who have had any of three measures of ever being sexually-experienced (1. ever had a chlamydia or gonorrhea test, or 2. have a prescription for oral contraceptive, or 3. received Depo-Provera in the last year) *but* have not had a chlamydia test in the last 12 months—to evaluate needs to meet HEDIS requirements. He contacts those patients needing a test by that confidential method already selected by the patient: usually private cell phone, sometimes secure messaging, rarely a letter to home.

5.4.2.2   Opportunities

Electronic medical records simplify collection and processing of data for quality improvement and risk identification within a practice population. Clinical decision support allows prompts to clinicians to improve practice during a visit and for proactive practice quality improvement.[11]

In addition, teens' comfort and facility with computers make automated medical, behavioral history collection easier[12-16] and sometimes preferable. Interviews through interactive computer programs on sensitive topics may be perceived as more confidential and less judgmental[17,5] than by human interviewers.[18,19] Functions that interviewing software should perform include:

- Obtaining a thorough health and behavioral history
- Summarizing interview response data for clinician's and educator's use
- Identifying and prioritizing problem areas and health needs
- Providing appropriate health advice and local referrals
  - Age-specific anticipatory guidance
  - Pertinent, succinct health education videos
  - Understandable take-home materials

5.4.3   Facilitating Communication with Adolescent Patients

Adolescents comfort with information and communication tools and devices and their growing ubiquity may facilitate health care. Most messaging (cell phone, short messaging services (SMS or texting)) between clinic and adolescents is free of office visit charges and confidential billing issues. Useful functions for adolescent care include providing answers for confidential clinical matters and appointment reminders. Use of electronic communication tools, such as cell phones, e-mail, secure electronic messaging and text messaging is covered in Chapter 23.

5.4.4   Improving Access to Teen Health Information

When children reach the age to consent to certain confidential services (varies by state), laws regarding proxy access to patient health information apply. At this point, parents/guardians lose their right to access a child's (adolescent) record (unless there are issues of patient competency). The impact of this has many dimensions. In addition to adolescent privacy issues, there may be health issues that the parent/guardian has not disclosed to the child. Communication and information access plans should notify caregivers and patients about local laws and practice policies regarding proxy access to teen PHI, including the age at which a teen can legally consent to procedures/treatments (which is also the age at which the teen alone is allowed direct access to the medical record regarding those procedures/treatments).

Direct access by teens is impacted by the Children's Online Privacy Protection Act, which requires "verifiable parental consent" for online transactions (i.e., direct access) for children under the age of 13. In addition, unanticipated disclosures may result from business/insurance notifications of care (as in Case Study 1).

5.4.5   Educating Teens About Health

Appropriate anticipatory and routine health guidance may be provided by a variety of information technology and media within the clinic setting (audio-visual materials, computer-based interactive multimedia, and/or vetted Internet sites).[20,21]

Video reinforcement can enhance teens' understanding and retention of a clinician's advice. With skeptical teens, it may help with medical compliance. In one study, patients watching anticipatory guidance from videos gained 57% more knowledge than those reading printed handouts.[22] In another study, compliance with treatment improved 50% when medical advice was followed by video viewing in the clinic.[23–25]

Computer-assisted instruction games can influence patient attitudes, beliefs, feelings, and knowledge, even on sensitive health subjects.[26–28]

Internet sites (See Table 5.1) are used by teens to obtain health education and information, with three fourths of all teens using the World Wide Web for health education and information, and two thirds using it for health information for school-related projects.[29]

Major considerations[30] for selecting and implementing adolescent health education hardware, software, video, and multimedia for use in the clinic setting include:

- Patient benefits and impacts on health outcomes
- Staffing and administrative requirement
- Cost (purchase vs. rental) and space
- Content quality, accuracy, and currency
- Accessibility, usability, and appropriateness for use by adolescents
- Hardware/software requirements for office systems vs. dedicated systems

5.4.6 Protecting Teens from IT-Enhanced Risks

The ubiquity of information and communication technology has paradoxically created health risks to adolescents. While teens have increased access to information and to family and peers, they also are at risk from:

- Time displacement from other physical and social activities
- Exposure to inaccurate health information, including messages that glorify inappropriate sexuality, violence and use of alcohol, tobacco, and illicit drugs

Table 5.1 Useful Internet sites with reliable health information for adolescents[31,32]

Site	Sponsor	Types of information	URL
Teen growth	TeenGrowth.com, Tampa, FL	Various health and safety	TeenGrowth.com
TeenHealth.org	Nemours foundation	Physical and mental health issues (including Spanish)	TeensHealth.org
Go Ask Alice	Columbia University	Alcohol, drugs, fitness, emotional health, sexuality, and relationships	goaskalice.columbia.edu
National Institute on Drug Abuse	National Institutes of Health	Data on drugs of abuse	nida.nih.gov
Teen Matters	So. Carolina Share	Mental health	Teen-Matters.com

- Access to purchase of alcohol, tobacco, illicit drugs, and firearms as well as information to enable their use and misuse
- Exposure to inappropriate and/or harmful online relationships
  - Exposure to online predators (one in five teens get an unwanted sexual solicitation)
  - Cyber-bullying
- Distraction from activities (such as driving) during use of mobile devices (cell phones and texting)

Such "new" risk behaviors are often omitted in medical screenings, and therefore may not addressed. Guidance in reducing these behaviors (through identification and counseling) in conjunction with novel applications of IT may reduce risks:

- Monitoring and limiting
  - Television, gaming, online, and computer time
  - Internet-based purchases (i.e., credit cards)
- Providing guidelines (including teen online behavior contracts)
  - Appropriate and inappropriate information exchange
    - Types of identifying information that should not be divulged
  - When to contact an adult about a problem
    - Obscene and/or threatening messages
    - Requests for personal meetings
  - When not to use IT (cell phones in the car)
- Specific applications
  - Television/computer time monitors
  - Linking online/computer time to physical activities and health monitoring
  - Providing direction to sources of reliable health information (MEDLINEplus)
  - Lockout and blocking of specific Internet sites[33]
  - Providing feedback to Internet service providers

5.5 Conclusion

Adolescent medicine provides challenges in clinical data management because of:

- The changing clinical information needs as children transition to adults
- The security and privacy needs for information access as children grow to the age of majority and deal with sensitive health issues
- The need to consider these issues in designing and implementing health information systems that address the needs of adolescent patients

References

1. Haggerty RJ. The new morbidity. In: Haggerty RJ, Roghmann KJ, Pless IB, eds. *Child Health and Community*. New York: Wiley; 1975.
2. Paperny DM. Computers and information technology: implications for the 21st century. *Adol Med: State Art Rev.* 2000;11(1):183–202.

3. Litzelman DK, Dittus RS, Miler ME, et al. Requiring physicians to respond to computerized reminders improves their compliance with preventive care protocols. *J Gen Intern Med.* 1993;8:311–317.
4. Schubiner H, Tzelepis A, Wright K, et al. The clinical utility of the safe times questionnaire. *J Adolesc Health* 1994;15:374–382.
5. Paperny DM, Aono JY, Lehman RM, et al. Computer-assisted detection and intervention in adolescent high-risk health behaviors. *J Pediatr.* 1990;116(3):456–462.
6. Gans JE, Alexander B, Chu RC, et al. The cost of comprehensive preventive medical services for adolescents. *Arch Pediatr Adolesc Med.* 1995;149:1226–1234.
7. Rathbun J. Development of a computerized alcohol screening instrument for the university community. *J Am Coll Health* 1993;42(1):33–36.
8. Deisher RW, Paperny DM. Variations in sexual behavior of adolescents. In Kelley VC, ed. *Brenemann – Practice Pediat.* New York: Harper & Row; 1982.
9. Elster AB. Confronting the crisis in adolescent health: visions for change. *J Adolesc Health* 1993;14(7):505–508.
10. HealthMedia Corp., Lafayette CO. Available at: http://www.HealthMediaCorp.com. Accessed December 14, 2008.
11. Paperny DM, Hedberg V. Computer-assisted health counselor visits: a low-cost model for comprehensive adolescent preventive services. *Arch Pediatr Adolesc Med.* 1999;153(1):63–67.
12. Greist J. A computer interview for suicide risk prediction. *Am J Psychiatr.* 1973;130:1327.
13. Grossman S. Evaluation of computer acquired patient histories. *JAMA* 1971;215:1286.
14. Havel RD, Wright MP. Automated interviewing for hepatitis B risk assessment and vaccination referral. *Am J Prev Med* 1997;13(5):392–395.
15. Space L. The computer as psychometrician. *Behav Res Meth Instruct.* 1981;13:595.
16. Stout R. New approaches to the design of computerized interviewing and testing situations. *Behav Res Meth Instruct.* 1981;13:436.
17. Millstein S, Irwin C. Acceptability of computer-acquired sexual histories in adolescent girls. *J Pediatr.* 1983;103(5):815–819.
18. Fisher LA, Johnson T, Porters D, et al. Collection of a clean voided urine specimen: a comparison among spoken, written, and computer-based instructions. *Am J Public Health.* 1997;67:640–644.
19. Slack WV. Computer-based interviewing system dealing with nonverbal behavior as well as keyboard responses. *Science.* 1971;171:84–87.
20. Rosen D, Elster A, Hedberg V, Paperny D. Clinical preventive services for adolescents: position paper of the Society for Adolescent Medicine. *J Adolesc Health.* 1997;21(3): 203–214.
21. Paperny DM. Computerized health assessment and education for adolescent HIV and STD prevention in health care settings and schools. *Health Educ Behav.* 1997;24(1):54–70.
22. Paperny DM. Automated adolescent preventative services using computer-assisted video multimedia. *J Adolesc Health.* 1994;15(1):66.
23. Gagliano, M. A literature review on the efficacy of video in patient education. *J Med Educ.* 1988;63:785–792.
24. Paperny DM. HMO innovations. Video-enhanced medical advice. *HMO Pract.* 1991;5(6):212–213.
25. Paperny DM. Pediatric medical advice enhanced with use of video. *Am J Dis Child.* 1992; 146(7):785–786.
26. Bosworth K, Gustafson D, Hawkins R, et al. Adolescents, health education and computers: the Body Awareness Resource Network (BARN). *Health Educ Microcomput.* 1983;14(6):58–60.
27. Paperny DM, Starn JR. Adolescent pregnancy prevention by health education computer games: computer-assisted instruction of knowledge and attitudes. *Pediatrics.* 1989;83(5):742–752.
28. Krishna S. Clinical trials of interactive computerized patient education: implications for family practice. *J Fam Pract.* 1997;45(1):25–33.
29. Kaiser Family Foundation. *Generation Rx.com: How Young People Use the Internet for Health Information*, Kaiser publication 3202.

30. Paperny DM, Zurhellen W, Spooner SA, et al. "W415; Advanced Clinical Computing Strategies." American Academy of Pediatrics Annual Meeting, 6-hour Workshop sponsored by Section on Computers & Other Technologies. Washington, DC; 1999.
31. Society for Adolescent Medicine: SAM Website. Available at: http://www.adolescenthealth.org/. Accessed December 14, 2008.
32. Skinner H, et al. Using the Internet to engage youth in health promotion. *Promot Educ.* 1997;4(4):23–25.
33. Top Ten Reviews, Inc., Internet pornography statistics; Internet Filtter Learning Center, 2009. Website (Last accessed 3/17/90): http://www.internet_filter_review.topten reviews.com/internet_pornography_statistics.html

Chapter 6
Children with Developmental Disorders and Other Special Needs

Larry W. Desch and Paul H. Lipkin

Objectives

- To define and describe the evolution of ideas regarding children with special health care needs (CSHCN)
- To describe the use of information technology in managing patients and educating families of CSHCN

6.1 Introduction

In the past half-century in the United States considerable changes have occurred, both in public opinion and legislation, regarding children and adults who have disabilities or special needs. Laws such as the Rehabilitation Act (especially Section 504) and the Americans with Disabilities Act (ADA), have led to guarantees of civil rights and protections for people with disabilities.[1,2] Important legislation, including the Education for Handicapped Children Act[3] and the Individuals with Disabilities Education Act,[2] specifically protect children with disabilities.[4,5] Many of these laws are still important because of the various rights and entitlements that were established, including access to technology. The Technology-Related Assistance for Individuals with Disabilities Act[6] established consumer-driven service delivery in all states to improve access to "assistive technology devices and services" including information and communication management tools.

The definition of children with special health care needs (CSHCN) has been formalized by both the federal Maternal and Child Health Bureau (MCHB) and the American Academy of Pediatrics (AAP) and has been nearly universally accepted. CHSCN are "those who have or are at risk for a chronic physical, developmental, behavioral or emotional condition and who also require health and related services of a type or amount beyond that required by children generally".[7]

CSHCN make up a sizeable and growing minority of children in the United States. Improved medical care for CSHCN has increased their survival and prevalence. According to the 2003 American Community Survey from the US Census

C.U. Lehmann et al. (eds.), *Pediatric Informatics: Computer Applications in Child Health,* Health Informatics,
© Springer Science + Business Media, LLC 2011

Bureau, 15% of children (3.7 million) in the US have some type of disabling condition,[8] ranging from mild learning disabilities to severe physical disabilities. The National Survey of Children's Health,[9] estimates that nearly 8% of children in the US have two or more problematic behaviors (with two thirds requiring ongoing professional treatment).

During the past 50 years, treatments for CSHCN have also radically changed, increasing the need for access to specialty care and improvements in the quality of primary care. The greatest need for this population has been coordinated primary and specialty care. Since 1985, the AAP has been promoting the Medical Home as a model for CSHCN. In response to increasing interest from the federal government (especially the MCHB) in the past 15 years, the AAP has articulated the Medical Home model,[10] two components of which are (1) early detection and referral of children with or at risk for special health care needs and (2) care coordination between the primary care provider and all specialists (e.g., medical, allied health, and educational). The potential for informatics and health information technology in facilitating these functions is great, and we illustrate these in a two-part case study.

6.2   Developmental Surveillance, Screening, and Referral

6.2.1   Case Study: Part 1

Jeffrey was born at term and had an unremarkable neonatal course. A newborn hearing screen performed on day two of life identified a hearing impairment in one ear. A faxed note and email was automatically sent from the hospital nursery to the primary care physician's office. The pediatrician sent an electronic referral to an audiologist to have a Brain Auditory Evoked Response (BAER) confirmatory text, which was reported as normal.

At 5 months of age, Jeffrey's mother noticed that he "didn't seem to move his left hand as well as his right," but thought she would "wait and see" before mentioning it to her pediatrician. One week prior to the 6-month visit, an automated e-mail was sent to the parents reminding them to complete an online developmental questionnaire on the practice Website. It was then on this online form that his mother related her concern about his left hand.

Just prior to seeing Jeffrey for the 6-month visit, his pediatrician reviewed Jeffrey's electronic medical record (EMR) and noted the flagged entry on the questionnaire, indicating a possible developmental problem. The flagged entry also informed the pediatric staff to give the parents a secondary questionnaire in the office waiting room, which verified the developmental concern. During the visit, his pediatrician confirmed through examination and developmental testing that the left hand in fact did not move as well as the right and that referrals were needed. Her office staff completed the appropriate EMR referral forms which were sent electronically to the state's Early Intervention (EI) program as well as to the local neuro-developmental specialist.

Therapists form the state EI program evaluated Jeffrey within 45 days of referral (as mandated by federal law), assured by the program's computerized tracking
system that provided timely reminders. By 7 months of age, Jeffrey was receiving
occupational and physical therapy services weekly and developmintal therapy and
monitoring monthly. Therapists educated his parents about infant motor development
by using several accredited health information Websites. Through these, his parents
found information on organizing health records and "coordinated care plans," and
wondered if there were better ways to collect these records by using a computer.

The first part of the Case Study suggests examples of how information technology can be used for CSHCN. The 2006 AAP recommendations on Developmental
Surveillance and Screening aims for the early identification of children with
developmental disorders and includes a clinical algorithm specifically designed for
incorporation into an EMR and medical informatics system.[11,12] (see Fig. 6.1)
In the hypothetical Case Study, parental concern over a problem was discovered
through developmental surveillance at the 6 month visit, which was verified by
screening and further medical and developmental evaluation. Surveillance was

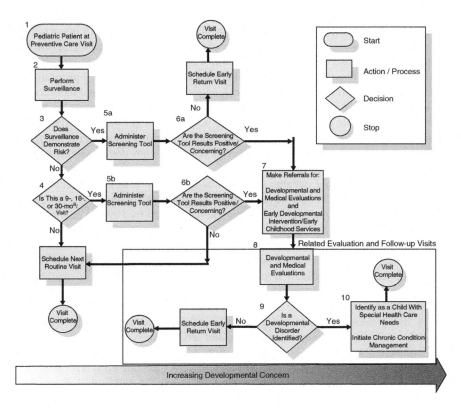

Fig. 6.1 The American Academy of Pediatrics Developmental surveillance and screening algorithm[12]

performed using a standardized developmental questionnaire through the office Website for use at the visit. At present, there are only a few standardized developmental surveillance and screening instruments that are adaptable to an EMR or include specific EMR-compatible software, such as the Ages and Stages Questionnaires[13] and the Parent's Evaluation of Developmental Status (PEDS).[14] Other tools, such as the Achenbach Child Behavior Checklist[15] have undergone extensive evaluation for EMR incorporation. Nonstandardized tools, which typically consist of questions on milestone achievement that the physician asks the parent during a health maintenance visit or could be on an office website, are best suited for surveillance.

Regardless of the implementation (paper, Web-based, using an EMR or other software), the reliability of a developmental test depends on evaluation of the validity, the sensitivity and specificity of the instrument,[12] the size and appropriateness of its normative population needs and the applicability of the test and its implementation to the practice population. Finding information on test validity is not a problem for commonly used questionnaires, but their availability in electronic (or EMR-compatible) versions may be limited due to development costs and royalty issues, but this will change as demand for EMR-compatible standardized instruments increases.

As in the Case Study (and as is recommended[12]), detection of a developmental problem should lead to a referral for Early Intervention (EI). All states have systems for EI,[4,5] including computerized data collection, but not all state agencies use collected data for more than internal administrative functioning.[16] In one example, in the state of Illinois, prevalence tracking of diagnoses by geographic regions has been used to allocate resources and funding.[17] At one time, Illinois had the only system in the US in which specialty pediatricians assisted the state EI program with determining appropriate services and service levels for the infants and toddlers who qualified for the program. In this program, these physicians had access to summaries of the entire state database of services to help ensure equity and standardization of decisions regarding the types and frequencies of therapy services provided.

It is possible that EI databases and other large state agency databases (e.g., Special Education, Medicaid) and subsets may be used to monitor programs and therapies being given to individual patients through linkage to public health agencies and/or private practice EMRs.[18,19] However, a major hurdle is the issue of privacy protection (HIPAA).[20] The Illinois project, although terminated by Federal administrators of EI because of concerns that it was "intrusive" on the parents' and clinical teams' decision-making for the children, remains an example of how large administrative databases can be used to assist in individualized clinical decisions for CSHCN.

The collection of accurate prevalence statistics for CSHCN is challenging. One approach has been to use state Medicaid data or data from large health care systems (such as Kaiser-Permanente). Research by the Institute for Child Health Policy using these data sets has found that this administrative data "disproportionately identifies children with injuries and tends to miss children with chronic well-controlled conditions."[21] Children with temporarily incapacitating injuries are sometimes inappropriately counted as CSHCN. Specialized questionnaires to collect and analyze the data have been devised, evaluated and demonstrated to be much better at correctly identifying CSHCN.[22,23]

Surveillance of more severe types of problems (such as birth defects) may be more standardized. An example of this is the Birth Defects Monitoring Program (BDMP) of the Centers for Disease Control. Although 34 states are involved in this program, reliability and validity of data collection vary. Although there is standardized collection of birth records, only 11 of these 34 states have active case-finding, without which many CSHCN might be excluded because their birth defects would not discovered until days or months after birth.[24] A report from the Centers for Disease Control and Prevention (CDC)[24] using BDMP data, for example, found that cleft lip/palate was the most common birth defect, followed by Trisomy 21. The key to achieving accurate results (reliable data) is to use programs that have been designed and standardized for a particular purpose (e.g., the BDMP) as opposed to "routine information systems" such as uncontrolled population registers or general child health surveys to monitor the prevalence of disabilities in children.[25]

Standardized surveillance and monitoring are useful to determine variations in incidence or prevalence. Data on variations may help identify or rule out causative agents. In one example, data from the Metropolitan Atlanta Congenital Defects Program did not reveal a significant seasonal variance in birth defects,[26] while in other examples, data have revealed seasonal variation of premature births in the United States, which have led researchers to look for causation, such as infectious diseases.[27,28]

An example of information technology to improve detection and coordination among public health agencies and private health services is a project of the Genetic Services branch of the federal Maternal Child Health Bureau. In this project, grants are given to 25 states to improve the integration of the newborn metabolic screening results systems (and their linked genetic referral systems) to other maternal and child health systems within each state. In cooperation with the federal Public Health Informatics Institute, a qualitative assessment named "All Kids Count" has been developed to assess these state innovations and to implement a "business/policy case addressing these innovations."[29]

The integration of information at the state level may improve decision-making and funding for agencies dealing with CSCHN which can improve outcomes for these children and families. Families have been found to be enthusiastic about integrated information systems, feeling that they might assist in coordination of health care, but need to be central in the planning, development, and implementation of such systems to maximize their value and impact.[30]

6.2.2   Case Study: Part 2

In looking for a specialist for Jeffrey, his pediatrician was able to get information and to set up an appointment through the secure Web site of the local children's hospital (of which she was also an attending pediatrician) via secure e-mail service. Jeffrey would be seen in the Neurodevelopmental Diagnostic Clinic within 1 month.

While waiting for the appointment, Jeffrey's parents began to notice that he seemed to have periods of "hiccups" several times per day that were increasing in frequency. After several days, they took him to the emergency department (ED) of the local children's hospital. Since the pediatrician's office EMR linked directly to the hospital EMR, the ED physician could access the office notes (after Jeffrey's parents gave consent). From these, the diagnosis of probable seizures was quickly made and the appropriate Pediatric Neurologist was contacted. She saw Jeffrey in the ED and admitted him with a diagnosis of infantile spasms and mild left hemiplegia. On further testing, Jeffrey was found to have had a stroke in-utero due to Factor V Leiden deficiency, an inherited coagulation disorder. He was started on ACTH treatment by the specialist, who used clinical decision support from a Neurology Website to determine the appropriate dosing.

While in the hospital, the parents were able to learn more about his diagnoses using the hospital's online digital patient library which connected them to patient information from the National Library of Medicine[31] using an information prescription[32] from Jeffrey's pediatrician. The neurologist had a number of patients from different parts of the country with similar problems, and Jeffrey's parents were able to meet other parents whose children had similar disorders using the hospital's computerized videoconference system and Internet services. The parents were also able to locate Internet resources to help the rest of their family. They arranged a tele-psychiatry videoconference for their teenage daughter Laura, who had been treated for depression and anxiety in the past and was now having more difficulties as a result of the parents' anxiety about Jeffrey and their need to devote so much time to his medical care.

Jeffrey responded well to the ACTH therapy but had adverse effects from this medication (which had been reported in the computerized medication database). Jeffrey's parents and pediatricians were aware and well-prepared for these with information from the database. The effects were mild and did not require discontinuation of therapy.

On Jeffrey's discharge from the hospital, his neurologist prepared a discharge summary and a care coordination plan which were sent directly to his pediatrician's office EMR. This care-coordination plan was particularly useful to the pediatrician because it contained an emergency care plan so that she and the parents knew exactly what to do in the case of increasing seizures (which occurred several months later).

Since Jeffrey's seizures were unusual in their clinical appearance and in the EEG findings, his pediatric neurologist contacted a British expert on unusual seizure types who had recently presented an Internet-based teleconference on new medications for seizures. Through review of the history and video EEG (via a secure online connection) and a virtual office visit with Jeffrey, his parents, and the primary-care pediatrician, the expert observed some unusual skin changes in both Jeffrey and his parents that had previously gone unnoticed. He diagnosed a second disorder, tuberous sclerosis, as a possible cause of Jeffrey's seizures.

Jeffrey's care management plan and its coordination was soon revised by his primary care pediatrician with input from all participants. These were then shared with his pediatrician's and neurologist's EMRs and subsequently to a shared database with decision support for use by his physical and occupational therapists select appropriate tools for monitoring his developmental progress. Many of these assessment tools included computer adaptive testing methods, which lessened the time it took to administer them.

6.3   Care Coordination

The management of chronic illness, both physical and mental, has changed radically in the past 20 years. Although most of this change is due to therapeutic advances, there have also been important changes in care delivery, with shared care becoming the norm. With this, there is an increasing need for coordination of care and coordinated chronic condition management.[33,34]

An essential facet of coordination of care for CSHCN is easily accessible shared information. In the Case Study, the pediatrician and the hospital both had EMR systems that were connected which shared the patient's electronic health record (EHR). An EHR has been defined as an electronic record that extends "the notion of an EMR to include the concept of cross-institutional data-sharing."[35] For any patient with a chronic disease or condition (such as CSHCN), an EHR is a necessity to ensure substantial care coordination.

There are many roadblocks to successful implementation of an EHR (Chapters 15–17) and health information exchange (HIE) (Chapter 31).

- Data in multiple EMRs are often stored in proprietary data formats, causing incompatibility between systems.[36]
- With many CSHCN, there is a need for storing large amounts of complex non-textual data (e.g., EEG, MRI images, video recordings (such as gait lab analyses)). Data compression and other techniques have addressed some of these issues,[37] and it is very important to note that multiple data types may need to be integrated for CSCHN care coordination.
- Data is frequently incomplete and in print formats. When print documents are scanned, they are frequently only readable by humans (and therefore unusable by electronic systems for searching or analysis).
- The management of privacy and sharing of nonmedical information is very complex. The Family Educational Rights and Privacy Act and other laws[38] require explicit signed consents which make sharing difficult, however public health agencies (such as the CDC) are finding methods to access de-identified data for public health monitoring[39] or to use encrypted data and electronic consent (e.g., electronic signatures).

Until these barriers can be overcome effectively, paper documentation, carried by parents/caretakers, remains the pragmatic "repository" of shared information for CSHCN. Beyond bulky original paper documentation, paper-based systems to summarize information in standard fashion for coordinating care have been developed.[40,41] Copies of such summaries may be stored on secure Internet sites for retrieval. Completed paper forms can also be scanned and stored on portable media

(Flash memory, CD or DVD) that may be helpful in emergent situations where a CSHCN is taken to an ED by nonfamily members (such as school personnel). A standardized "Emergency Information Form for Children with Special Needs" has been developed jointly by the AAP and the American College of Emergency Physicians[42] for this purpose.

Limitations of these methods include maintenance of changing information over time. Paper records cannot be linked to office or hospital EMR systems. Although parents of CSHCN may be very accurate in providing and updating medication histories[43] and are essential in reconciling these histories when a CSHCN is moved to a new environment (admission to an ED or hospital or discharged to home), this information exchange is still fraught with the problems of privacy and security and with ensuring that all the medical providers and hospitals appropriately receive updates as they occur. One possible solution is to have knowledgeable and willing parents update medical providers by e-mail, who must then update their respective EMRs. Another solution could be the use of electronic personal health records (PHR) that could be linked to update hospital or outpatient EMR's.

Secure electronic mail can be helpful in care coordination. This is already being used widely despite concerns that have been raised about privacy by school and agency administrators. Physicians concerned about the appropriateness of e-mail communication with patients and families may choose to employ secure messaging systems specifically designed for patient communication that require a unique user ID and password (See Chapter 24). One recent study[44] suggests that much of the concern over security is unwarranted if appropriately designed e-mail systems with alerts and reminders for the patients and their families about what is and is not permissible to put into the email messages (such as emergency messages and sensitive content) are used. Such guidelines may help allay the fears of administrators.

6.4   Acute Care of CSCHN

Acute care for CSHCN is responsible for a large percentage of pediatric emergency and inpatient care. In Utah, up to 24% of the children who used emergency medical services were CSHCN and most were subsequently hospitalized.[45] Hospital data from New Jersey from 1983 to 1991 showed an increase in admissions (56%) and hospitalization days (42%) used by patients "with developmental disabilities,"[46] with "moderation" of increases and sometimes decreases in the hospitalization charges when care coordination was used.

Health information technologies that may benefit CSHCN in inpatient care by decreasing medical errors include computerized provider order entry (CPOE), evidence-based order sets and clinical decision support systems (CDS):

- *Computerized provider order entry* (Chapters 19, 26) in conjunction with other information support for the medication process (See Chapters 25–28) aids providers (physicians, primary and specialized nurses and allied health personnel) in accurate prescribing. Only 11% of hospitals had CPOE in early 2006 (with 24% in progress).[47]

- *Evidence-based, condition-specific order sets*, in conjunction with CPOE, define efficient standard inpatient care for children for a variety of conditions (including acute exacerbations of chronic disease) from the time of admission. Standard order sets are part of most paper-based hospital systems and transition to CPOE provides an opportunity to review them for evidence, impact, and usefulness. Multidisciplinary input in order set development is essential. At the Mayo Clinic, for example, the "Order Set/Protocol Advisory Group" consists of 3–4 physicians (with a physician chair) as well as professionals from nursing, pharmacy, quality assurance, and EMR/IT areas.[48] Efforts to encourage structured creation of order sets based on evidence[49,50] are feasible in large institutions, and the possibility of sharing order sets with smaller institutions exists, but this has yet to happen for CSHCN.
- *Automated safety alerts* have been used for inpatient medication use in both adults and CSHCN.[51] Clinical data (from EMRs) that might indicate a problem (drug allergy, drug–drug interaction, dosage error, etc.) with a prescribed drug (from CPOE) are important to CSHCN since they are frequently on multiple drugs, which puts them at higher risk for medication errors.[52] The development and use of electronic tools such as alerts and trigger tools[53] for vulnerable populations may help decrease the incidence of medication errors.

6.5 The Medical Home

There have been and will continue to be great opportunities for informatics and information technology to play a central role in the implementation of Medical Home models to provide chronic, comprehensive, and family-centered care coordination for CHSCN, with ongoing projects in urban (the Pediatric Alliance for Coordinated Care (PACC) in Boston)[54] and rural (the MO-PEDS program in Missouri)[55] areas.

During the past decade research has been done with CSHCN and their families to evaluate their ongoing care. Primarily funded by the AHRQ, using nationally-based survey instruments such as the Medical Expenditure Panel Survey (MEPS) and the National Survey of Children with Special Health Care Needs (NSCSHCN), this research has only been made possible by information technology to enable the survey implementations and data analyses. Results of analyses of the MEPS survey show that (in 2004) twice as many CSHCN in the US were reported to see a specialist compared to other US children (26% vs. 13%),[56] while results of NSCSHCN analyses found that many children with special needs did not receive the therapy services and assistive devices that they needed, such as hearing aids or glasses, especially if they were below the federal poverty level or had more severe disabilities.[57]

Concerns have been raised regarding financial disincentives to providing comprehensive services for patients in managed care, including Medicaid managed care.[54] Information technology can help pediatricians persuade managed care organizations by providing EMR data on the types of patients seen, by use of ICD9-CM codes to justify the type and amount of work done for CSHCN and to improve reimbursement. Managed care databases that share patient information among primary care physicians, specialists, and hospitals can reduce duplicate work and improve patient care.[54]

Other functions that information technology can provide to enhance the care of CSHCN include the following:

- **Integrated growth charts**, which have advantages over paper systems,[58] and for which modules which incorporate data for CSHCN such as those with Trisomy 21, Turner syndrome, those born prematurely, and other CSHCN may be adapted for use in a pediatric EMR system.
- **Patient data entry for visits** such as assisted interviewing, is also becoming more commonplace[59] and has been shown to be helpful in identifying behavioral problems in teens. A self-entry system for patient data from adult rheumatology has been described and could be used with teenagers with rheumatic disorders.[60]
- **Electronic diaries** for recording of daily pain scores have also been found to be very useful, often leading to more compliance in keeping records, when compared to paper diaries.[61]
- **Mental health assessment and testing** to identify learning disability, intellectual disability and depression exist, some with the ability to export data to EMRs in mental health offices. Such tools may be used to screen siblings and family for secondary mental health problems.[62]
- **Streamlining reliable assessment tests**[63,64] for outcomes assessments using "computer adaptive testing" (CAT) versions for those tests[65] can be used to reduce the number of questions needed to make an accurate assessment.[66]
- **Decision support** or expert systems may help a clinical therapist select a proper assessment tool for individual patients or for program evaluations.[67].
- **Telemedicine** (Chapter 20) combines information and communication technology to provide care at a distance for review of patient self-assessment tools, monitoring medical interventions[68] or for chronic disease management where accurate and reliable patient data may produce better outcomes.[69] Real-time video teleconferencing that interfaces specialists for CSHCN with remote physicians provides needed expertise with high acceptance.[70]

6.6 Future Needs

The medical care of CSHCN is challenging, time-consuming and costly.[71] However, investment in health information technology for the care of CSHCN can help improve outcomes and show a positive return on investment, even for the high need, high-cost populations which is CSHCN.[72,73] To realize these benefits fully for CSCHN, pediatricians must participate in planning of health care IT in integrated systems by:

- Educating IT professionals of the unique and special needs of CSHCN
- Participating in the design and adoption of IT tools that facilitate data collection from patients, improve access to care and allow timely analysis of patient outcomes
- Demonstrating to policy makers and other stakeholders by using IT to collect data on unmet needs that low reimbursements and related issues have led to difficulties in providing adequate care for CSHCN
- Serving as local and national champions to garner grassroots support for the needs of CSHCN to be represented in IT development that supports the Medical Home and all its functions in providing chronic care management

The growing population of CSHCN will require resources, expertise and development of information tools to improve the health and to protect the rights of this vulnerable group of children.

References

1. Rehabilitation Act of 1973 (Section 504), PL 93–112. (1973). 29 U.S.C. §§ 701 et. seq.
2. Americans with Disabilities Act (ADA), Public Law 101–336 (1990), 42 U.S.C. § 12101 et. seq.
3. Education for All Handicapped Children Act, Public Law 94 142 (1975) 20 U.S.C. § 1400 et. Seq.
4. Duby JC. Role of the medical home in family-centered early intervention services. *Pediatrics.* 2007;120(5):1153–1158.
5. Lipkin PH., Schertz M. Early intervention and its efficacy. In: Accardo PJ, Capute AJ, eds. *Capute & Accardo's Neurodevelopmental Disabilities in Infancy and Childhood.* 3rd ed. Baltimore, MD: P.H. Brookes; 2008:519–552.
6. Technology-Related Assistance for Individuals with Disabilities Act, Public Law 100–407 (1988), 29 U.S.C. §§ 2201 et. seq.
7. McPherson M, Arango P, Fox H, et al. A new definition of children with special health care needs. *Pediatrics.* 1998;102(1 Pt 1):137–140.
8. US Census Bureau website. Accessed June 15, 2006.
9. Newacheck PW, Kim SE. A national profile of health care utilization and expenditures for children with special health care needs. *Arch Pediatr Adolesc Med.* 2005;159(1):10–17.
10. American Academy of Pediatrics Medical Home Initiatives for Children With Special Needs Project Advisory Committee. The medical home. *Pediatrics.* 2002;110(1 Pt 1):184–186.
11. Biondich PG, Downs SM, Carroll AE, Shiffman RN, McDonald CJ. Collaboration between the medical informatics community and guideline authors: fostering HIT standard development that matters. *AMIA Annu Symp Proc.* 2006;(12):36–40.
12. American Academy of Pediatrics Council on Children With Disabilities, Section on Developmental and Behavioral Pediatrics, Bright Futures Steering Committee, and Medical Home Initiatives for Children With Special Needs Project Advisory Committee. Identifying infants and young children with developmental disorders in the medical home: an algorithm for developmental surveillance and screening. *Pediatrics.* 2006;118(1):405–420.
13. Squires J, Bricker D, Potter L. Revision of a parent-completed development screening tool: ages and stages questionnaires. *J Pediatr Psychol.* 1997;22(3):313–328.

14. Glascoe FP. Parents' evaluation of developmental status: how well do parents' concerns identify children with behavioral and emotional problems? *Clin Pediatr (Phila).* 2003;42(2):133–138.
15. Rescorla LA. Assessment of young children using the Achenbach System of Empirically Based Assessment (ASEBA). *Ment Retard Dev Disabil Res Rev.* 2005;11(3):226–237.
16. Kogan MD, Newacheck PW, Honberg L, Strickland B. Association between underinsurance and access to care among children with special health care needs in the United States. *Pediatrics.* 2005;116(5):1162–1169.
17. Janet G. Director of CFC-Illinois, Illinois Department of Human Services, personal communication, 2007.
18. Clements KM, Barfield WD, Kotelchuck M, Lee KG, Wilber N. Birth characteristics associated with early intervention referral, evaluation for eligibility, and program eligibility in the first year of life. *Matern Child Health J.* 2006;10(5):433–441.
19. Farel AM, Meyer RE, Hicken M, Edmonds LD. Registry to referral: using birth defects registries to refer infants and toddlers for early intervention services. *Birth Defects Res A Clin Mol Teratol.* 2003;67(9):647–650.
20. Banks DL. The health insurance portability and accountability act: does it live up to the promise? *J Med Syst.* 2006;30(1):45–50.
21. Shenkman E. Identification tools. AHRQ user liason program. Available at: www.ahrq.gov/news/ulpcshcn2.htm on 7/25/06.
22. Newacheck PW, Strickland B, Shonkoff JP, Perrin JM, McPherson M, McManus M, et al. An epidemiologic profile of children with special health care needs. *Pediatrics.* 1998; 102(1 Pt 1):117–123.
23. Westbrook LE, Silver EJ, Stein RE. Implications for estimates of disability in children: a comparison of definitional components. *Pediatrics.* 1998;101(6):1025–1030.
24. Centers for Disease Control and Prevention (CDC). Improved national prevalence estimates for 18 selected major birth defects–United States, 1999–2001. *MMWR Morb Mortal Wkly Rep.* 2006;54(51):1301–1305.
25. Johnson A, King R. Can routine information systems be used to monitor serious disability? *Arch Dis Child.* 1999;80(1):63–66.
26. Siffel C, Alverson CJ, Correa A. Analysis of seasonal variation of birth defects in Atlanta. *Birth Defects Res A Clin Mol Teratol.* 2005;73(10):655–662.
27. Boggess KA. Pathophysiology of preterm birth: emerging concepts of maternal infection. *Clin Perinatol.* 2005;32(3):561–569.
28. Meis PJ, Goldenberg RL, Mercer BM, et al. The preterm prediction study: risk factors for indicated preterm births. Maternal-Fetal Medicine Units Network of the National Institute of Child Health and Human Development. *Am J Obstet Gynecol.* 1998;178(3):562–567.
29. Saarlas KN, Hinman AR, Ross DA, et al. All Kids Count 1991–2004: developing information systems to improve child health and the delivery of immunizations and preventive services. *J Public Health Manage Pract.* 2004;S3–15 (suppl).
30. Hastings TM. Family perspectives on integrated child health information systems. *J Public Health Manage Pract.* 2004;S24–29(suppl).
31. National Library of Medicine. MEDLINEplus Website. Available of at: http://medlineplus.gov/. Accessed June 9, 2008.
32. Ritterband LM, Borowitz S, Cox DJ, Kovatchev B, Walker LS, Lucas V, Sutphen J. Using the internet to provide information prescriptions. *Pediatrics.* 2005 Nov;116(5):e643–e647.
33. Cooley WC. Redefining primary pediatric care for children with special health care needs: the primary care medical home. *Curr Opin Pediatr.* 2004;16(6):689–692.
34. American Academy of Pediatrics Council on Children with Disabilities. Care coordination in the medical home: integrating health and related systems of care for children with special health care needs. *Pediatrics.* 2005;116(5):1238–1244.
35. AHRQ-Agency for Healthcare Research and Quality. National Resource for Health Information Technology, Knowledge Library-Electronic Medical/Health Records. Available at: http://healthit.ahrq.gov. Accessed July 25, 2006.

36. Ferranti JM, Musser RC, Kawamoto K, Hammond WE. The clinical document architecture and the continuity of care record: a critical analysis. *J Am Med Inform Assoc.* 2006;13(3): 245–252.
37. Lowe HJ. Multimedia electronic medical record systems. *Acad Med.* 1999;74(2):146–152.
38. Association of State and Territorial Health Officials. Position Statement: Accessing school health information for public health purposes. Available at: http://www.astho.org. Accessed July 25, 2006.
39. Centers for Disease Control and Prevention (CDC). Mental health in the United States: health care and well being of children with chronic emotional, behavioral, or developmental problems–United States, 2001. *MMWR Morb Mortal Wkly Rep.* 2005;54(39): 985–989.
40. Nickel RE, Desch LW. *The Physician's Guide to Caring for Children with Disabilities and Chronic Conditions.* Baltimore, MD: P.H. Brookes; 2000.
41. American Academy of Pediatrics. National Center for Medical Home Initiatives for CSHCN website-Care Coordination Tools. Available at: http://www.medicalhomeinfo.org/. Accessed July 25, 2006.
42. American Academy of Pediatrics. National Center for Medical Home Initiatives for CSHCN website-Emergency Medical Resources. Available at: http://www.medicalhomeinfo.org/tools/ emer_med.html. Accessed July 25, 2006.
43. Porter SC, Kohane IS, Goldmann DA. Parents as partners in obtaining the medication history. *J Am Med Inform Assoc.* 2005;12(3):299–305.
44. White CB, Moyer CA, Stern DT, Katz SJ. A content analysis of e-mail communication between patients and their providers: patients get the message. *J Am Med Inform Assoc.* 2004;11(4):260–267.
45. Suruda A, Vernon DD, Diller E, Dean JM. Usage of emergency medical services by children with special health care needs. *Prehosp Emerg Care.* 2000;4(2):131–135.
46. Walsh KK, Kastner T, Criscione T. Characteristics of hospitalizations for people with developmental disabilities: utilization, costs, and impact of care coordination. *Am J Ment Retard.* 1997;101(5):505–520.
47. Conn J. Hard(ly) wired. CPOE systems still a rarity at U.S. hospitals. *Mod Healthcare.* 2006;36(3):32–33.
48. Paul C, MD, email communication, 4/11/06.
49. Chisolm DJ, McAlearney AS, Veneris S, Fisher D, Holtzlander M, McCoy KS. The role of computerized order sets in pediatric inpatient asthma treatment. *Pediatr Allergy Immunol.* 2006;17(3):199–206.
50. McAlearney AS, Chisolm D, Veneris S, Rich D, Kelleher K. Utilization of evidence-based computerized order sets in pediatrics. *Int J Med Inform.* 2006;75(7):501–512.
51. Galanter WL, Polikaitis A, DiDomenico RJ. A trial of automated safety alerts for inpatient digoxin use with computerized physician order entry. *J Am Med Inform Assoc.* 2004;11(4): 270–277.
52. Slonim AD, LaFleur BJ, Ahmed W, Joseph JG. Hospital-reported medical errors in children. *Pediatrics.* 2003;111(3):617–621.
53. Takata GS, Mason W, Taketomo C, Logsdon T, Sharek PJ. Development, testing, and findings of a pediatric-focused trigger tool to identify medication-related harm in US children's hospitals. *Pediatrics.* 2008 April;121(4):e927–e935.
54. Palfrey J, Haynie M. Managed care and children with special health care needs: creating a medical home. Strategies for Managed Care: An Update from the Committee on Child Health Financing. AAP News. (insert); 12(2), 1996 (Summary); 1996. Available at: http://www.aap. org/advocacy/mmcmdhom.htm.
55. Farmer JE. Comprehensive Care for Children with Special Health Care Needs. Available at: http://www.hsc.missouri.edu/~MO-PEDS/. Accessed July 25, 2006.
56. Newacheck PW, Kim SE. A national profile of health care utilization and expenditures for children with special health care needs. *Arch Pediatr Adolesc Med.* 2005;159(1):10–17.

57. Dusing SC, Skinner AC, Mayer ML. Unmet need for therapy services, assistive devices, and related services: data from the national survey of children with special health care needs. *Ambul Pediatr*. 2004;4(5):448–454.
58. Rosenbloom ST, Qi X, Riddle WR, et al. Implementing pediatric growth charts into an electronic health record system. *J Am Med Inform Assoc*. 2006;13(3):302–308.
59. Stevens J, Kelleher KJ, Gardner W, Chisolm D, McGeehan J, Pajer K, Buchanan L. Trial of computerized screening for adolescent behavioral concerns. *Pediatrics*. 2008 June;121(6):1099–1105.
60. Williams CA, Templin T, Mosley-Williams AD. Usability of a computer-assisted interview system for the unaided self-entry of patient data in an urban rheumatology clinic. *J Am Med Inform Assoc*. 2004;11(4):249–259.
61. Palermo TM, Valenzuela D, Stork PP. A randomized trial of electronic versus paper pain diaries in children: impact on compliance, accuracy, and acceptability. *Pain*. 2004;107(3):213–219.
62. Van Riper, M. The sibling experience of living with childhood chronic illness and disability. *Annu Rev Nurs Res*. 2003;21:279–302.
63. Ostensjo S, Bjorbaekmo W, Carlberg EB, Vollestad NK. Assessment of everyday functioning in young children with disabilities: an ICF-based analysis of concepts and content of the Pediatric Evaluation of Disability Inventory (PEDI). *Disabil Rehabil*. 2006;28(8):489–504.
64. Wong V, Au-Yeung YC, Law PK. Correlation of Functional Independence Measure for Children (WeeFIM) with developmental language tests in children with developmental delay. *J Child Neurol*. 2005;20(7):613–616.
65. Haley SM, Raczek AE, Coster WJ, Dumas HM, Fragala-Pinkham MA. Assessing mobility in children using a computer adaptive testing version of the pediatric evaluation of disability inventory. *Arch Phys Med Rehabil*. 2005;86(5):932–939.
66. Haley SM, Ni P, Ludlow LH, Fragala-Pinkham MA. Measurement precision and efficiency of multidimensional computer adaptive testing of physical functioning using the pediatric evaluation of disability inventory. *Arch Phys Med Rehabil*. 2006;87(9):1223–1229.
67. Law MC. *All About Outcomes: An Educational Program to Help You Understand, Evaluate, and Choose Adult Outcome Measures*. Thorofare, NJ: Slack, Inc; 2001.
68. Gringras P, Santosh P, Baird G. Development of an Internet-based real-time system for monitoring pharmacological interventions in children with neurodevelopmental and neuropsychiatric disorders. *Child Care Health Dev*. 2006;32(5):591–600.
69. Pare G, Jaana M, Sicotte C. Systematic review of home telemonitoring for chronic diseases: the evidence base. *J Am Med Inform Assoc*. 2007;14(3):269–277.
70. Karp WB, Grigsby RK, McSwiggan-Hardin M, et al. Use of telemedicine for children with special health care needs. *Pediatrics*. 2000;105(4 Pt 1):843–847.
71. Newacheck PW, Kim SE. A national profile of health care utilization and expenditures for children with special health care needs. *Arch Pediatr Adolesc Med*. 2005;159(1):10–17.
72. Kaushal R, Jha AK, Franz C, Jaggi T, et al. Return on investment for a computerized physician order entry system. *J Am Med Inform Assoc*. 2006;13(3):261–266.
73. Frisse ME. Comments on return on investment (ROI) as it applies to clinical systems. *J Am Med Inform Assoc*. 2006;13(3):365–367.

Chapter 7
Pediatric Emergency and Pediatric Critical Care Considerations

Mark A. Del Beccaro, Howard E. Jeffries and George R. Kim

Objectives

- To outline information needs, workflow, and communication in pediatric emergency medicine (PEM) and pediatric critical care (PCC)
- To list functions of health information technology tools within PEM and PCC settings
- To describe PICU health IT implementation (CPOE) within one pediatric academic institution

7.1 Introduction

Pediatric emergency medicine (PEM) and pediatric critical care (PCC) provide care for all children in all states of distress. The primary distinction between the two is that PEM must be prepared to locate, stabilize, and transfer children in extremis to appropriate care. Therefore, PEM must extend beyond any single or group of institutions and into the regional community. Thus, PEM and PCC have similar and distinct information needs and workflows, many of which are high-risk.

7.2 PEM and PCC: Common Information Needs

Since both PEM and PCC deal with all children in all states of health or distress, they have common information needs that center on the needs of children.

7.2.1 Core Functionality

- **Prevention and surveillance**: If mortality, morbidity and distress in children can be prevented by any means (including education, early detection and intervention, or surveillance/screening), these should be incorporated into a system-wide approach to providing PEM/PCC services. Included in planning is the creation

C.U. Lehmann et al. (eds.), *Pediatric Informatics: Computer Applications in Child Health,* Health Informatics,
© Springer Science + Business Media, LLC 2011

and maintenance of local emergency readiness protocols,[1,2] rapid response and triage systems,[3] public information centers,[4] and research networks.[5]

- **Recovery and maintenance of viability**: The variability of the needs of children has given rise to training programs[6] (education/certification), protocols[7,8] and standards for resuscitation, stabilization, and transport of children of differing ages and medical needs in the field. The "platinum half-hour"[9] refers to the need for speed of delivery of resuscitative care to a child or infant quickly after a physiologic insult.
- **Real-time monitoring**: The need for second-to-second updating of vital signs and other indicators of physiologic functioning implies a core data set for children and infants for collection, communication, and trending. This also implies the need for a knowledgebase of what is normal in each population and the differences in response and tolerances to stressors such as trauma, blood loss, temperature, and exposure, as well as preparedness to respond to those differences in a child-appropriate fashion.

7.2.2   Core Knowledge

- **Normal values**: Norms for vital signs (blood pressure, pulse, respirations) and responses (Glascow Coma Score) vary across the age spectrum. In addition, there are special indicators (Apgar Scores) which may apply in different situations (birth). Laboratory values (hemoglobin, blood glucose) and changes over time may have different meanings at different ages and states of health, and these must be interpreted correctly in the context of the patient and the situation (birth, trauma, illness).
- **Vulnerabilities**: Smaller children have differences in the distribution of body surface area, which makes them vulnerable to heat loss. Smaller absolute losses of blood may well be fatal if not appreciated in the field. A major difference in pediatric and adult arrests is that most pediatric arrests are due to respiratory failure as opposed to cardiac failure, which may shift the order of resuscitation protocols in the two populations. In addition to vulnerabilities in the field, children have vulnerabilities within care environments, to preventable errors and adverse events, as a consequence of the complexity of pediatric critical and emergency care.
- **Tolerances**: Children have differential tolerances to stressors in comparison to adults. Adults may present with progressive signs of deterioration, where in children, sympathetic responses may sustain blood pressure and pulse (and appear to be stable) to the point of exhaustion and present as a sudden arrest that may be preventable.
- **Pediatric standards**: Pediatric-specific resuscitation standards and equipment may not be available, in which case, knowledge of appropriate protocols to follow is necessary. Pediatric equipment adjustments (such as smaller paddles and voltages for defibrillation[10]) may or may not be required to prevent additional

harm to children. Equipment that is routinely used in adult care (esophageal obturator airways[11] (or other devices that may cause pressure necrosis) and automatic external defibrillators[12]) may be contraindicated in children.

7.2.3 Core Data

- **Personal identifiers**: Accurate identification of patients is needed to link patients to appropriate care. Their management includes handling of privacy issues.
- **Real-time vital signs**: The high potential for arrest with the need for immediate response requires continuous monitoring of vital signs, at the bedside or remotely.
- **Standard terminology**: In addition to accurate descriptions, calculated indicators are available to communicate physiologic status or predict outcomes (Glasgow Coma Score,[13] Apgar Score,[14] PRISM/PIM Scores[15]) that must be validated and standardized for performance.

7.3 PEM and PCC: Workflow and Information

PEM and PCC are high-risk workflows of variable complexity that involve a great breadth, depth, rate, and scope of information that must be quickly organized to provide effective care (the range and number of problems that must be considered and managed simultaneously, the level of physiologic and descriptive detail that must be measured and shared, the invasiveness of diagnostic and therapeutic modalities and the types of rapid complex clinical decisions that must be made), in highly distractive environments. Communication and information use patterns in PEM and neonatal ICU environments have been studied, with physician preferences in PEM[16] and neonatal ICUs[17] for trend information (flow sheets) and direct (face-to-face) communication with colleagues (physicians and nurses) that are different from those in adult environments. In addition, there is need for overviews of patient locations (whiteboards)[18] for larger emergency departments, observation units (under 24h) run by emergency staff[19] and for surge or disaster[20] management.

Pediatric EDs are vulnerable to medication reconciliation failures,[21] while PICU and NICU workflows have vulnerabilities[22-24] in medication, documentation[25] and total parenteral nutrition ordering.[26] Studies in pediatric EDs[27-29] have also shown vulnerabilities to medication delivery errors, with weight based dosing posing a significant risk unique to pediatrics in the ED setting when compared to a general adult ED.[30] These challenges are opportunities for improvement that health information technology, such as CPOE, decision support, structured documentation, results review, and enhanced communication in these high-paced environments.[31]

7.3.1 PEM Workflow and Information Distinctions

The management of PEM patients and information generally consists of three phases:

- *Pre-hospital/pre-emergency-department*: This topic is broad and beyond the scope of this text[32] and many field communications issues are already standardized. Pediatric EDs, PICUs, and NICUs are parts of regional emergency networks that are connected and coordinated for patient allocations that are regulated. Each part of the network is accessed through a central communication network that connects community providers with emergency medical and transport services. ED information systems must communicate with the field on multiple levels (voice, telemetry, visual) and with other nodes in the network and must be able to maintain an audit trail of communications.
- *Emergency department management*: Patients transported to the ED are triaged and admitted according to the acuity of their need. Patient information is collected and entered into the ED information system for identification, diagnostic testing and therapy, and billing. ED patient identifiers and data are linked to inpatient systems as required. ED information systems must match the pace of clinical work.
- *Disposition*: Patients may be discharged home, observed in the ED or in a "short-stay" unit, admitted to an inpatient floor or higher level of care (critical care unit or operating room), transferred to another facility or in some cases, they may die in the ED. Each of these cases is associated with ED creation, organization, and communication of information for care transition. ED information systems must be able to facilitate the packaging of information in each of these diverse outcomes.

7.3.2 PCC Workflow and Information Distinctions

PICU management can similarly be divided into three phases:

- *Pre-PICU management*: Patients may come from a variety of sources, including the pediatric ED, the pediatric inpatient floor, the operating room or post-anesthesia recovery room, another critical care unit (such as the NICU) or in some institutions direct admissions from field responses—often "life flight" scenarios. In each case, the pre-PICU care of the patient must be summarized and organized according to a problem list for management in a PICU information system.
- *PICU management (NICU covered in Chapter 4)*: This topic is broad and beyond the scope of this text, but IT is essential to managing the large volume of data used in PCC.[33]
- *Post-PICU management*: This is similar to ED disposition, however, the volume of information that must be processed may be much larger, since the pre-PICU management must be summarized in addition to that from a prolonged PICU stay.

7.4 Linking PEM/PCC Information Needs to IT Tools

The goal of health information technology (HIT) design and implementation in PEM/PCC is to support the core functionalities, to coordinate communication and data flow, to inform and support clinician decisions for timely and effective response and to reduce information failures and errors. Central tools in achieving these goals include:

- *Data/knowledge level management tools*
  - A usable electronic clinical information infrastructure: to collect, organize, and distribute timely information for multiple uses from disparate sources (bedside nursing, laboratory, imaging)[34]
  - Search engine: to allow users to locate patients, test results, providers quickly[35]
  - Customized record and trend views and dashboards: to provide users with overviews of information and to "drill down" to specific levels of detail ("Overview, zoom and filter, details on demand")[36]
  - Clinical decision support: to guide care and trigger appropriate user actions
- *Patient level management tools*
  - Electronic medical records: to document and review patient course (Chapter 18)
  - Computerized order entry: to initiate and document care actions (Chapter 26)
  - Medication administration tools (Chapter 28): to track and control medication delivery
  - Picture archiving and communication systems: to allow point-of-care visualization of imaging results for clinical use and education[37]
- *Care unit level management*
  - Central monitors: to monitor physiologic measures for multiple patients[38]
  - Electronic whiteboards: To locate/organize patient workflow[18]
- *Beyond the unit*
  - Communications networks: to communicate, to assess and allocate regional resources
  - Telemedicine, Virtual ICUs: to provide expertise and control remotely[39]
  - Surveillance systems: to alert care systems of possible hazards or threats at the hospital and community levels[40,41]

7.5 Case Study: Seattle Children's Hospital

7.5.1 EMR Implementation and Deployment

The Seattle Children's Hospital in Seattle, Washington implemented a hospital-wide commercial EMR in several stages. In July 2002 Children's deployed laboratory and imaging results viewing, radiology workflow, demographic/visit data and document transcription, with limited online documentation. By November 2003 a rapid

("Big Bang") deployment brought CPOE, including the electronic medication administration record (eMAR) to all inpatient units (including psychiatry and rehabilitation units), ICUs, ED and pre and post operative areas. Since then, the hospital has expanded from 200 to 250 inpatient beds. All orders except chemotherapy are entered by clinicians, with chemotherapy orders entered by pharmacists (based on physician orders entered on paper templates). By June 2006, hospital ambulatory specialty clinics (approximately 25 different clinics with 150,000 visits that year) went live with all orders including future visit orders, electronic prescriptions and fee sheet orders.

7.5.2   CPOE in Pediatric Critical Care

Children's also published one of two studies that evaluated implementation of a commercial CPOE in academic PICUs[42,43] with different findings with regard to mortality. The Children's deployment and study benefited from the shared experience of the University of Pittsburgh, and found that many of the same issues in PICU with regard to CPOE were also important in the pediatric ED. Lessons learned included:

- *The presence of an EMR/CPOE does not guarantee perfect communication*: Communication and workflow failures are frequently root causes in medical errors. CPOE may: (1) remove informal but critical communication between nurses and physicians during ordering ("technology does not replace talking") and (2) reduce workflow efficiency by requiring more operators during critical situations (such requiring an additional physician to order medications while resuscitation is progressing).
- *Order set design is crucial*: Order sets and prescripted choices for completing single orders are powerful ways to supply decision support. These standards for care must be accessible to users: (1) users must know they exist (education) and (2) users must be able to find them (search mechanism with knowledge of the proper terminology to find them quickly). This is especially true in high-stress patient situation where nonstandard (verbal) orders may contribute to a high chance of medical errors.[44] Order sets must be based on published evidence and must be organized to guide provider choices and actions based on patient attributes.

By "go live" Children's had over 20 ICU and 20 ED specific order sets covering general and specific conditions, including standard admit, intubation and tumor lysis order sets for the PICU and new leukemia patient, diabetic ketoacidosis, fractures, dehydration, and four different fever order sets based on age or condition (neonate or cancer for example) in the Pediatric ED. Order sets configure the appropriate routes, frequencies and other details to minimize effort (clicks) and to standardize care. Orders can be generated from the ED or PICU within 10 min and are immediately routed to the appropriate areas (nursing, laboratory, radiology, pharmacy, etc.). In both PICU and Peds ED, additional order sets were designed and implemented within 2 weeks of the system "go live" based on additional provider needs.

- *Implementation is iterative and break-the-glass functionality is essential*: While order sets are a very effective way to reduce errors and streamline care, even in arrest situations, they may need modification by clinicians to optimize care. These modifications may range from being able to add specific orders to order sets to being able to override lockout rules to emergency medications when needed. The existence of recurrent modifications may indicate the need for adjustments in baseline order sets.
- *Clinical workflow evaluation is important*: Interventions that improve speed and accuracy of clinician data use and entry are important. Evaluation of these aspects may be based on studies of task times, error rates and user feedback. Examples of important process streamlining include:
  - *Rapid Registration/Preregistration.* The ability to establish orders quickly for new patient arrivals or transports is essential. Establishment of a record with minimum data set (name, birth date, etc.), even as a "John Doe" allows patients to be "in the system" on arrival for tests, drugs and access to EMR/CPOE systems.
  - *Order "sentences."* Specification of nonstandard orders (those not already in an order set) must be fast (minimum number of choices, clicks or keystrokes to enter). An example is the order for a urine sample: instead of a sequence of selections: (1) test (urinalysis), (2) source (bag, catheter, suprapubic tap, or clean catch), (3) urgency (routine or stat), and (4) indication (text entry), the user should be given a selection of single phrase orders (sentences) at a single click. The same model is used for medications and other orders, using standardized weights, routes or medical conditions.
  - *Calculators*: Inline and dedicated calculators for complex critical care processes such as continuous infusions[45] and total parenteral nutrition[46] reduce arithmetic errors associated with the cognitive burden of manual computation. Alerts, reminders and automated dose-range checks can be performed, with great time savings and reduction of errors.
  - *System response time and security*: Network and workstation capacity must be anticipated for normal to high work loads, and these must not be underestimated. In both studies of CPOE in PICUs, this has been an issue. Included in this planning is time required for security (logging into the system, selecting the patient, etc.). Clinician expectations for rapid access to a chart are high with short wait times (1 min from log in to access a patient record) before they are tempted to perform a workaround (typically a verbal order).
  - *Time and frequency*: In the ED, most orders have a frequency of once (i.e. single orders). However, if orders are delayed until a patient is admitted to the floor or ICU, they may be specified in terms of a frequency (such as every 12h). However, this may be interpreted as every 12h per the routine floor schedule, which may result in overdosing or a missed dose of an essential medication. Clear policies must be established to avoid this type of error.

○ *Duplicate and conflicting orders*: Medication reconciliation to avoid duplication should occur when a patient is transferred between care units. However, duplicate medication orders may also occur when an order is changed, or if there are different orders for different contingencies (such as two orders for acetaminophen: one for fever and one for pain). Such scenarios allow for overdosing. In the ICU, depending on the CPOE system, titrations of continuous infusions may pose similar problems (Changing an infusion rate may mean discontinuing the first rate, followed by ordering the new rate). Standards for addressing these issues are in development.

• *It's about culture change*: The biggest factor that contributes to success with CPOE is the recognition that HIT adoption is cultural change. With strong leadership, all of Seattle Children's was involved in the design, build, implementation, and post "go-live" support of the system after months of preparation and universal training on the system. The driving force of patient safety requires institutional "buy in" as the fundamental first step.

7.6   Areas of Research and Development

Progress in invasive and noninvasive monitoring of patients provides opportunities and challenges for ED/critical care information systems to incorporate new data into decision support tools. Outcome prediction models based on noninvasive monitoring[47] may allow real time decision making in trauma. Trigger tools[48,49] may help in identifying and averting errors in critical care. Patterns such as heart rate variability may help predict sepsis in critically ill children and infants.[50]

Communication handoffs are another area of investigation to improve safety in critical care. An understanding of the daily care plan goals by all team members is an essential component to the management of complex, critically ill patients.[51] Clinical information systems should provide the centralized repository of these daily goals as document that changes as the patient's conditions change and serves as the basis for care decisions. However, the adoption of this form of technology, does not eliminate the need for face to face communication, and in fact may increase it, in order to provide the necessary context.[52]

7.7   Conclusion

The challenges of PEM and PCC pose new opportunities for the application of information technology and systems design to better handle critically ill children in all types of situations, outside and within the hospital. The ability of technology to extend pediatric-specific emergency care into remote areas and to reduce errors within hospitals will improve outcomes.

References

1. American Academy of Pediatrics Committee on Pediatric Emergency Medicine, Frush K. Preparation for emergencies in the offices of pediatricians and pediatric primary care providers. *Pediatrics*. 2007;120(1):200–212.
2. Hazinski MF, Markenson D, Neish S, et al. American Heart Association Emergency Cardiovascular Care Committee. Response to cardiac arrest and selected life-threatening medical emergencies: the medical emergency response plan for schools. A statement for healthcare providers, policymakers, school administrators, and community leaders. *Pediatrics*. 2004;113(1 Pt 1):155–168.
3. Haller JA Jr. The evolution and current status of emergency medical services for children. *Surg Clin North Am*. 2002;82(2):263–271.
4. Klein KR, Herzog P, Smolinske S, White SR. Demand for poison control center services "surged" during the 2003 blackout. *Clin Toxicol (Phila)*. 2007;45(3):248–254.
5. Miller SZ, Rincón H, Kuppermann N. Pediatric emergency care applied research network. Revisiting the emergency medicine services for children research agenda: priorities for multicenter research in pediatric emergency care. *Acad Emerg Med*. 2008;15(4):377–383.
6. American Academy of Pediatrics. Neonatal Resuscitation Program. Available at: http://www.aap.org/nrp/nrpmain.html. Accessed May 23, 2008.
7. American Heart Association. PALS Course Guide. ISBN 0-87493-527-X; 2006.
8. Hunt EA, Walker AR, Shaffner DH, Miller MR, Pronovost PJ. Simulation of in-hospital pediatric medical emergencies and cardiopulmonary arrests: highlighting the importance of the first 5 minutes. *Pediatrics*. 2008;121(1):e34–43.
9. Gausche M, Seidel JS. Out-of-hospital care of pediatric patients. *Pediatr Clin North Am*. 1999;46(6):1305–1327.
10. Deakin CD, Bennetts SH, Petley GW, Clewlow F. What is the optimal paddle force during paediatric external defibrillation? *Resuscitation*. 2003;59(1):83–88.
11. Pons PT. Esophageal obturator airway. *Emerg Med Clin North Am*. 1988;6(4):693–698.
12. König B, Benger J, Goldsworthy L. Automatic external defibrillation in a 6 year old. *Arch Dis Child*. 2005;90(3):310–311.
13. Martin C, Falcone RA Jr. Pediatric traumatic brain injury: an update of research to understand and improve outcomes. *Curr Opin Pediatr*. 2008;20(3):294–299.
14. Odd DE, Rasmussen F, Gunnell D, Lewis G, Whitelaw A. A cohort study of low Apgar scores and cognitive outcomes. *Arch Dis Child Fetal Neonatal Ed*. 2008;93(2):F115–120.
15. Slater A, Shann F, ANZICS Paediatric Study Group. The suitability of the Pediatric Index of Mortality (PIM), PIM2, the Pediatric Risk of Mortality (PRISM), and PRISM III for monitoring the quality of pediatric intensive care in Australia and New Zealand. *Pediatr Crit Care Med*. 2004;5(5):447–454.
16. Fairbanks RJ, Bisantz AM, Sunm M. Emergency department communication links and patterns. *Ann Emerg Med*. 2007;50(4):396–406.
17. Brown PJ, Borowitz SM, Novicoff W. Information exchange in the NICU: what sources of patient data do physicians prefer to use? *Int J Med Inform*. 2004;73(4):349–355.
18. Aronsky D, Jones I, Lanaghan K, Slovis CM. Supporting patient care in the emergency department with a computerized whiteboard system. *J Am Med Inform Assoc*. 2008;15(2):184–194.
19. Zebrack M, Kadish H, Nelson D. The pediatric hybrid observation unit: an analysis of 6477 consecutive patient encounters. *Pediatrics*. 2005;115(5):e535–542.
20. Kanter RK. Strategies to improve pediatric disaster surge response: potential mortality reduction and tradeoffs. *Crit Care Med*. 2007;35(12):2837–2842.
21. Porter SC, Manzi SF, Volpe D, Stack AM. Getting the data right: information accuracy in pediatric emergency medicine. *Qual Saf Healthcare*. 2006;15(4):296–301.
22. Kaushal R, Bates DW, Landrigan C, et al. Medication errors and adverse drug events in pediatric inpatients. *JAMA*. 2001;285:2114–2120.

23. Koren G, Zohar BZ, Greenwald M. Tenfold errors in administration of drug doses: a neglected Iatrogenic disease in pediatrics. *Pediatrics*. 1986;77:848–849.
24. Menke JA, Broner CW, Campbell DY, et al. Computerized clinical documentation system in the pediatric intensive care unit. *BMC Med Inform Decision Making*. 2001;1:3
25. Carroll AE, Tarczy-Hornoch P, O'Reilly E, et al. Resident documentation discrepancies in a neonatal intensive care unit. *Pediatrics*. 2003;111:976–980.
26. Miller SZ, Rincón H, Kuppermann N. Pediatric emergency care applied research network. Revisiting the emergency medicine services for children research agenda: priorities for multicenter research in pediatric emergency care. *Acad Emerg Med*. 2008;15(4):377–383.
27. Folli HL, Poole RL, Benitz WE, et al. Medication error prevention by clinical pharmacists in two children's hospitals. *Pediatrics*. 1987;79:718–722.
28. Leape LL, Brennan TA, Laird N, et al. The nature of adverse events in hospitalized patients. Results of the Harvard Medical Practice Study II. *N Engl J Med*. 1991;324(6):377–384.
29. Kozer E, Scolnik D, Macpherson A, et al. Variables associated with medication errors in pediatric emergency medicine. *Pediatrics*. 2002;110:737–742.
30. Selbst SM, Fein JA, Osterhoudt K, Ho W. Medication errors in a pediatric emergency department. *Pediatr Emerg Care*. 1999;15(1):1–4.
31. Potts AL, Barr FE, Gregory DF, Wright L, Patel NR. Computerized physician order entry and medication errors in a pediatric critical care unit. *Pediatrics*. 2004;113(1 Pt 1):59–63.
32. Woodward GA, King BR, Garrett AL, Baker MD. Prehospital care and transport medicine. In: Fleisher GR, Ludwig S, Henretig FM, Ruddy RM, Silverman BK, eds. *Textbook of Pediatric Emergency Medicine*. 5th ed. Philadelphia, PA: Lippincott Williams & Wilkins; 2006:93–134.
33. Vaidya V, Pon S. Information technology in the PICU. In: Nichols DG et al., eds. *Rogers Textbook of Pediatric Intensive Care*. London/Philadelphia, PA: Walter Kluwer/Lippincott Williams & Wilkins 2008;124–135.
34. Dinh M, Chu M. Evolution of health information management and information technology in emergency medicine. *Emerg Med Australas*. 2006;18(3):289–294.
35. Feied CF, Smith MS, Handler JA. Keynote address: medical informatics and emergency medicine. *Acad Emerg Med*. 2004;11(11):1118–1126.
36. Shneiderman B. The eyes have it: a task by data type taxonomy for information visualizations. In: Proceedings of the IEEE Symposium on Visual Languages. Washington, DC: IEEE Computer Society Press; 1996:336–343.
37. Halsted MJ, Perry LA, Perry DJ, Benton C. Development of an interactive model for teaching emergency pediatric radiography: preliminary report. *J Am Coll Radiol*. 2005;2(8):701–703.
38. Shin DI, Huh SJ, Lee TS, Kim IY. Web-based remote monitoring of infant incubators in the ICU. *Int J Med Inform*. 2003;71(2–3):151–156.
39. Wetzel RC. The virtual pediatric intensive care unit. Practice in the new millennium. *Pediatr Clin North Am*. 2001;48(3):795–814.
40. Bourgeois FT, Olson KL, Brownstein JS, McAdam AJ, Mandl KD. Validation of syndromic surveillance for respiratory infections. *Ann Emerg Med*. 2006;47(3):265.
41. Bradley CA, Rolka H, Walker D, Loonsk J. BioSense: implementation of a national early event detection and situational awareness system. *MMWR Morb Mortal Wkly Rep*. 2005;54(suppl):11–19.
42. Han YY, Carcillo JA, Venkataraman ST, et al. Unexpected increased mortality after implementation of a commercially sold computerized physician order entry system. *Pediatrics*. 2005;116(6):1506–1512. (correction published Pediatrics 2006;117:594).
43. Del Beccaro MA, Jeffries HE, Eisenberg MA, et al. Computerized provider order entry implementation: no association with increased mortality rates in an intensive care unit. *Pediatrics*. 2006;118:290–295.
44. Kozer E, Seto W, Verjee Z, et al. Prospective observational study on the incidence of medication errors during simulated resuscitation in a paediatric emergency department. *BMJ*. 2004;329:1321–1326.

45. Lehmann CU, Kim GR, Gujral R, Veltri MA, Clark JS, Miller MR. Decreasing errors in pediatric continuous intravenous infusions. *Pediatr Crit Care Med*. 2006;7(3):225–230.
46. Lehmann CU, Conner KG, Cox JM. Preventing provider errors: online total parenteral nutrition calculator. *Pediatrics*. 2004;113(4):748–753.
47. Shoemaker WC, Wo CCJ, Lu K, et al. Outcome prediction by a mathematical model based on hemodynamic monitoring. *J Trauma*. 2006;60:82–90.
48. Resar RK, Rozich JD, Simmonds T, Haraden CR. A trigger tool to identify adverse events in the intensive care unit. *Jt Comm J Qual Patient Saf*. 2006;32(10):585–590.
49. Sharek PJ, Horbar JD, Mason W, et al. Adverse events in the neonatal intensive care unit: development, testing, and findings of an NICU-focused trigger tool to identify harm in North American NICUs. *Pediatrics*. 2006;118(4):1332–1340.
50. Griffin MP, Lake DE, O'Shea TM, Moorman JR. Heart rate characteristics and clinical signs in neonatal sepsis. *Pediatr Res*. 2007;61(2):222–227.
51. Pronovost P, Berenholtz S, Dorman T, Lipsett PA, Simmonds T, Haraden C. Improving communication in the ICU using daily goals. *J Crit Care*. 2003;18(2):71–75.
52. Arora V, Johnson J. National patient safety goals: a model for building a standardized hand-off protocol. *Jt Comm J Qual Patient Saf*. 2006;32(11):646–655.

Part III
The Pediatric Data-Knowledge-Care Continuum

Chapter 8
Complexity in Healthcare Information Technology Systems

Willa H. Drummond, Jeffrey M. Ferranti, Christoph U. Lehmann and Donald E. Lighter

Objectives

The reader will be able to:

- Understand that the implementation of a healthcare computer/human system is a complexly interacting change agent that will alter the status quo
- Organize a logical approach to evaluating human/computer/healthcare interaction problems in pediatric environments
- Participate effectively in local, cross-disciplinary, team-based process improvement efforts

8.1 Introduction

Changes in healthcare processes are implemented with the goal to improve care through improved patient safety, reduction in costs and work load, and improved communication. However, change often triggers unintended consequences that may cause stress to other healthcare system components, sometimes to a point of outright failure. Change that improves a process in one hospital will not necessarily succeed in another. This chapter discusses how health information technology (HIT) as a change agent affects health care delivery in predictable as well as unpredictable ways. We will explore the complexity of existing health care structures using evaluative scenarios of IT implementations. HIT implementations add complexity that may break existing workflow processes and interrupt care delivery in unexpected ways.

8.1.1 Health IT as Change Agent

The implementation of IT systems in health care changes the delivery of clinical care in ways that can have unexpected negative consequences.[1-3] An IT system may destabilize the workflow of a clinical site such as a physician's office, hospital, or inpatient unit (i.e. ICU) with cascading downstream effects on associated processes.

C.U. Lehmann et al. (eds.), *Pediatric Informatics: Computer Applications in Child Health,* Health Informatics,
© Springer Science + Business Media, LLC 2011

A recovery room implementation of an IT system may unexpectedly slow down transfer processes. Consequently, the number of cases admitted from the operating room may exceed the number of unoccupied beds in the recovery room, resulting in canceled surgeries and dissatisfied patients and providers.

Change may interrupt the healthcare process at multiple levels, requiring analysis, subsequent modifications and interventions to respond to the interruptions. Change (especially IT implementation) can make existing latent failures of the care system more pronounced, because previously established work-arounds no longer function. One example is the implementation of a CPOE system in a hospital where the admission, discharge, and transfer (ADT) process is not working effectively. Previously, providers were able to order on paper, even if the patient's medical record number was not yet available. With CPOE system, the patient must be registered and must "be in the system" in order for a provider to place an order. The work-around (the piece of ordering paper) has effectively been rendered useless without being replaced by another "break-the-glass functionality" for quick interventions in critically ill patients.

IT implementations in health care venues can fail on many levels.[4-7] In "worst case" scenarios, poorly designed or implemented IT systems may impact an entire healthcare system and may lead to a removal of the HIT system, as occurred at Cedars-Sinai Hospital.[4, 8-10] In health care, unanticipated consequences may not only have a negative effect on the institution and the providers, but may be dangerous and detrimental to the health of patients.[11-13]

8.2   Scenario A: Change and Consequences

Summary: This case study explores the failure of a quality improvement (QI) initiative in a neonatal critical care unit. The scenario highlights how important human factor analysis is to the success of every change process involving human systems, while illustrating how HIT may sometimes become an obstacle to optimum patient care.

8.2.1   Quality Improvement Goal: Achieving Optimal Oxygen Saturation

Newborn Intensive Care units (NICU) struggle with managing the oxygen saturation of premature infants in an optimal range. Too much oxygen may cause blindness; too little causes brain injury. In this scenario, two NICUs within the same health system implemented a QI protocol to improve oxygen management in premature infants that had been successfully used in other institutions (Fig. 8.1).

Nurses set the oxygen alarm limits on the patient's monitor as per physician order. The percent of time that the oxygen saturation limits were set as ordered during random audits was selected as outcome measure. In the first 3 months, the intervention failed completely in NICU B, while NICU A could show some moderate success (Fig. 8.2).

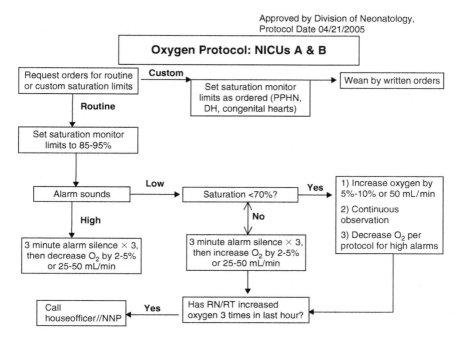

Fig. 8.1 Oxygen saturation management protocol

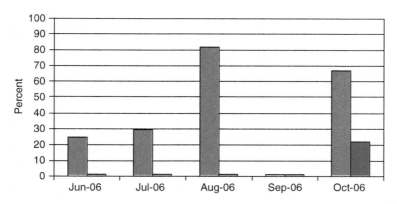

Fig. 8.2 O_2 saturation within accepted limits – intervention was initiated in May 2006

8.2.2   Formative Evaluation of the QI Initiative's Results

After it became apparent that the protocol implementation had failed, an analysis of the process was conducted and revealed multiple problems:

1. High Work Load: The new, more stringent oxygen saturation limits created more monitor alarms, requiring the staff to adjust supplemental oxygen more frequently, adding additional workload for already busy nurses. A high patient census and many labile patients, whose saturations always fluctuate, further magnified the staff work load.
2. Lack of "Buy-in": Several influential staff members did not believe in the protocol's premises. Maintaining oxygen saturation in a more narrow range was not seen as beneficial to patients' outcome, so the required titration of oxygen was considered a useless chore. Some staff members were unsure if all babies would benefit from this protocol or only smaller premature infants.
3. Regulations: Pressured to save time in order to comply with work-hour rules,[14] residents quickly learned to ignore the time-consuming titration protocol steps and reverted to increasing the oxygen to 100% at the beginning of a desaturation episode, leaving the nurse or respiratory therapist to titrate the FiO_2 back down.
4. Ambiguity: Users were unclear if this protocol applied to all patients or if there were legitimate exceptions. The resulting confusion led to inconsistent protocol application and measurement errors.[15]
5. Negative Impact of Hospital IT: One of the major obstacles discovered in the course of the failure analysis, was the impact of a newly implemented respiratory therapy clinical documentation system designed entirely for adult patient care. This system was designed in response to a JCAHO mandate, and required the respiratory therapists (RT) to document their work using a remote computer terminal – effectively pulling the RT away from the patient bedside for extended periods of time. The reporting system added a significant documentation burden. The time spent documenting could be more than twice as long as the actual patient encounter. This HIT system effectively interrupted RTs' workflow, increased their work load, and made it impossible for them to aid in the implementation of the care optimization protocol.
6. Workflow and Layout: NICU B had been recently renovated, modernized, and enlarged, using a custom architectural design focused on solving lighting, noise, and privacy problems. Sound dampening walls, floors and translucent partitions were used to quiet the environment and to create visual and auditory privacy between the bed spaces (Fig. 8.3). Nurses in the new cubicles could not see, or hear, much of what was happening elsewhere in NICU B.

The new bed space arrangement was very different from the former layout of the NICU B (Fig. 8.4), and from the layout of NICU A. Both NICU A and the previous design of the NICU B had a floor plan that aligned the beds in rows along counters, about 4 ft apart. While noisy and very unpleasant for parents, visual and auditory access to all the bed spaces was excellent with the previous design.

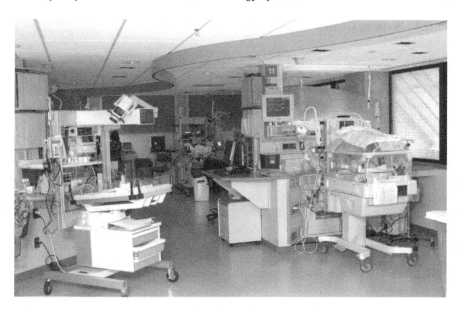

Fig. 8.3 The renovated NICU B has partial visual and auditory isolation of the staff and parents who are in the semi-closed bed spaces. At the time of the picture, the unit is 100% occupied. Note the acoustically dampening, translucent partition above the headwall and the muted south-facing exterior window in the upper right corner. The space in the view contains 7 caregivers, 11 babies, and 2 parents

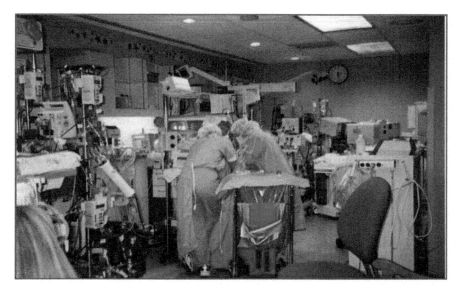

Fig. 8.4 Previous configuration of NICU B. The space is open, without any noise damping designs. All patients are visually accessible from any location in the room. Providers are easily visible

8.2.2.1 System Change

In the NICU scenario, a failure mode or root cause analysis[16] conducted by the team implementing the oxygen saturation management protocol revealed that the failure in NICU B was multifactorial. The finding was not unexpected: In complex environments such as a NICU, failures usually can be attributed to a number of individual problems.

Failure could not be blamed on a single group of people or a single process but responsibility was distributed throughout people, work flows, beliefs, conflicting interests, IT systems and physical design solutions.

Several factors contributing to failure were beyond anybody's control (such as existing wall structures). However, the many factors identified made this problem a "target-rich" human factors engineering situation. A multifaceted "system change," which focused on several of the identified problems, resulted an immediate consensus for action on many variables.

The problem was split into multiple tasks assigned to different people in order to address the list of contributing factors, simultaneously. The oxygen saturation management protocol was suspended in September 2006 to allow revisions, educational efforts, and involvement of staff nurses in focus groups. When the protocol was reintroduced in October 2006 after most of the failure causes had been addressed, improvement in NICU B compliance with resetting the monitor alarms occurred (Fig. 8.2).

8.2.3 Root Cause Analysis

While this book is focused on health information systems in pediatrics, many of the failures in implementing these systems – and the root cause of problems in these scenarios – can be traced to poor Human Factors Engineering. To make this point, we selected a scenario that had HIT systems as a minor variable. (Note, that in Scenario A the only HIT systems were the oxygen saturation monitor and the respiratory care department charting system) to emphasize the complexity of the environment, the important role that work flow, beliefs, conflicting interests, complexity of care and physical layout may play. Medicine is already complex and difficult to navigate – introducing an HIT system to this mix will raise the complexity dramatically.

The root causes of the failure of our oxygen saturation management protocol were multifactorial:

- Increased workload (increased number of alarms requiring checking and protocol based responses)
- Physical layout (Verification of alarms from a different cubicle in NICU B)
- Conflicting tasks (RT charting workflow)
- Beliefs (Lack of protocol buy-in related to the deeply ingrained belief of many nurses and physicians that a pink baby is good)

- Conflicting interests (time spent with adjusting oxygen takes providers away from other patients, and pushes 80-hour rule boundaries for residents, coping)
- Ambiguity (Unclear to users on which patients to implement the protocol)

The implementation failure of an apparently simple protocol to facilitate an evidence based "practice change," was unexpected by the implementers and revealed a complicated "systems" problem. While the required workflow changes resulted in a total "failure" of the Protocol in NICU B, NICU A produced fairly good process compliance results that were improving monthly. In retrospect, the difference between the success rates in the different NICUs is not unexpected. Had the implementers done a Failure Mode and Effect Analysis (FMEA) (Chapters 9, 29), many of the failures might have been discovered in advance. "Tribal knowledge" of existing structures, work arounds, beliefs, obstacles, and conflicts can be highly predictive of failures to be experienced later. Human factors analysis of HIT problems often uses techniques emerging from ethnographic research.[16]

Health care environments are under constant ethical, regulatory, and financial pressure to improve performance, which paradoxically can have the unintended consequence of materially decreasing system performance. NICU B's redesign was a response to new regulatory and oversight requirements by JCAHO (for formal quality improvement initiatives), HIPAA (for privacy) and the AAP/ACOG (for improved perinatal infrastructure quality standards).[17-19] Physical design changes usually result in workflow adaptations. Change instituted to improve one performance measure may result in negative effects on other performance measures. The NICU B redesign specifically, and very successfully, addressed recommendations for decreasing ambient noise, for modifying lighting environments geared to patient needs, and for increasing parental involvement.[18-22] These changes affected the ability of providers to monitor alarms effectively and to regulate oxygen saturations more tightly.

8.2.3.1 Human Factors Engineering

"Human Factors Engineering" includes physical, sensory and psychological stressors, body mechanics problems, fatigue, time pressure, workflow and physical space design, computerized alarms, control systems (knobs, system status feedback to users, cognitive design), shift work, heavy lifting, repetitive stress injuries (Ergonomics) and human–computer interaction. Most Human Factors Engineering (HFE) research has focused on avionics (pilots, planes' controls and cockpit design, and cockpit crew teamwork), military venues, corporate offices, transportation situations, and nuclear power plants.

Very little HFE research is available for health care settings,[23] and even less for intensive care unit environments. Research has focused on single devices, such as physiologic monitors, anesthesia machines, gas connectors, and controls. However, HFE lessons learned in avionics and military research may be applicable to hospitals.

The multidisciplinary, continuous, team-based work in intensive care units has many commonalities with previously studied cockpit and military environments; the lessons are of interest for redesigning health care settings as computers are installed.

HFE in avionics is the study of the interaction of pilots and crew, crews' teamwork and communication strategies, and the study of cockpit design and human interaction with cockpit controls, visual dashboards, alarms, and errors (Fig. 8.4). HFE studies the complex human–machine (computer) interactions that modern aircraft and cockpit situations create. Changes based on the HFE have drastically reduced errors, making flying one of the safest modes of transportation today. For health care, many lessons can be learned from the 40-year evolution of the culture of safety developed by the airline industry.[24, 25]

Battleships' (HFE) situations that relate to team performance under stress have been studied for a century. In the closed and isolated battleship environment, perfect teamwork of the militarily trained crew is imperative, driven by need for instantaneous coordinated response during attack and defense actions. Military HFE research includes the impact of noise, sleep deprivation, severe psychological stress, need for both acoustic and visual communication strategies, as well as coordinating human emergency responses in situations of life threatening uncertainty that occur intermittently and unexpectedly.

For those familiar with health care, the comparison between battleship situations and the ICU or emergency department in modern hospitals is obvious, suggesting that HFE lessons learned from battleship environments may be important in hospital settings.

Specific HFE research regarding appropriate designs for ICU workspaces, machines, and workflow is in its infancy, especially for the newborn and pediatric intensive care units (PICU). An extensive literature search (by WHD) in 2007 found no articles that are pertinent to the Human Factors problems in NICU or PICUs, except those mentioned in the second case study (Scenario B).

General lessons can be transferred to health care environments from HFE research in avionics (pilots, teamwork, cockpit physical design, alarms, and error signals), and in battleships (physical spaces, extreme time pressure and need for accuracy, teamwork despite noise, shift work, and fatigue). Corporate office HFE research contributed information about lighting, noise, ergonomic considerations (especially in the use of computers), financial optimization, and human responses to psychosocial isolation in cubicles. HFE research in the safety critical areas of nuclear power plants and air traffic control contributed understanding about alarms, alerts, information flow, human–machine errors and their consequences, and "latent errors."[25, 26]

Unique challenges in hospital settings (not found in avionics or battleship environments) are the steady, piecemeal addition of new treatment and monitoring machines to ICUs of all types. These additions of machines (like a new type of ventilator or a new "smart pump" system) that are designed to perform the same tasks as existing equipment but may require different adaptors, training on a new user interface, and recognition of a new set of alarms and new charting caveats, add to the complexity of the health care environment. Further, the frequent presence of "visitors" in the workspace, even during crisis situations may hinder providers from performing optimally. Human Factors Engineering and its' sub-field Ergonomics, which deals with machine-related physical stresses on the human body, have never been specifically studied for NICUs or PICUs. Thus, current knowledge is derived from research in other venues that may have conceptual overlap with NICU and PICU environments. Caution is warranted when extrapolating site-specific findings to other "similar" environments.[26]

NICUs and PICUs are complex environments with missions that are constantly changing and evolving in real-time. Important ICU issues include the impact of lighting and noise on human cognition, and the need to differentiate multiple alarms with a response speed measured in seconds (Fig. 8.4). Many user interfaces being applied in health care were designed for office or bench workers, not the ICU caregivers. The law does not require that new medical equipment be tested in the complex, multimachine environment with the intended users. Flaws in design are thus often not recognized until the equipment is widely used.[6–8] Federal and state pressure to computerize clinical healthcare quickly has resulted in installation and use of software products that were not designed for intensive care environments and have not been extensively tested in these venues.[27]

8.2.3.2 Contribution of Health IT to Noise Pollution

Research of auditory alarms in complex environments such as power plants, airplanes, and battle ships, has shown that most humans cannot reliably differentiate more than six different, simultaneous auditory alarms.[26, 28] A NICU is a very noisy environment, largely due to a cacophony of auditory alarms, not only from the eight required monitor alarms,[19] but also from a variety of bedside medical devices with individual alarms such as ventilators, warmers, and syringe pumps. Multisource human speech, beepers, telephones, overhead paging, and local intercom conversations all add to the noise level. Not only are patients and providers suffering from generalized auditory overload, but also nursing staff are hampered in the difficult task of identifying critical alarms from false alarms and background noise, and responding efficiently and effectively.

Approximately 90% of the alarms are false in Pediatric critical care venues. This means that despite a visual or auditory alarm that requires the attention of a nurse, the patient is actually fine in the majority of events. Nevertheless, the provider is expected to identify the source of the alarm, quickly assess the situation, and take corrective action. Speed is essential, because the alarm may signal a true life-threatening situation.

Measurements in NICUs have recorded transients noise levels to as high as *120–130 db*.[29, 30] Decreasing auditory overload has become a primary design consideration NICU and PICU renovations, mainly to reduce the noise associated stress on neonates. Research on acoustic overload has shown that noise also has important effects on human performance and cognition.[31] Long term exposure to constant noise at levels that are common to a busy NICU (~85 + dB) can temporarily or permanently deafen those exposed; even levels as low as 80db "can have detrimental effects on performance."[31] Less cognitive information can be processed under continuous noise overload conditions. Novel, random intermittent noises inhibit efficiency in most tasks, especially complex ones, where vigilance, multitasking, and judgmental sorting performance are required and interruptions are frequent.[32–35]

8.2.3.3 Human Factors: Social Environment and Individual Psychology

Poorly designed and implemented Health IT systems may add to the high cognitive burden of pediatric intensive care unit providers, including distraction and physical absence from the bedside.[23–24]

Documentation of clinical care in health IT systems is often cumbersome and may require up to 40% more time than paper systems.[36] Health IT systems that have poor response times, frequent outages and cause interruptions in workflow (for example by forcing providers to leave the bedside or carespace to document) have been recognized as problematic. Computer screens that can be viewed by visitors from neighboring bed spaces in crowded ICUs result in the loss of privacy.

Caregiver interactions with Health IT systems are currently designed to be performed with one clinician paying full attention to one computer. The constant interruptions in a medical environment make this use design realistically impossible.[36, 37] Interruptions take a special toll on care tasks that require undivided attention to manage complex mental processes (i.e. managing fluids, calculations, drug infusions and complicated treatment devices like ECMO or computerized ventilators), or complicated human situations such as confronting the death of a patient, and comforting the parents as a baby dies.

Successful implementation of Health IT in critical care environments requires participation of clinical users in design, implementation, evaluation, and management. Without participation and buy-in (including from night, weekend, and holiday shift workers), information technology efforts in ICUs are usually viewed as time-consuming, distracting, and without obvious direct benefit to the care staff, or their patients.

Additional challenges for pediatric providers include the disenfranchisement of Pediatric patients in device and IT system development. Devices, workflow support and software products that are appropriate for the Pediatric subgroups, if they exist, are usually more expensive than for the adults. While drug manufacturers are federally incentivized to test new medications on pediatric populations, the same is not true for devices and software applications. For a variety of reasons including cost savings, institutions may thus elect to implement devices and computer systems designed and tested only for adults, potentially resulting in adverse events and dangerous conditions in children.

8.2.4 Summary

Changes in difficult, complex, and fast-paced "safety critical" environments such as ICUs, including computerization, must be handled carefully. Team-based preliminary planning, user engagement, adaptive preparations and testing are needed before adding more tasks that affect the caregivers' job characteristics, coping strategies, time pressures and control matrix. Failures often result when the changes are made in ways that disempower the clinical staff or added work without perceived benefit for the patient. Poor change management is characterized by low user involvement throughout the new system's development lifecycle from planning forward, as happened in Scenario A.

Good system design and implementation practice includes rapid prototyping, user-based planning and testing, ongoing outcomes surveillance with feedback to the users (Fig. 8.2), with problem resolution and retesting in the target environment.[7] Large-scale user buy-in should precede an actual "protocol institution," new device "go live," or computer system "roll out."

Identified design criteria for ICU software systems include extreme speed (milliseconds matter), easy error detection and recovery, ease of complete clinical data capture, rapid recovery from system interruptions, and quick clinical information return to the bedside caregivers via automated, intuitive, easily visualized user interfaces.

Good Health IT design for NICUs and PICUs is often constrained by financial and regulatory considerations (state and federal laws, outdated building codes and legal standards for floor space allotments and other support infrastructure). These external pressures are currently adding ever-increasing demands on clinical caregivers (doctors, nurses, and respiratory therapists) for non-patient care related tasks such as performance reporting.

8.3   Scenario B: A Tale of Two PICUs

In this scenario, we will explore how complexities in pediatric care environments may cause problems in the implementation of Health IT with unintended consequences. First, we must discuss a prevalent and very powerful notion: Backed by a number of studies in institutions that developed a home-grown Computerized Provider Order Entry (CPOE) system, many lay people and health care professionals believe that CPOE systems will decrease medical errors and improve patient safety.[1, 2] However, this notion may not always be correct. A quarter of these studies have been conducted by only five organizations.[36] Implementation of technology may bring to light an existing, interrelated *web* of operational dependencies in heath care environments. CPOE may interrupt these dependencies, disrupting carefully designed and well implemented care processes, leading to clinical problems and many unanticipated consequences, both negative and positive.[2, 3, 8, 24, 38]

8.3.1   Problem Statement

Infants and children represent a unique patient type. Children's medical needs differ greatly from those of adults, and the information systems that support children's needs require tailored designs and implementations. Epidemiology of Adverse Drug Events (ADEs) in children reveals that most events originate at the drug ordering stage, with the smallest and most critically ill patients at highest risk.[4, 8–12, 39–42] Dosing errors are extremely common in pediatrics. Children less than 2 years of age and ICU patients are particularly susceptible.[39, 40] Given this evidence, it is easy to understand why people believe that CPOE has potential for stopping these errors at the source. Medical centers often implemented emerging technology in an urgent fashion in the hopes to reduce medical errors and improve outcomes.

Initial studies of CPOE were promising, but few addressed the complex socio-technical challenges involved in a successful pediatric implementation. A study of an adult population showed that CPOE alone decreased incidence of medication errors by 64%; CPOE with clinical decision support can decrease error rates by 83%.[43] These successes must be put into perspective: Medication events most likely prevented by CPOE such as illegible orders are also least likely to cause real patient harm in a paper order environment, diminishing the effectiveness of CPOE. One study suggested that pediatric CPOE system could have prevented 76% of poten-tially harmful medication errors.[41] The Ohio State University showed that CPOE dramatically improves operational efficiency, pharmacy turnaround times, and radio-logy procedure completion times.[44] Similar operational improvements in the NICU increased efficiency in delivering essential therapies to critically ill newborns.[45]

The primary impetus for implementing pediatric CPOE remains patient safety and not efficiency or cost reduction. Several pediatric inpatient studies reported decreases in serious Adverse Drug Events (ADEs) and medication errors after the implementation of CPOE.[42, 46–48] A study of pediatric ICU patients found a 95% reduction in medication errors and a 40% reduction in potential ADEs.[48, 49] Although this literature is encouraging, very few studies have looked at direct clinical outcome measures such as mortality to assess the true impact of CPOE on pediatric patients.

When the 1999 Institute of Medicine (IOM) report concluded that between 44,000 and 98,000 people die each year from iatrogenic injury, physicians started seeking innovative ways to improve the safety of patients, including children.[49] Several investigators concluded that deaths might be decreased by lowering the rate of potential Adverse Drug Events (ADEs).[50–52] Similar to drug studies, most of the initial safety literature focused on adults, so early findings were not easily generalized to Pediatric populations. Until the Scenario B publications, CPOE research was limited to mainly "home-grown," CPOE utilities,[53–55] as opposed to commercially purchased, essentially free-standing systems, "interfaced" to connect to older "core" hospital information systems. The need to build interfaces generates a novel problem space. Interfaces present software-based speed and accuracy problems (e.g. decimal place and data type transforms, matching of catalogues).

Despite the lack of data on Pediatric systems and commercial systems, in 2003 an American Academy of Pediatrics (AAP) Policy Statement on the prevention of medication errors officially recommended the use of "computerized systems" wherever feasible.[56] More recently the IOM encouraged use of CPOE, clinical decision support, bar coding, and smart pumps in all care settings to help prevent medication errors.[57] These mandates have prompted physician practices and hospitals to (perhaps in part prematurely) implement electronic "solutions" without fully understanding how to specify, purchase, and implement, test and maintain Health IT systems that can manage the complex operational interdependencies that have profound impact on safe patient care.[58-64]

The human culture of inpatient Pediatric environments has evolved to a safer level: Today physicians, pharmacists, and allied health personnel work synergistically to deliver care. This coordinated "symphony" delivers complex, time-sensitive care to many pediatric patients simultaneously and is often called "workflow." In the inherently dynamic period of childhood, these providers work collaboratively to identify risk factors and prevent harm. In many cases, the introduction of new technology interrupts communication, redirects efforts, and places unanticipated stress on these delicate human systems, sometimes with untoward consequences. Change magnifies inefficiencies, demolishes existing work-arounds, and disrupts the delicate workflow balance that stabilizes a complex Pediatric ward.

Scenario B addresses the interrelationship of human factors and technology in a Pediatric ward, and describes the occult workflow problems that technology exposed. Children create distinctive challenges for medication ordering.[64, 65] Pediatric patients have threefold the risk of adults for suffering harm from a medication error. Pediatricians must calculate medication doses based on weight, age, gestational age, and indication, increasing the risk of cognitive and mathematical errors (e.g. the tenfold overdose error).[64] Pediatric pharmacists often work with adult formulations, and must manually compound suspensions and intravenous dilutions for use in pediatric patients. Children experience rapidly changing weights and sequentially changing laboratory normative values, which increases risk for incorrect dosing. The immature renal and hepatic systems in children and neonates inconsistently clear drugs, and limited physiologic reserve makes infants more likely to be harmed by even modest medication errors.[64-66] Computer systems with inappropriate normal values and adult-based decision support modules increase error risk. Efficient communication between providers helps mitigate this risk, but technology often constitutes a barrier to human interaction.

8.3.2 Scenario B: Situation Analysis

Two published studies from major children's hospitals with very different results on PICU mortality[8, 9] raise a key question: How can two Pediatric CPOE implementations, using the same commercial system, produce completely different patient mortality outcome results?

8.3.2.1 Review: Comparison of the Case Details

The Pittsburg Children's Hospital[8] is a nationally recognized 235 bed tertiary pediatric care facility admitting about 12,000 pediatric patients per year; 25% of the admissions are directly to the hospital's Pediatric ICU (PICU). Pittsburg

Children's Hospital implemented CPOE in December of 2002, becoming one of the first children's hospitals to use a commercial CPOE system. Shortly after implementation, Upperman published a series of articles discussing pediatric CPOE at Pittsburgh Children's Hospital, outlining the Pediatric implementation methodology and reporting the impact of Pediatric CPOE on medical errors and adverse drug events.[47, 67] Over a 9 month study period he found that harmful adverse drug events decreased from 0.05 events per 1,000 doses to 0.03 events per 1,000 doses (p = 0.05). Based on this initial experience, it appeared that the Pittsburgh implementation was modestly successful in decreasing ADEs.

When Dr. Han later published a follow-up article describing an unexpected increase in PICU patient mortality after the Pittsburg CPOE implementation, the report was surprising and made national headlines.[8] Han had analyzed a high risk subset of ICU patients who were transported to the PICU, rather than studying the whole inpatient Pediatric population or the whole PICU population. The subset results showed a 3.86% *increase* in risk adjusted mortality after the CPOE system was implemented; odds ratio of 3.28 [95% CI 1.94–5.55].

The negative findings of the Han paper were not solely related to technology. In fact, the technology itself likely was a minor cause of the increased mortality. Table 8.1 lists the confounding factors that played a prominent role in Pittsburg PICU's increased mortality.

Table 8.1 Confounding factors in Pittsburg PICU's increased mortality

Implementation problem	Assessment of risk	Possible prevention strategy
Order entry		
Unable to enter orders on critically ill patients prior to transport arrival	Delay in delivery of critical medications and tests likely to cause patient harm	Establish "virtual" beds so admission orders can be entered before arrival. Use paper orders in emergency situations
Order entry slow and cumbersome (1–2 min per order)	Slow order entry delays delivery of care. Clinicians are not at bedside when interacting with the computer	Streamline screen design Place workstations at bedside Build extensive order sets
Physicians locked out of system while pharmacy processes order	Delay in medications administration may cause harm Physicians are unable to respond to acute deteriorations common in transported PICU admissions	Allow for simultaneous order entry by several providers incorporating concurrency into the data structure
No Pediatric ICU specific order sets available at "go live"	Inefficient order entry Inconsistent care Slow, cumbersome order entry in emergency situations	Evaluate clinical services' emergency workflow and build order sets that reduce effort and streamline work flow

(continued)

Table 8.1 (continued)

Implementation problem	Assessment of risk	Possible prevention strategy
All new medication orders require activation from nursing	Orders remain pending until nursing approval resulting in delayed care. Nurses are forced away from the bedside to perform cumbersome medication activation procedures	Careful workflow analysis prior to implementation will identify potential workflow concerns Allow medication to activate upon ordering
Workflow		
Face to face communication between doctor and nurse decreased noticeably	Unaware of placed orders, nurses did not sign off on medication orders in a timely fashion. This compounded the delay in therapy secondary to the order activation procedure and led to delay in patient	CPOE training must educate providers that CPOE is a tool, not a substitute for personal interactions with nursing and other allied health professionals. Clinical decision support that pages providers if orders remain unacknowledged
Technical		
Limited wireless bandwidth	Frequent system hangs and long order processing times delay patient care	Careful technical analysis and testing under maximal load is essential prior to "go live"
Concurrent deployment of clinical applications platform	The adult focused clinical applications platform may have conflicted with CPOE reducing performance	Implement critical systems one at a time and ensure adequate error testing and quality assurance
Implementation occurred over a 6 day period on all units ("Big Bang" approach)	Rapid implementation did not allow for identification and repair of critical system problems before moving to other units	Implementation is an iterative process. Begin with general pediatric floors and correct all identified problems Implement subsequent units over months Continuous support during critical "go live" phases is required
Institutional		
Pharmacy was moved out of the ICU and into centralized location without prior time delay and process throughput testing	Long lag time between medication ordering and delivery to bedside	Unit based pharmacies have been independently associated with faster drug administration and lower ADE rates. In pediatric ICUs unit-based pharmacies can be life saving in the event of system failures Simultaneous implementation and physical layout changes must be avoided

After the Pittsburg report, DelBeccaro et al. published the Children's Hospital of Seattle's experience implementing the same commercially available product in their PICU. Like Han, Del Beccaro evaluated the mortality rates of Pediatric patients before and after CPOE installation, finding no change in mortality for both transported critical care patients and for pediatric patients in general (nonsignificant trend towards mortality reduction).[9] DelBeccaro attributed the discrepancies in mortality in both studies to multiple socio-technical differences in the implementation methodologies. Table 8.2 is the 18 variable evaluation matrix used for making specific situational comparisons.

Although there are many similarities between the Seattle and Pittsburgh situations, there are also key differences. The study populations were quite different. Pittsburgh had four times more inter-facility transport patients than Seattle. Transported patients are more complex and at increased risk for error (due to increased complexity, and need to transfer information). Lower patient ages are an independent risk factor for mortality. Pittsburg had a much lower median patient age than Seattle did (9 versus 87 months), adding a second major risk factor. The population incidence of several life-threatening conditions such as Asthma, Cancer, Pneumonia, and Sepsis also differed. Admitting a patient from a general pediatric floor into an ICU is much lower risk than admitting a Pediatric critical care patient transport from an outside hospital. The significantly lower risk in the Seattle cohort makes a comparison of the studies difficult.

Pittsburg researchers used a more rigorous statistical analysis than the Seattle group, which used unadjusted mortality rates. The unadjusted mortality rates did not correct for the group differences or pre- and post-differences; nor did the researchers adjust data for other confounding factors. In contrast, the Pittsburg researchers controlled for multiple confounding factors using logistic regression reported as an adjusted Odds Ratio.

Even though the two reports differ in patient population variables, disease profile, risk factors, and statistical rigor, making comparison difficult, the two studies provided valuable insights into the socio-technical complexities of Pediatric CPOE implementations.[67] These reports are a unique pair of case studies for developing a "systems analysis" approach to complex Pediatric Informatics problems. Improvements in process time through Hospital IT systems are much more readily detectable in fast-paced ICUs where every second counts, and where small inefficiencies can be tremendously important to critically unstable patients. The differences in the studies were not entirely due to patient population variables. Human Factors adaptations in the Seattle implementation were: (1) improving communication post-CPOE, creating PICU specific "Order Sets" with new "order sentences"; (2) altering workflows to guarantee immediate on site availability of emergency medications; and, (3) instituting effective processes for patient preregistration. Workflow factors were not "inherently" related to the CPOE technology, but related more to preexisting institutional practices, protocols, and culture. Seattle paid close

Table 8.2 Evaluation matrix to compare POE implementation

	Children's Hospital of Pittsburgh	Children's Hospital of Seattle
Hospital characteristics		
Affiliation	University of Pittsburgh	University of Washington
Annual Admissions	235 pediatric beds	250 pediatric beds
	12,000 admissions/year	11,000 admissions/year
	3,000 PICU admissions/ year	1,100 ICU admissions/year
	~734 transport admissions to PICU/ year	~110 transport admissions to PICU/year
Study characteristics		
Study period	13 months pre, 5 months post	13 months pre, 5 and 13 months post
	10/1/2001 until 3/31/2003	10/1/2002 until 12/31/2004
Study population	Children admitted via *inter-facility transport*	All children
	1942 total *transport* admissions	2,533 PICU admissions (transport and in-house)
	1102 inter-facility transport admissions to PICU	284 inter-facility transport admissions to PICU (much smaller cohort than in Pittsburgh)
Severity of illness metric	PRISM score (median 4)	PRISM score (median 4.57)
Demographic differences in the study populations	Median age: 9 months	Mean age: 86.76 months (patients much older than in Pittsburgh)
Technical		
CPOE system	Cerner power orders	Cerner power orders
	Cerner millennium 7.8 platform	Cerner millennium 7.8 platform
Implementation period	6 days	14 h
Pharmacy	Emergency medications difficult to obtain due to centralized pharmacy and inefficient medication approval process	Emergency medications available immediately
Infrastructure	Network reliability problems	No network problems
Registration	Inability to preregister patients	Allow for preregistration of patients
Time for Order set Completion	1–2 min per order	<5 min for entire order set
ICU specific order sets	0	16
Training and support	Mandatory 3 h tutorial and practice session	Mandatory 2–4 h tutorial and practice session
	Hands on support during implementation, phone support thereafter	24/7 in house support for 14 days after "go live"
		"Super User" training

(continued)

Table 8.2 (continued)

	Children's Hospital of Pittsburgh	Children's Hospital of Seattle
Study results		
Methodology	Retrospective design	Retrospective design
Comparison of "pre" and "post" groups	There are no statistically significant differences between the groups except for the number of patients with CNS disease (288 pre, 89 post)	There are multiple differences in the pre and post groups. Most notably age (90.5 versus 83.25 mos) and the incidence of asthma, cancer, pneumonia, and sepsis
Mortality rate	Mortality statistics (inter-facility transfers to PICU): Pre 2.80% (39/1394) Post 6.57% (36/548)	Mortality rate (all patients): pre 4.22–post 3.46% Mortality rate (Inter-facility transfers to PICU) Pre 9.60–post 6.29%
Factors affecting mortality	Patients younger, history of prematurity, direct admission to PICU	Not evaluated
Adjusted for confounding factors	Yes	No
Conclusion	Unadjusted mortality rate is significantly higher in the "post" CPOE group. This conclusion is likely the result of multiple socio-technical factors rather than an isolated CPOE system	There is no significant change in unadjusted mortality between the "pre" and "post" CPOE groups. However, this comparison of unadjusted mortality rates may be invalid due to significant differences between the pre and post groups, and the failure to adjust for confounding factors

attention to recognizing work flow changes needed for system adaptation to change generated by IT implementation.

One of the fundamental differences between the two PICU CPOE installations was the substantial preliminary effort by Seattle in building pediatric ICU order sets. At Pittsburgh, a single order took 1–2 min. In Seattle, an entire "pre-built" set of admission orders could be entered in 5 min. Even though clearly faster than Pittsburgh, *5 min is still a fivefold increase in provider effort compared to paper versions of the same order set.* Accounts from both hospitals support the time saving value of pre-built order sets versus single order entry. In the future, formal time, effort, and workflow analyses must be used to specify and build more efficient archival software, better user interface utilities, team workflow support, and user-friendly process modification capabilities. Health IT is a rapidly advancing, interdisciplinary informatics research and development area.[12, 67]

8.3.3 Pediatric Health IT Implementation: Learning from Each Other

We are only beginning to understand the complex interrelationship between human factors and technology. Even though it is more difficult to publically discuss failures than successes, it is incumbent upon centers who have implemented pediatric CPOE to thoroughly define the human factors and workflow processes that predict success or failure and to report their experiences. In Pediatric Informatics, we must learn from each other, and from our failures and successes. The Seattle group had the benefit of visiting Pittsburgh before beginning their own CPOE implementation. That visit provided valuable and explicit lessons, especially for identifying stumbling points that can hamper smooth implementations. One of the fundamental problems faced by Children's Hospital Pittsburg was the inefficient "stat" ordering of urgent, life saving therapies. Life-threatening events, where seconds count, are a daily occurrence in all hospitals and must be addressed by CPOE implementers. Often times, Health IT systems are not **flexible** enough to deal with these emergency situations. Hospital based implementation teams must assure that "break-the-glass" functionality is available to users that allows them override system deficiencies in critical care situations.

Armed with real world observational and experiential data, Seattle Children's was able to navigate the workflow, communication, socio-technical challenges of their commercial CPOE with less difficulty than their predecessors. Through continued communication and collaboration, hospitals will continue to learn from prior implementations and vendors will improve commercial products for children. The aggregate effort will increasingly improve the positive safety profile of inpatient Pediatrics.

A roadmap outline of the specific problem elements that contributed to the divergent results in the "Tale of Two PICUs" is summarized in Table 8.3.

8.3.4 Information Technology and Complexity in Pediatric Care Environments

The following paragraphs discuss the challenges that the combination of existing complexities in Pediatric care environments and the introduction of health IT solutions can generate. The list of issues discussed here is by no means exhaustive, it is meant only to allow users to reflect on the complexity and unforeseen problems encountered by teams attempting to implement information technologies.

Table 8.3 Critical factors impacting outcomes in POE implementation

Communication Factors
- Technology does not replace the need for face to face bedside communication with nursing and other care team members

Workflow issues
- Patient movement and transfers
- Paper management in a mixed CPOE/Paper environment
- Patient flow through the OR and PACU

Demographics and Patient identification
- Name changes are more common in pediatrics
- Multiple gestations add to the complexity of Newborn ICU Patients
- Entering orders on unborn patients is particularly challenging

Human factors
- Lack of human factors engineering for safety critical systems
- Time pressured humans coupled with unintuitive systems

Pharmacy factors
- Medication reconciliation in the electronic age
- Medication scheduling conflicts
- Attention to units of measure/proper unit conversions
- Weigh based dosing/computerized rounding
- Decision support is critical

CPOE factors
- CPOE causes providers to be much more explicit which can lead to errors
- Many decisions previously absorbed by the culture of medicine must now be detailed by the provider
- Temporal reasoning/complex dosing schedules/contingent orders
- Tocsin toxicity – low signal to noise ration of clinical alerts

Implementation Challenges
- Mixed adult/children's hospitals versus dedicated children's hospitals

8.3.4.1 Communication

Maintaining good interdisciplinary communication after a HIT implementation is absolutely vital to success. Technology often depersonalizes the care delivery process or disrupts existing chains of communication. With CPOE, physicians can place orders from other wards, call rooms, homes. All too often, computer ordering becomes the primary focus for physicians, and previous simultaneous communication with nursing and pharmacy disappear. For example, if a medication is changed in the CPOE system, but the revised order is not verbally communicated to nursing, it is likely that the patient will continue to receive the original order until the bedside nurse notices hours to days later that the order was changed, or that the floor stock in the patient's computerized medication "bin" is depleted, or that an unanticipated medication is waiting to be administered.

Many institutions have not installed a companion electronic medication administration record (eMAR) concurrently with CPOE implementation. Amazingly, in 2008, not all vendors even offer both components for an ordering-to-administration integrated inpatient medication management. The resulting temporal and cognitive disconnect between the paper MAR and the computerized CPOE orders is an error-prone system that is frustrating and labor intensive for clinical caregivers. Neither complex technological solutions nor cumbersome medication reconciliation procedures using extensive human work-arounds (including hiring additional nursing/pharmacy staff) have entirely mitigated the risk of communication glitches and medication delivery failures.[60] Currently, the safest procedure is to maintain effective direct methods for nurse, physician, and pharmacist communication.

In a paper-based world, the bedside nurses receive a visual cue when a physician writes an order in the bedside chart. CPOE eliminates this cue because physicians can enter orders from remote locations unobserved by the nurse. On a general Pediatric ward, this scenario can cause a delay in therapy and possible harm to the patient. In an ICU, this problem is magnified by patient acuity and the large number of time-sensitive orders.

Before any CPOE system is implemented, all care providers must understand that CPOE is not a replacement for effective interpersonal communication between care team members. Physicians must continue to notify bedside nurses of changes in management. Strong verbal communication is one of the critical factors that differentiated the successful CPOE implementation in the scenario outlined above.

8.3.4.2 Workflow Issues: Patient Movement and Multiple Transfers

The dynamic, "real-time" nature of the critical care transport process between units, to radiology or operating rooms, or by ambulance between institutions, places unstable patients at high risk for serious error. Monitoring patient movement and documenting transfers while responding to new orders in near real-time is vital for in inpatient critical care venues and any HIT system must respond to this need. Tracking of inpatients in "real-time" is one of the most challenging aspects of a pediatric critical care CPOE implementation. Orders and medication delivery must follow patients through a number of off-unit venues, including hallways and other unusual areas, especially during surge capacity situations.

Based on hospital policies and patient needs, transfers may require that orders be temporarily suspended or modified. Some transfers require discontinuation of all existing orders. Other situations require that all existing orders be continued, despite a physical move. Effectively managing the dynamic needs of critically ill patients moving from the Emergency Room to an ICU, to OR, and back, via the Radiology facility, followed by a second trip to the OR can be extremely challenging for computer and human systems designers and implementers of CPOE/medication reconciliation utilities. Obviously, policies must be developed to manage transfer situations within every CPOE implementation and providers must be educated when to suspend, discontinue, or maintain orders. Even with well-designed policies, transfer processes are error-prone events.

Vended systems designed for use in the emergency department or operating room (Specialty Systems) rarely have the temporal reasoning tools required to handle movement from one hospital computer system to another, smoothly. Frequently, they are not integrated with other hospital IT systems. Subsequently, knowledge of orders may be lost, threatening safe patient care (e.g., the provider is unaware of a medication administered in the operating room and orders another dose). Developing a process for reconciling computerized orders in the peri-transport period is extremely challenging for nearly all existing systems. Specialty systems that are capable of integrating the many inpatient processes needed to manage very sick patients quickly and accurately, remain nonexistent. "Work-arounds" that involve time-consuming interaction of humans (nurses, pharmacists) with several "specialty systems" can fall hopelessly behind he patient's changing condition and location, particularly at change of shift times.

8.3.4.3 Coupled or Linked Orders

Many types of medication administrations occur in proper temporal synchronization for maximal benefit to the patient. CPOE implementation often leads to uncovering of hidden temporal synchronization (separate tasks that are completed on paper simultaneously seemingly as a single task). Breaking these combined orders apart introduces novel, inherent workflow inefficiencies and increases complexity and costs, especially in hospitals that have mixed electronic and paper based records. For example, when an order is placed for a bronchodilator to treat an asthmatic attack, a message must be sent to the pharmacy to dispense the drug, and a separate parallel message must be sent to the Respiratory Therapist to administer the drug to the patient. Drug administration requires dispensing of ordered devices for the specific situation and patient. If any of these communications fail, there will be a delay in care delivery. In a second example, incomplete implementation of medication ordering systems can result in uncoupling of connected orders.

Many CPOE implementations exclude cytotoxic chemotherapeutic agents (a common practice work-around with many CPOE systems due to the complexity of chemotherapy agents), so these agents continue to be ordered on paper. Simultaneously, ancillary drugs that must be ordered at the same time such as rescue medications, anti-emetics, and hydration are managed by CPOE. This separation, which requires a multiple orders (chemotherapy on paper, rescue medication on paper), wastes caregiver time, slows the order delivery to the bedside, and, most importantly, may lead to patient harm due to risk of omission errors as a result of decoupling.

In an ideal world, all medication orders (delivery and administration) would be maintained, temporally organized, routed, confirmed, and cross-checked with a "completed delivery" message within a single CPOE system. Coupled orders would remain linked in the system (such as chemotherapy and rescue medications). Status of any particular order would be immediately accessible to all members of the care team, as would be the current physical location of the patient (including rare locations such as "in the elevator"). Response time for "STAT" calls should be measured in seconds.

8.3.4.4   Demographics and Patient Identification

Patient name changes are very common in pediatrics due to social, legal, and practical factors. Newborns often retain their mother's last name until the birth certificate is created. Admission names may be changed according to local rules during the baby's neonatal admission. This may lead to confusion of identity and incorrect resulting in the complex collection of inpatient archival, clinical, and laboratory databases.[67] Names are key identifiers in nearly all clinical database systems. Neonatal and Pediatric intensive care patients often have the same last names, due to multiple births and family groups involved in auto accidents, etc. In these situations, it is relatively easy to succumb to error and place an order on an incorrect patient.[68] The risk increases when orders are placed away from the patient's bedside, where physicians lose visual identity cues. In the paper world, "name alerts" were pasted in bold red letters on the bedside charts, name cards are on the beds, and the nurse and parents nearby conducted independent, redundant checks. CPOE eliminates many of these geo-spatial safety checks. Thus, CPOE systems require increased vigilance by nurses, pharmacists, and physicians to ensure safe ordering and care delivery practices.

8.3.4.5   Registration, Lack of Registration and HIT

In perinatal medicine, caregivers often must order medicines for, or send blood samples from, an unborn baby (or babies) while preparing for an emergent delivery. The perinatal situation is analogous to the problem that Pittsburgh faced when trying to enter orders on transport patients prior to the patient's arrival. Many CPOE systems are not capable of permitting orders on a patient that has not been admitted yet. Due to billing requirements and antifraud protection, many admitting systems that feed patient information into CPOE systems do not allow admission of a patient that has not yet arrived. Entering identities for babies not yet born, or for other unidentifiable individuals (unconscious emergency room patient) is a particularly perplexing problem for which future HIT developers need standardized procedures that are not yet (2008) functionally specified.

Efficient processes must be developed to deal with the complex but common "pre-admit" dilemma in Pediatric and Perinatal medicine, before hospitals implement a new technology. Possible solutions include creating "phantom" medical record numbers, or using a paper based process for arrest situations, unborn babies, and incoming, possibly unidentified, critical care transports. In this work-around, the paper orders could be entered into CPOE once the child has been formally admitted and/or stabilized. In practice, this solution is very time consuming, delays information flow, eliminates the benefits of a CPOE system, is very error prone at every step and distracts critical caregivers. (In practice, critical admit records are often reconstructed from handwritten notes on paper towels and scrub pants.)

It is critical to identify and consider such key issues prior to implementation to facilitate a seamless transition to a computerized workflow in any environment. Speed of medication administration to the critical patient could serve as process-based quality indicator.

8.3.5   Engineering Pediatric HIT Systems

Existing CPOE systems were created without much attention to human factors and usability metrics.[68] A physician's workflow varies depending on specialty, patient census, and acuity factors that are often unpredictable and uncontrollable. Experts in Human Factors Engineering can optimize computer utilities, including user interfaces to accommodate the variability in work load.

Vended CPOE systems that are flexible and easily configurable, still require the user, who is usually a novice in both CPOE and in the psychology of effective interface design for healthcare users to build the clinical cognitive content and visual manifestation for a particular care setting. In situations with time pressure, the nonintuitive, workflow unaware, and cognitively incorrect computer systems may lead to significant delays in patient care, especially with novice users.

Quality clinical content creation and inpatient user interface design is a science. It is only perfected through experience, testing, and iterative tuning, plus an institutional commitment to ongoing maintenance and user-based improvement cycles. Appropriate design experts often have advanced degrees in Psychology, Art, Music, Math, or Library Science as well as in Health Informatics, Computer Science, or Business Administration. Especially in interface design, is essential that we learn from other professionals' and institution's experience to avoid duplication of known errors that jeopardize patient safety and frustrate providers.

Unfortunately, trained experts in optimizing healthcare software architecture, user interface design and front end human factors situations are rarely employed during CPOE installations. Applied expertise from HFE professionals could revolutionize the usability of many clinical systems through improving system efficiency and enhancing user satisfaction by using iterative refinement techniques.

8.3.5.1   Prescribing and Medication Administration

Understanding the interaction between pharmacy and electronic order entry is one of the most complex obstacles faced when implementing a new technology. Since most institutions have not yet implemented a full electronic medication administration record (eMAR), users interact with a system based both on paper and on CPOE. The partial implementation increases the risk for transcription and omission errors and makes the medication reconciliation process in hospitals more difficult. Well built clinical order sets enhance productivity, streamline the order entry process, and provide concrete clinical guidance and standardization at the point of care.

Efficient verbal communication can solve this problem only partially. The required scheduling of a medication at ordering remains unsolved. Traditionally, nurses have been in charge of these tasks.[69] Physicians are usually unaware of important information required to schedule a task: (1) order schedules are often inconsistent with the other medications on the MAR, or would require the nurse to wake the child unnecessarily, or must be changed due to vascular access problems; (2) scheduled procedures; (3) family situations such as breast feeding or "skin to skin" encounters, and; (4) the need to coordinate one patient's care with a second patient assigned to the same nurse, or, with; (5) other bedside processes (e.g. auditory screening, ultrasounds, etc.).

These medication "scheduling" conflicts were easily resolved on paper, when nurses had the authority to reschedule doses as needed, or to call physicians or pharmacies to negotiate amended orders. On paper, nurses were looking at the original, official version of the orders, and could physically apply an amendment. For time critical orders (i.e. for platelets), the negotiation might require workflow changes in other departments' workflow (e.g. the blood bank). In these situations, effort is reduced and accuracy improved with end-to-end synchronous communication in a single system between the bedside nurse and involved ancillary staff. In CPOE, a physician's offsite orders that conflict with bedside schedules and situations cannot easily be amended by other providers thus causing delay in medication administration and additional work to alter the medication administration workflow.

8.3.5.2 Medication Reconciliation

The best human/computer system interaction process is for medication reconciliation is currently unclear. Traditionally "reconciliation" occurred at the bedside once per shift, between two nurses reviewing all the orders (of all types) in chronological sequence, in the paper chart, while checking all the medications, tubes, and other equipment at the bedside. CPOE increases the possibility of missed orders due to poor screen display, order fragmentation, and poor temporal sequencing of reports. A full electronic MAR with fully developed temporal reasoning capabilities that can be installed and integrated with other medication-related hospital information utilities (i.e. blood bank, laboratory, supply chain, and nutritional product management) is urgently needed for children undergoing inpatient care. Without such an eMAR, increased risks of "new types" of medication errors from partially integrated, adult designed, add-on systems will persist.[67, 70]

8.3.5.3 Unit of Measures

Correct and appropriate units of measure are critical in Pediatric medication ordering. Particular attention must be paid to the default ordering unit of measure, and to the proper unit of measure conversion calculations. In adults, Ampicillin is traditionally ordered in grams. In children, this medication is most often ordered in milligrams, although it may be dispensed in 1 or 2 g vials. CPOE systems must be aware of these conversions so that the provider can dose medications in familiar units without introducing missing leading "0," extraneous trailing "0," decimal point and human calculation errors. Pediatric CPOE systems should be capable of calculating the appropriate dose and rounding for the dispensable form.

8.3.5.4 Clinical Decision Support

Robust clinical decision support is a desired component of any CPOE implementation. Well designed and fully integrated "decision support" improves both physician choices and hospital financial performance.[71, 72] Most current CPOE systems do not offer advanced clinical decision support. For Pediatrics, even simple dose range checking utilities may not be part of the standard package. Due to changing tolerance to medications with chronologic and gestational age and growth in children, dose range tables are significantly more complex than in adult patients.

8.3.5.5 Mandatory Detail

CPOE systems force hospital-based providers to make explicit decisions about issues that are neither their responsibility nor their area of expertise. For example, using CPOE, a physician cannot simply order an "OG tube" and trust the nurse to select the appropriate size for the infant or child from the unit stocks. Instead, the physician is required to make a decision that is in the scope of practice for a nurse and order an OG tube of a specific size.

The ordering physician must know whether or not the CT scan requires contrast; previously this was in the scope of practice for the board-certified radiologist.

Simple procedures such as ordering Erythromycin may now require an in depth knowledge of its various salt forms (e.g. Erythromycin Stearate, Erythromycin Estolate, Erythromycin Ethylsuccinate, Erythromycin Propionate, or Erythromycin Thyocinate). Many such decisions were previously absorbed by the team-based knowledge.

The doctor ordered an OG tube, and the nurse decided, based on her practice experience and visual judgment of her baby's size and condition that "8 French" was the appropriate size. Similarly, the pharmacist interpreted the physician order and chose the Erythromycin salt from the hospital pharmacy's standard stocks, based on standard pharmacy procedures. With CPOE, front end clinicians have to make these decisions. Lack of sub-domain knowledge may result in delays, errors, inefficiencies, and frustrated caregivers.

8.3.5.6 Volume of Orders

The critical care environment is a challenge to any order entry system. Rapid prescribing and administration of emergency shock and trauma medications requires computerized "temporal reasoning," which is currently a research area in Computer Science.[73–75] Existing computer systems are not usually designed to deal with the temporal reasoning of complex dosing schedules and conditional orders written to titrate vasopressor medications, insulin, emergency fluids, and/or intravenously administered anticoagulants, sometimes simultaneously.

8.3.5.7 Volume of Data

All critical care patient data (laboratory, monitoring, and treatment machines, drug and fluids administration) have temporal and logistical complexities caused by interactions of several hundred different data items that each could be observed as frequently as several times each minute (automated monitoring and drug administration machines). The complex data represented by ICU patient variables contain time-dependent, variant, repeated measures with many missing ("null") values.

Missing medical data can be critical. Clinician-initiated attempts that fail to return values (laboratory results or diagnostic information), or products, (e.g. medications), must be recognized and managed by medical software for hospital-based applications. A valueless (Null value) datum with a time stamp (indicating that an order sent to pharmacy did not return a medication), is conceptually very different from an absent attempt (at diagnosis, treatment, or other intervention). Absent value situations have legal implications on "failure to diagnose" and "failure to treat" malpractice issues.

8.3.5.8 Temporal Reasoning in Health Care[74–76]

In critical care, any change has the potential to cause deterioration of the patient. However, iterative and simultaneous changes in titrations of ventilator support, fluid and vasoactive medication, gas flow, and electrolyte supplementation are a constant part of a critical care process called "stabilizing the patient." Stabilizing is a time dependent (temporal reasoning) process.

Conceptual temporal reasoning is difficult to model, especially for Pediatric ICUs in part because of the temporal intensity of the data and the need for speed and complex representations.[77] Multiple simultaneous patient care processes create human time-pressure, and a multivariate, mixed effect data model that must be managed in an information system. The involvement of humans in the complex, simultaneous processes often results in extensive pollution of sequenced data by important, unavoidable, or "subliminal" human process and point-of-view interactions such as variable narratives, forgetting, jargon, nonverbal communications, and faulty date and time recording, both in typed and written records. Supporting the total clinical data management situation in intensive care units will require very advanced models for satisfactory computerized decision support.[76–78]

Computerized temporal logic is required for dealing with synchronicity and many types of partial time overlap calculations (e.g. medication delivery in NICUs and PICUs) Complex temporal reasoning problems are processed easily by normal human beings, without recognizing the complexity of translational semantics and human social nuances. For example teaching a computer to process the query "Did you start the vancomycin before or after you talked to the surgeons?," can require very complex processing, even when not occurring in real-time.[75, 76]

8.3.5.9   Clinical Trends

Tracking changes over time is a very important component of clinical decision making in Pediatrics. Decisions concerning conservative treatment versus surgery (i.e. for premature patent ductus arteriosus), discharge prediction (e.g. for funding and planning purposes), and ultimate outcome prediction (i.e. speed of normalization of brain function after a perinatal hypoxemic/ischemic episode), all require temporal reasoning.[74, 75] Existing information systems for "charting" and "ordering" have limited capabilities of recording time elements. For example, in expressing plans for follow-up, some systems provide "month" with only a single character to list a time (the provider might want to choose days or more than 9 months for a follow up appointment). Some systems require a duration unanchored to a beginning or ending date and time point (e.g. elapsed minutes of chest compression during resuscitation efforts). Many archival hospital databases do not have provisions for inclusion of multiple, sequential occurrences of the same procedure or disease (e.g. sequential fetal and cranial ultrasounds, sepsis and suspected sepsis episodes, x-rays, and serial eye exams).

8.3.6   General Discussion

Lessons from avionics, nuclear power plants, and military subsystems on battleships underscore the importance of socio-technical factors in safe system implementation. The medical literature has reinforced these lessons through a series of well respected articles by Leape.[25, 51, 52, 79, 80] Brilliant, single situation "systems analyses"[2, 7-9, 23, 72] provide examples of the complex interaction between human factors and technology at every level in healthcare.[67]

The growing literature dissecting past HIT errors should serve as a warning beacon to reorient planning for a HIT implementation to consider ergonomics, human factors, and time-sensitive workflow processes that healthcare computerization may change. While technology holds tremendous promise, it has also proven its excellent capacity to interrupt processes, disable communication, increase burden to providers and potentially worsen existing conditions unexpectedly. Research in human factors must be refocused on the healthcare industry. System designers must adopt the same strict controls that have been defined around overall aviation safety by the FAA and around the development and assurance testing of computerized medical devices by the FDA.

Dissecting complicated health IT problems requires a multidisciplinary team of experts (Table 8.4). This team must be adept at identifying potential failure modes

Table 8.4   HIT implementation – required team member experiences

Experiences required
Medical informatics
Nursing informatics
Clinical care delivery in intensive care units (doctors and nurses)
Clinical and regulatory compliance and education
Marketing, business development and contracting
New information technology introduction
Healthcare enterprise change management
Software/electrical engineering
User-focused design of software architectures databases, and programs
Financial and strategic planning

early in the functional design process and actively create installation, software, and human system strategies that enhance safety and minimize risk. Dr. Reason's model for human error[81] explains: "The most important distinguishing feature of high reliability organizations is their collective preoccupation with the possibility of failure. They continually rehearse familiar scenarios of failure and strive hard to imagine novel ones." Although difficult to maintain, preoccupation with failure is what distinguishes safe system implementations from tragic scenarios. In Pediatric Informatics, it is essential that we learn from each other's mistakes. Han's courage in reporting the system failures that occurred in Pittsburgh has helped countless other institutions that are struggling through complex system implementations. Safety is best achieved by embracing the lessons learned in practice, found in the literature and in the current media[4] and respecting the socio-technical complications inherent in computerized healthcare.

8.3.6.1   Transitional Planning for Implementations

Having discussed at great length how health IT implementation can interrupt, modify, break, or alter existing clinical processes, we must stress that these changes also represent potential to improve care delivery processes. Prior to any implementation, all providers must understand and cognitively "walk through" changes. They must understand how and when they will generate or receive orders, whether the orders will be on paper or electronically. A "cognitive walkthrough"[82, 83] that involves all key personnel, including staff users, from the care delivery team is an extremely powerful tool for uncovering implementation oversights and gaps in adapting to proposed new care process. Such an exercise is helpful in identifying functional problems at "handover" points (care transition) like nursing change of shift, physician to physician sign-out rounds, and communications between nurses, social work, aftercare planning staff and health unit coordinators.

Implementers, not physicians, must be aware of which orders are transmitted electronically and which orders must be sent on paper. Often laboratory orders, blood products, and specialized treatments are managed by an entity outside the hospital that is not a part of existing inpatient CPOE system. Thus, these items must be managed by (a) some parallel paper process, or (b) by a freestanding computer system in a different hospital department, or (c) an independent external computer system (diagnostic laboratory, blood bank, etc.). External systems may have a standardized messaging interface that the legacy hospital system cannot support. It is important to identify and think through all possible parallel and interactive human, technical, and business processes well before CPOE implementation, otherwise the implementations runs the risk of preventing providers from performing needed actions and jeopardizing patient care. Hundreds of staff members may need to be retrained for navigating the two (or more) partial processes.

8.3.6.2   Gap Analysis

New clinical information technology projects have historically routinely overlooked key issues, people, and departments (e.g. Medical Records, or Admissions) in the initial financial/installation planning. Such oversights are a common cause of severe failures. Many implementation problems may be mitigated prospectively if they are well framed during prespecifications functional assessment evaluation including all department and roles within the institution. The assessment component should include at least a 24-h observational visit to the physical departmental spaces (including weekend and holidays to check for alternative workflows), meetings with: (1) key people (the nurses and RTs) of the care units; (2) the supporting departments (Pharmacy, Laboratory, Radiology, Admissions, Clinical Engineering); and (3) the Information Technology managers and staff, who potentially would be involved with any new system installation. The proposed scope of the new installation is important in organizing the focus and composition of the teams responsible for planning, specifications development, contracting, installation, education, and management. The discovery process must address the stake holders' needs and prioritize requirements to withstand the contract development and budget negotiation processes.

Functional specification discovery and development is best undertaken *early* in the overall process, to assure that all the important participants, technical needs and workflow concerns are discovered (A good rule for implementation could be: "Fail often but EARLY"). Functional specifications are easily developed as a log of the walk throughs. A good example of formal functional specifications setting effort is the Certification Commission on Health Information Technology (CCHIT). CCHIT's documents are publicly available.[84]

Complex inpatient human systems and immature, not integrated CPOE, EMR, and HIT products often prevent us from achieving the goal of safer patient care. New software architecture, system designs, and workflow processes are all needed to mange the parallel, multiaxial, temporally overlapping real-time "workflow" in health care. When the target units are Pediatric Intensive Care Units, the list of main considerations to guide the overall process should include the areas and situations outlined in Table 8.5.

Table 8.5 Planning new information systems for pediatric critical care

Existing Bedside Medical Devices
- Inventory
- Technical specs (ports, models, fixed or portable…)
- Driver protocols needed?

Space
- Consider optimal install configurations for decreasing the frequent ICU crowding concerns
- Single room, pod, or other bed space arrangements

Configuration of physical bed spaces: (photographs needed)
- Electrical
- Current data management strategies – how are flowsheets or COWs (computers on wheels) used?
- Wireless management – data ports location?
- Staff expectations for wireless?
- Bandwidth considerations?

Workflow: (stopwatch, observation check list)
- Informal brief observations by a clinical informaticist
- Formal study, conducted by workflow management engineers
- Walk through mockups by clinical staff, all shifts

Target unit team structure
- How do nurses work in the environment?
- How does the nursing staff cover for each other?
- How do they deal with "offsite" needs (supplies, feeds, medications?)
- Do they use a formal team structure for care, for coverage, for parent communication, for emergencies' management?
- What are nursing concerns about new technology?
- How do the doctor teams gather their daily data? Who does the "Daily Note" and how are data obtained?
- Does the unit use nurse practitioners or physician assistants? Will they interact with the new system? How? Where?
- Consider other staff "visitors" and team members (e.g. consultants, social work, pharmacists, others) their roles and likely interactions with the new system
- Remember HIPAA and the "80 hour rule"
- Consider parents roles and physical spaces

Education
- Does the Unit have a nurse educator?
- Does the hospital have a nurse educator?
- How is education and "in service" for new things usually managed? Is staff paid for educational hours?
- If the data are never to be printed, how will providers be notified of data?
- How much provider time and attention does the system take from (or add to) rounds?

Installation setup: evaluate the target ICU's needs for Hardware
- Note existing terminals and lab links, are wires and data ports
- Inventory bedside lab devices and their data output methods
- Note existing servers for other vendors' systems (e.g. partial vital signs automated systems, doctor note systems, computerized provider order entry systems (CPOE), nurse charting systems)
- Check location, number, speed, and maintenance considerations of printers

(continued)

Table 8.5 (continued)

Cabling and network Installation and management
- Seek input from the hospital IT department
- Bandwidth consideration
- Real-time speed is critical for critical caregivers

Unit specification data configuration setup
- Collect blank source documents
- Bedside flowsheets
- Lab reports
- Order forms
- Respiratory flowsheet
- Technical checking documents
- Reports' samples
- Daily note samples
- Fluids and drugs charting
- Ancillary documents like visit and educational auditing logs
- Transfer forms
- Pharmacy change orders

HIS vendor requirements
- Methods, costs, control, personnel needed from installing hospital?
- Observe how clinicians access HIS (and from where, for what information)

References

1. Campbell EM, Sittig DF, Ash JS, Guappone KP, Dykstra RH. Types of unintended consequences related to computerized provider order entry. *J Am Med Inform Assoc.* 2006;13:547–556.
2. Ash JS, Berg M, Coiera E. Some unintended consequences of information technology in health care: the nature of patient care information system-related errors. *J Am Med Inform Assoc.* 2004;11:104–112.
3. Tenner E. *Why Things Bite Back: Technology and the Revenge of Unintended Consequences.* New York: Vintage Books; 1996.
4. InjuryBoard Online. Bay Pines VA Medical Center; 2004. Available at: http://www.injuryboard.com/view.cfm/Topic=9905. Accessed December 24, 2008.
5. Obradovich JH, Woods DD. Users as designers: how people cope with poor HCI design in computer-based medical devices. *Hum Factors.* 1996;38:574–592.
6. Leveson NG, Turner CS. An investigation of the Therac-25 accidents. *Computer.* 1993;18–41.
7. Cook RI, Woods DD. Adapting to new technology in the operating room. *Hum Factors.* 1996;38:593–613.
8. Han YY, Carcillo JA, Venkataraman ST, et al. Unexpected increased mortality after implementation of a commercially sold computerized physician order entry system. *Pediatrics.* 2005;116:1506–1512.
9. Del Beccaro MA, Jeffries HE, Eisenberg MA, Harry ED. Computerized provider order entry implementation: no association with increased mortality rates in an intensive care unit. *Pediatrics.* 2006;118:290–295.
10. Gaba DM, Howard SK, Small SD. Situation awareness in anesthesiology. *Hum Factors* 1995;37:20–30.

11. Menke JA, Broner CW, Campbell DY, McKissick MY, Edwards-Beckett JA. Computerized clinical documentation system in the pediatric intensive care unit. *BMC Med Inform Decis Mak*. 2001;1:3.
12. Sittig DF, Ash JS, Zhang J, Osheroff JA, Shabot MM. Lessons from "Unexpected increased mortality after implementation of a commercially sold computerized physician order entry system". *Pediatrics*. 2006;118:797–801.
13. Cunningham SN, Deere S, Symon A, Elton RA, McIntosh N. A randomized, controlled trial of computerized physiologic trend monitoring in an intensive care unit. *Crit Care Med*. 1998;26:2053–2060.
14. Carpenter RO, Spooner J, Arbogast PG, Tarpley JL, Griffin MR, Lomis KD. Work hours restrictions as an ethical dilemma for residents: a descriptive survey of violation types and frequency. *Curr Surg*. 2006;63:448–55.
15. Adam S. Standardization of nutritional support: are protocols useful? *Intensive Crit Care Nurs*. 2000;16:283–9.
16. Van den Heuvel LN, Lorenzo DK, Montgomery RL, Hanson WE, Rooney JR. *Root Cause Analysis Handbook: A Guide to Effective Incident Investigation ABS Consulting*. Rothstein; 2005:ISBN #1-931332-30-4.
17. Joint Commission. Quality Improvement Initiatives 2007 Hospital/Critical Access Hospital National Patient Safety Goals; 2007. Available at: http://www.jointcommission.org/PatientSafety/NationalPatientSafetyGoals/07_hap_cah_npsgs.htm. Accessed December 24, 2008.
18. Yang JA, Kombarakaran FA. A practitioner's response to the new health privacy regulations. *Health Soc Work*. 2006;31:129–36.
19. American Academy of Pediatrics, American College of Obstetricians and Gynecologists. *Guidelines for Perinatal Care*. 5th ed. Washington, DC: American Academy of Pediatrics; 2002.
20. Kock NF. *Process Improvement and Organizational Learning: The Role of Collaborative Technologies*. New York: Idea Group Publishing; 1999:ISBN 1878289586.
21. Drucker PF. *Managing in a Time of Great Change*. New York: Truman/Talley Books/Plume; 1995.
22. Gilbert A. The patient-monitor system in intensive care: eliciting nurses' mental models. In: Harris D, ed. *First International Congress on Engineering Psychology and Cognitive Ergonomics*. Brookfield, VT: Ashgate; 1993.
23. Staggers N. Human factors: imperative concepts for information systems in critical care. *AACN Clin Issues*. 2003;14:310–319.
24. Leape LL. Error in medicine. *JAMA*. 1994;272:1851–1857.
25. Tsang PS, Vidulich MA. *Principles and Practice of Aviation Psychology*. Lawrence Erlbaum; 2002:ISBN 0805833900.
26. Sternberg RJ. *Practical Intelligence in Everyday Life*. Boston, MA: Cambridge University Press; 2000:ISBN 0521659582.
27. Lehmann CU. Medical information systems in pediatrics. *Pediatrics*. 2002;111(3):679.
28. Howard Hughes Medical Institute. Whitepaper: brain scans that spy on the senses; 2007. Available at: http://www.hhmi.org/senses/e110.html. Accessed December 24, 2008.
29. Patterson RD. Auditory warning sounds in the work environment. *Phil Trans R Soc Lond B*. 1990;327:485–492.
30. Cohen S, Weinstein N. Nonauditory effects of noise on behavior and health. *J Soc Issues*. 1981;37:36–70.
31. Jones DM, Broadbent DE. Noise. In: Salvendy G, ed. *Handbook of Human Factors*. New York: Wiley; 1987:623–649.
32. Poulton EC. Continuous intense noise masks auditory feedback and inner speech. *Psychol Bull*. 1977;84:977–1001.
33. Morrison WE, Haas EC, Shaffner DH, Garrett ES, Fackler JD. Noise, stress and annoyance in a pediatric intensive care unit. *Crit Care Med*. 2002;31:113–119.
34. Brixley JJ, Tang Z, Robinson DJ, et al. Interruptions in a level one trauma center: a case study. *Int. J Medical Inform*. 2008; 77:235–241.

35. Collins S, Currie L, Patel V, Bakken S, Cimino JJ. Multitasking by clinicians in the context of CPOE and CIS use. *Stud Health Technol Inform.* 2007;129(Pt 2):958–962.
36. Poissant L, Pereira J, Tamblyn R, Kawasumi Y. The impact of electronic health records on time efficiency of physicians and nurses: a systematic review. *J Am Med Inform Assoc.* 2005;12(5):505–516.
37. American Medical Informatics Association. A Roadmap for National Action on Clinical Decision Support; 2006. Available at: http://www.amia.org/inside/initiatives/cds/. Accessed December 24, 2008.
38. Patel VL, Cohen T. New perspectives on error in critical care. *Curr Opin Crit Care.* 2008;4:456–459.
39. Anderson BJ, Ellis JF. Common errors of drug administration in infants: causes and avoidance. *Paediatr Drugs.* 1999;1:93–107.
40. Fortescue EB, Kaushal R, Landrigan CP, et al. Prioritizing strategies for preventing medication errors and adverse drug events in pediatric inpatients. *Pediatrics.* 2003;111:722–729.
41. Kaushal R, Bates DW, Landrigan C, McKenna KJ, Clapp MD. Medication errors and adverse drug events in pediatric inpatients. *JAMA.* 2001;285:2114–2120.
42. Folli HL, Poole RL, Benitz WE, Russo JC. Medication error prevention by clinical pharmacists in two children's hospitals. *Pediatrics.* 1987;79:718–722.
43. Bates DW, Teich JM, Lee J, et al. The impact of computerized physician order entry on medication error prevention. *J Am Med Inform Assoc.* 1999;6:313–321.
44. Mekhjian HS, Kumar RR, Kuehn L, et al. Immediate benefits realized following implementation of physician order entry at an academic medical center. *J Am Med Inform Assoc.* 2002;9:529–539.
45. Cordero L, Kuehn L, Kumar RR, Mekhjian HS. Impact of computerized physician order entry on clinical practice in a newborn intensive care unit. *J Perinatol.* 2004;24:88–93.
46. Upperman JS, Staley P, Friend K, et al. The impact of hospitalwide computerized physician order entry on medical errors in a pediatric hospital. *J Pediatr Surg.* 2005;40:57–59.
47. King WJ, Paice N, Rangrej J, Forestell GJ, Swartz R. The effect of computerized physician order entry on medication errors and adverse drug events in pediatric inpatients. *Pediatrics.* 2003;112:506–509.
48. Potts AL, Barr FE, Gregory DF, Wright L, Patel NR. Computerized physician order entry and medication errors in a pediatric critical care unit. *Pediatrics.* 2004;113:59–63.
49. Kohn L, Corrigan J, Donaldson M. *To Err Is Human: Building a Safer Health System.* Washington, DC: National Academy Press; 1999.
50. Leape L, Bates D, Cullen D. Systems analysis of adverse drug events. *JAMA.* 1995;274:35–43
51. Leape LL, Lawthers AG, Brennan TA, Johnson WG. Preventing medical injury. *Qual Rev Bull.* 1993;19:144–149.
52. Bates D, Cullen D, Laird N. Incidence of adverse drug events and potential adverse drug events: implications for prevention. *JAMA.* 1995;274:29–34.
53. Kim GR, Chen AR, Arceci RJ, et al. Error reduction in pediatric chemotherapy: computerized order entry and failure modes and effects analysis. *Arch Pediatr Adolesc Med.* 2006;160(5):495–498.
54. Lehmann CU, Kim GR, Gujral R, Veltri MA, Clark JS, Miller MR. Decreasing errors in pediatric continuous intravenous infusions. *Pediatr Crit Care Med.* 2006;7(3):225–230.
55. Lehmann CU, Conner KG, Cox JM. Preventing provider errors: online total parenteral nutrition calculator. *Pediatrics.* 2004;113(4):748–753.
56. Committee on Drugs and Committee on Hospital. (2003) Prevention of medication errors in the pediatric inpatient setting. *Pediatrics.* 2003;112:431–436.
57. Committee on Identifying and Preventing Medical Errors. *Preventing Medication Errors. Quality Chasm Series.* Aspden P, Wolcott J, Bootman JL, Cronenwett LR, eds. Washington, DC: National Academy Press.
58. Kaushal R, Barker KN, Bates DW. How can information technology improve patient safety and reduce medication errors in children health care? *Arch Pediatr Adolesc Med.* 2001;155:1002–1007.
59. Koppel R, Leonard CE, Localio AR, Cohen A, Auten, R, Strom BL. Identifying and quantifying medication errors: evaluation of rapidly discontinued medication orders

submitted to a computerized physician order entry system. *J Am Med Inform Assoc.* 2008;15:408–423.

60. Matheny ME, Sequist TD, Seger AC, et al. A randomized trial of electronic clinical reminders to improve medication laboratory ordering. *J Am Med Inform Assoc.* 2008;15:424–429.

61. Tamblyn R, Huang A, Taylor L, et al. A randomized trial of the effectiveness of on-demand versus computer-triggered drug decision support in primary care. *J Am Med Inform Assoc.* 2008;15:430–438.

62. van der Sijs H, Aarts J, van Gelder T, Berg M, Vulto A. Turning off frequently overridden drug alerts: limited opportunities for doing it safely. *J Am Med Inform Assoc.* 2008;15:439–441.

63. Koren G, Barzilay Z, Modan M. Errors in computing drug doses. *Can Med Assoc J.* 1983;129:721–723.

64. Sullivan JE, Buchino JJ. Medication errors in pediatrics - the octopus evading defeat. *J Surgical Oncology.* 2004;88:182–188.

65. Goldmann D, Kaushal R. Time to tackle the tough issues in patient safety. *Pediatrics.* 2002;110:823–826.

66. Upperman JS, Staley P, Friend K, et al. The introduction of computerized physician order entry and change management in a tertiary pediatric hospital. *Pediatrics.* 2005;116:e634–e642.

67. Gray JE, Suresh G, Ursprung R. Patient misidentification in the NICU: quantification of risk. *Pediatrics.* 2006;117:e43–e47.

68. Patel VL, Cohen T. New perspectives on error in critical care. *Curr Opin Crit Care.* 2008;14:456–459.

69. Hughes D. When nurse knows best: some aspects of nurse/doctor interaction is a casualty department. *Sociol Health Illness.* 1988;19:1–22.

70. Buerhaus PI, Staiger DO, Auerbach DI. Why are shortages of hospital RNs concentrated in specialty care units. *Nurs Econ.* 2000;18:111–116.

71. Ash JS, Sittig DF, Poon EG, Guappone K, Campbell E, Dykstra RH. The extent and importance of unintended consequences related to computerized provider order entry. *J Am Med Inform Assoc.* 2007;14:415–425.

72. Evans RS, Pestotnik SL, Classen DC, et al. A computer-assisted management program for antibiotics and other antiinfective agents. *N Engl J Med.* 1998;338:232–238.

73. Combi C, Shahar Y. Temporal reasoning and temporal data maintenance in medicine: issues and challenges. *Comput Biol Med.* 1997;27:353–368.

74. Dolin RH. Modeling the temporal complexities of symptoms. *J Am Med Inform Assoc.* 1995;2:323–331.

75. Adlassnig KP, Combi C, Das AK, Keravnou ET, Pozzi G. Temporal representation and reasoning in medicine: research directions and challenges. *Artif Intell Med.* 2006;38:101–113.

76. Das AK, Musen MA. A formal method to resolve temporal mismatches in clinical databases. *Proc AMIA Symp.* 2001;130–134.

77. Wachter SB, Johnson K, Albert R, Syroid N, Drews F, Westenskow D. The evaluation of a pulmonary display to detect adverse respiratory events using a high resolution human simulator. *J Am Med Inform Assoc.* 2006;13:635–642.

78. Bardram JE. Temporal coordination: on time and coordination of collaborative activities at a surgical department. *Computer Supported Cooperative Work.* 2000;9:157–187.

79. Leape LL, Berwick DM. Five years after to err is human: what have we learned? *JAMA.* 2005;293:2384–2390.

80. Leape LL, Berwick DM, Bates DW. What practices will most improve safety?– evidence-based medicine meets patient safety. *JAMA.* 2002;288:501–507.

81. Reason J. Human error: models and management. *Brit Med J.* 2000;320:768–770.

82. Peute LW, Jaspers MM. Usability evaluation of a laboratory order entry system: cognitive walkthrough and think aloud combined. *Stud Health Technol Inform.* 2005;116:599–604.

83. Chan W. Increasing the success of physician order entry through Human Factors Engineering. *J Healthc Inf Manag.* 2002;16(1):71–79.

84. Certification Commission on Health Infromation Technology (CCHIT). Available at: http://www.cchit.org. Accessed December 24, 2008.

Chapter 9
Pediatric Care, Safety, and Standardization

Anne Matlow and John M. A. Bohnen

Objectives

- To distinguish between standard of care and standardized care
- To review cognitive and workflow tools to improve safety through standardization

9.1 Introduction

The Institute of Medicine (IOM) defines patient safety as "freedom from accidental injury due to medical care, or medical errors," and promotes the establishment of systems and processes to improve the reliability of patient care as one route to making health care safer.[1] In his recent book, Patient Safety, Charles Vincent offers two different approaches to achieving this aim, each founded in a distinct "vision of safety."[2] One vision highlights the expertise and skills that providers regularly channel into creating safe patient care, and promotes the adoption of new and enhanced skills such as teamwork training and mindfulness as keys to improving patient safety. The other vision recognizes the fallibility of human beings, and seeks to improve safety by replacing or supporting the health care provider using technical and procedural interventions such as standardization, guidelines, and information technology. The important role of information technology was underscored in the IOM's report, "Crossing the Quality Chasm."[3] Standardization of practice patterns is one aspect of clinical care that is very amenable to the use of informatics.[4] By reducing process variability, standardization can potentially reduce errors and make outcomes more predictable, thereby improving care processes. In this chapter we will explore various strategies currently being used to standardize care, and their impact on patient safety.

9.2 Standard of Care Versus Standardized Care

It is useful first to understand the distinction between "standard of care" and "standardization of care."

C.U. Lehmann et al. (eds.), *Pediatric Informatics: Computer Applications in Child Health,* Health Informatics,
© Springer Science+Business Media, LLC 2011

A standard of care is not a "guideline or list of options; instead it is a duty determined by a given set of circumstances that present in a particular patient with a specific condition at a definite time and place;... a measure of the duty practitioners owe patients to make medical decisions in accordance with any other prudent practitioner's treatment of the same condition in a similar patient."[5] In a legal sense, "the standard of care" includes but may surpass the lowest stratum of clinical care that provides patient safety and effective care; it is the primary yardstick used in medical malpractice litigation. Key elements within this definition include individualized patient care, physician assessment and judgment, and care comparable to that practiced by others in the profession.

In contrast, standardization of care refers to reducing variations in care processes. From a clinical care perspective, the ultimate goals of standardization are to reduce harm and improve the quality of care. From a hospital or payer point of view, standardization should facilitate financial accounting to help rein in overspending. Examples of methods used to standardize care include clinical practice guidelines (CPGs), bundles, and checklists. More recently, methodologies rooted in the business industry, such as Six Sigma and reliability science are being applied to the health care sector to improve quality and patient safety. We will discuss the successes and limitations of each.

9.3   Clinical Practice Guidelines (CPGs)

CPGs (also covered in Chapter 11) are "systematically developed statements to assist practitioners' and patients' decisions about appropriate health care for specific clinical circumstances."[6] They were first introduced in the USA in the 1980s as a cost containment strategy, at a time when Medicaid and Medicare programs were under pressure and variability in care was evident at many levels: institutional, departmental, practitioner, and individual patient. The impact of this variability on the quality of care, in addition to fiscal considerations, resulted in the establishment of the federally legislated Agency for Health Care Policy and Research (now known as the Agency for Healthcare Research and Quality), "to enhance the quality, appropriateness, and effectiveness of health care services and access to these services."[7] Development of CPGs was a specific mandate of this newly formed Agency. With the profile of CPGs elevated, many organizations developed CPGs as a tool to improve the quality of care.[8] Given endorsement by the American Medical Association, attention from the IOM, involvement of hospitals, insurers, and others, a new paradigm in medicine was clearly evident.[9]

CPGs generally are based on literature review by subject matter and domain experts who apply the tenets of evidence-based care. In its policy statement on classifying recommendations for CPGs, the American Academy of Pediatrics describes three steps in evidence – based CPG development: "1. determination of evidence quality in support of a proposed recommendation, 2. evaluation of the balance between anticipated benefits and harms when the recommendation is carried out, and 3. designation of recommendation strength."[10] Assignation of recommendation strength is based on 1. level of aggregate evidence quality, ranging from A to D, where A is the strongest evidence e.g. well designed trials, and on 2. benefit-harm assessment (preponderance of benefit/harm or a balance between them). An additional category exists for recommendations which may not be supported by evidence, but for which the benefits or harms are clearly evident. As stated by the AAP: "Guidelines are never intended to overrule professional judgment; rather they should be viewed as a relative constraint on individual clinician discretion in a particular clinical circumstance.... Clinicians should always act and make decisions on behalf of their patients' best interests and needs regardless of guideline recommendations. Guidelines represent the best judgment of a team of experienced clinicians and methodologies addressing the scientific evidence for a particular topic."

One has then to ask the obvious question, what evidence supports CPGs? Stated otherwise, do CPGs improve patient safety? Maybe! In a classic article, Grimshaw and Russell evaluated the impact, and determinants of the impact of 59 CPGs.[11] Twenty-four guidelines addressed specific clinical conditions, 27 dealt with preventive care and 8 focused on prescribing or support services. Fifty-five (93%) demonstrated significant improvement in processes of care, and of those that measured outcomes, 82% (9/11) demonstrated significant improvement in outcomes. The authors concluded that although specific CPGs can improve clinical practice, dissemination, and implementation strategies are critical success factors in determining whether the guidelines will be effective. Guidelines were more likely to be effective if they were developed internally, included a specific education intervention as part of dissemination, and included a patient-specific reminder at the time of consultation.

As an example of a dissemination strategy, "safety e-mail alerts" have been used successfully at the Rush University Medical Center to notify housestaff that new CPGs are available. The notification originates from the Chief of Staff, underscoring the leadership's commitment to the guideline. Personal accountability is incorporated into the process by requiring the residents to respond through the e-mail that the CPGs have been read; if no response is received after a period of time, the chief resident follows up.[12] By incorporating decision alerts into the electronic order entry, use of the CPGs has then been facilitated.

Example of a Clinical Practice Guideline (CPG)

Issue

Perioperative antibiotic prophylaxis should be administered within 60 min prior to the incision.

It is often administered too late, which increases the risk of surgical site infection.

Proposed Solution

Embed a pop-up into computerized surgical preoperative order sets, such that when the antibiotic is entered, the physician would be reminded that the drug should be administered within 60 min prior to the incision.

Some limitations of CPGs are listed in Table 9.1. The CPGs themselves may be problematic. Alternatively, problems with physician adherence may limit their applicability.[13] In a survey of pediatricians about their knowledge and practice of four CPGs (management of the febrile infant, neonatal hyperbilirubinemia, otitis media with effusion, and preventive care), Christakis et al.[14] found that knowledge of the guidelines ranged from 16–66%, assessment of mean helpfulness scores (1–10 scale, where 1 = "not at all helpful" and 10 = "extremely helpful") ranged from 3.67 to 6.67, and change in patient management based on the guidelines ranged from 19–36% for the four guidelines. More recent graduation from medical school and increased helpfulness scores were associated with more guideline-related behavior change by providers. Variability in actual implementation was recently further borne out in a review of compliance with the AAP's CPG on management of first urinary tract infection (UTI) in infants, in which recommendations include timely imaging, and adequate antimicrobial prophylaxis.[15] The authors reviewed Washington State's Medicaid data, on in-patients and out-patients diagnosed with a UTI within the first year of life, and found that overall, only 44%, 39.5%, and 51% of eligible patients received anatomic imaging, imaging for reflux and antimicrobial prophylaxis where warranted respectively.

In 2003, the Centers for Medicare and Medicaid Services embarked on a large pay-for-performance pilot project using the American College of Cardiology/American Heart Association guidelines for acute myocardial infarction. The goal of pay-for-performance programs is to tie financial incentives to adherence with guidelines.[16] However, Walter et al. have recently drawn attention to problems in using adherence to guidelines as a measure of quality of care.[17] Studying compliance with colorectal cancer screening guidelines, the authors identified the following as limitations to using adherence rates to guideline-based performance measures

Table 9.1 Limitations of clinical practice guidelines

Technical (guideline-related) limitations	Adaptive (physician-related) limitations
Recommendations are wrong	Users have limited knowledge
• Are open to subjective interpretation	• Lack awareness of guidelines
• Contain outdated content	• Lack familiarity with guidelines
Recommendations limit freedom of choice	• Users have implementation limitations
• Negatively influence resource allocation	• Disagree with recommendations
• Do not take patient preferences into account	• Lack self efficacy
• Reduce flexibility for special needs patients	• Lack outcome efficacy
Recommendations do not reach target audience	• Resist change (practice inertia)
Recommendations discourage research	
Recommendations increase costs of care	

as indicators of the quality of cancer screening: "(1) not properly considering illness severity of the sample population audited for adherence to screening, (2) not distinguishing screening from diagnostic procedures when setting achievable target screening rates, and (3) not accounting for patient preferences or clinician judgment when scoring performance measures."

It has been proposed that if CPGs were available at the point of care, enabling the clinician to access timely and relevant knowledge and support at the time of decision making, compliance with CPGs might be enhanced.[18] However, there are conflicting reports on the success of implementing point-of-care CPGs. Chin described the experience at Kaiser Permanente, Northwest region, embedding CPGs into the CPOE process on the computerized patient record. Ordering according to the CPG was designed as the default mode.[19] For example, the authors reported a marked increase in orders for upper gastrointestinal (UGI) series conforming to the guidelines when appropriate indications for the test were embedded in the order requisition. In contrast, Asaro et al. did not see improved compliance with a CPG for acute coronary syndrome that was embedded in their commercial CPOE system. They attributed this to the lack of co-embedded patient-specific decision support, and suggested that vendors consider the feasibility of incorporating patient-specific support in designing their systems.[20]

Clinical informatics affords us the opportunity to expand the cadre of CPGs available for use at the point of care. It is likely that some guidelines, perhaps those that are more generic, will be amenable to more rapid and successful incorporation and adoption through informatics. Only by capturing and understanding the barriers to use will future systems be able to be more capably designed.

9.4 Clinical Algorithms and Care Maps

Clinical algorithms (CAs) describe a diagnostic, therapeutic, or management approach to a given clinical problem, which is outlined by a detailed, step-by step account, often presented as a flow chart. They facilitate application of consistent care, save time for the user, expedite care, and provide the decision support to enable providers to function outside their usual knowledge or skill set.[21] Furthermore they provide a framework for thinking about clinical problems, and are particularly useful for the clinician who lacks mental models for this problem because he has not seen this problem recently or ever.[22] Although diagnostic, therapeutic, and management algorithms can theoretically be embedded into CPOE systems (Chapter 18), physician use may be the rate-limiting factor. For example, Margolis et al. reported that a barrier to the adoption of computerized CAs was the time required for what was considered a "lockstep recording procedure that was both irritating and tiring".[23] Fischer et al. recently reported their experience developing and using an algorithmic CPOE to select patients for treatment with activated protein C, which at that time was an investigational drug.[24] The embedded decision support was able to delineate whether the patient was a candidate for use of this drug based on specific inclusion criteria: if the patient was a candidate, the order was completed. An override capability was also incorporated. On review, 65% of patients received the drug through the computerized algorithm and in the rest, by overrides. There was no significant in-hospital mortality difference between the two groups. The authors concluded that anticipatory development of guidelines with a computer based algorithm should be considered for use of an unapproved drug when recommendations are imminent.

Example of a clinical algorithm (CA)

Issue

Gentamicin is a nephrotoxic drug.
  Gentamicin serum levels must be within a therapeutic range.
  The dosage should be adjusted if the peak level is >10 mg/L.

Proposed Solution

When a gentamicin level is elevated, the laboratory report has a tag that reads:
  "Serum gentamicin level elevated. Gentamicin is nephrotoxic.
  Adjust dosage and follow serum gentamicin levels and serum creatinine.
  Discontinuation or further dosage adjustment may be required."

Another tool that provides a framework for standardization of care is the care map. Care maps, also called critical care plans or clinical pathways, have been called the "blueprint of nursing management."[25] They define the care required for a designated group of patients, including interventions, time frames and expected outcomes. In their traditional paper form, standardized interventions are displayed across a daily timeline; outcome targets and the ability for documentation may or may not be included. Computerization of care maps that consider the complexity of medical care are under development.[26]

9.5   Bundles

The concept of "care bundles" originated in the USA at the Institute for Healthcare Improvement (IHI) as a means to improve health care outcomes. The IHI's recent 100,000 Lives Campaign has raised the profile of care bundles, as they were integrated into many of the campaign's interventions.[27] In the UK, care bundles were introduced as part of a national initiative to modernize critical care following the 1999 publication of the Department of Health's review, Comprehensive Critical Care.[28] Evidence to date suggests that they enhance the ability of CPGs to deliver safe and quality care.

Care bundles consist of selected CPGs or evidence-based protocols that have been grouped together as a unit to encourage their consistent and systematical application as part of specific treatment regimens. In theory, by grouping several evidence-based interventions together in a single protocol, it is more likely that caregivers will provide a complete set of interventions, and patient outcomes will improve. A bundle should contain no more than three to five practices or precautionary steps that are effected at the same time and in the same space.[27]

The success of the care bundle is based in part on its focus on goal achievement, which encourages development of the teamwork necessary for effective implementation.[29] Furthermore, the simplicity of the bundle should make it easy to implement and easy to audit compliance.[30] Three bundles in particular have been widely touted: the ventilator care bundle, the central line bundle, the sepsis bundle (comprised of the resuscitation bundle and the sepsis management bundle).[31] In both the UK and the USA, introduction of the ventilator bundle (prophylaxis against peptic ulceration, prophylaxis against deep vein thrombosis, daily cessation of sedation and elevation of the patient's head and chest to at least 30° to the horizontal) was effective in reducing the length of ventilation and ICU length of stay,[32] as well as reducing the incidence of ventilator associated pneumonia, respectively.[30] IHI's central line bundle which targets central line-related bloodstream infection consists of five components: hand hygiene, maximal barrier precautions, chlorhexidine skin antisepsis, optimal catheter site selection, and daily review of line necessity with prompt removal of unnecessary lines.[33] The IHI website is rife with success stories from organizations that have successfully implemented the central line bundle. For example, Regions Hospital in St. Paul, Minnesota, reported a progressive fall in catheter related blood stream infection rate from over 8 in the medical ICU and burn centre to 0 infections per 1,000 line days within 3 years after the bundle was implemented.[34]

It is to be noted that the six bundles in the 100,000 Lives Campaign were developed from evidence well founded in the adult population. A Pediatric Node, consisting of the Child Health Corporation of America (CHCA), the National Association of Children's Hospitals and Related Institutions (NACHRI), and the National Initiative for Children's Healthcare Quality (NICHQ) adapted the bundles for use in children.[35] For example, the pediatric central line bundle is divided into insertion and maintenance bundle elements, and is outlined in Table 9.2.[36] The pediatric ventilator care bundle excludes the daily "sedation vacation." Anecdotal evidence suggests that outcomes in pediatric care have been improved by use of the bundles.

The beauty of using the bundle lies not only with the framework for implementing multiple evidence based practices as part of a unit, but in the proposed strategy for measuring compliance. Rather than focusing on compliance with each individual component of the bundle, compliance is measured using the "all or nothing" approach, i.e. the rate at which *all* elements in the bundle are followed.[37] Although the journey to 100% compliance may be long, the end result is that more "best practices" are followed, with the likelihood of better patient outcomes.

Table 9.2 Pediatric central line bundle[36]

Central line insertion bundle elements	Maintenance bundle elements
• Hand hygiene	• Hand hygiene
• Use of transparent semipermeable dressings when possible/use of gauze only with bleeding/oozing	• Aseptic technique throughout (sterile gloves, dressing)
• Maximum barrier protection (sterile technique maintained throughout)	• Use of transparent semipermeable dressings when possible/use of gauze only with bleeding/oozing
• Skin preparation with antiseptic/detergent chlorhexidine 2%, except in those with a contraindication (e.g., patients less than 2 months of age)	• Replacement of dressing if damp, loosened or visibly soiled

Example of a Bundle

Issue

The Blood Stream Infection (BSI) bundle includes: hand hygiene, maximal barrier precautions, chlorhexiding skin antisepsis, attention to optimal catheter site selection and daily review of line necessity with prompt removal of unnecessary lines. The latter may need a regular reminder.

Proposed Solution

Integrate in CPOE that when a patient has an IV in place, there is a daily reminder: "Does this patient still need an IV?" that must actively be closed before being able to proceed with new orders.

9.6 Checklists

The aviation industry is a high reliability organization. Unanticipated and stressful situations that can arise in air travel necessitate consistent, specific, and coordinated activities in the airplane cockpit, and this has led to adoption of checklists as a means to reduce variability and enhance coordination, to counterbalance those times when relying on memory or sustained vigilance may be challenging.[38] Periods of urgent action and stress are not unfamiliar to healthcare professionals, and recently checklists have been introduced in healthcare to standardize practice and avoid reliance on memory. The items on the checklist often include evidence based recommendations.

Handoffs are situations in which important information is transmitted between practitioners. Handoffs are critical in providing optimal care to patients and with reduced work hours for residents have become more frequent.[39] Information not relayed may result in severe complications and poor patient outcomes. However handoffs often take place under time and space constraints. Types of handoffs include intrahospital patient transfer (e.g. between hospital wards, from the emergency department to the operating room), and interhospital patient transfer. Other types of handoffs relate to information communication at staff transition times (e.g. nursing shift change or off-hours medical coverage). In reviewing 176 reports of incidents resulting from the intrahospital transfer of critically ill patients in Australia, Beckman et al. noted that rechecking the equipment and the patient as well as using protocols were important in mitigating a negative outcome.[40] As a result, development and use of a pre-transport checklist was recommended. Recently, the Child Health Accountability Initiative (CHAI) pediatric collaborative reported that using a checklist to improve the accuracy of information communication on transferring patients from the emergency department to an in-patient unit resulted in fewer duplicate or missed laboratory tests, fewer early or late medications fell, and an increase in the rate of correct patient isolation and nursing satisfaction.[41]

Checklists have been used successfully in other vulnerable clinical situations vulnerable to errors of omission, for example in reducing the incidence of catheter-related blood stream infections(CR-BSI) in intensive care units,[42, 43] improving airway management in critical airway situations,[44] improving interprofessional communication in operating rooms,[45] and in discharging patients from out-patient surgery.[46]

Schwartz has raised the concern that a checklist might actually be a threat to patient safety. In responding to the inclusion of oxytocin and a nondepolarizing agent under the "drugs drawn up" heading of the checklist for cesarean delivery under general anesthesia,[47] he noted that these drugs are not mandatory elements of anesthesia, and that inadvertent use of these drugs in this clinical situation could be catastrophic.[8] Clearly all elements of a checklist should be carefully considered prior to inclusion.

9.7 Six Sigma and Reliability Science

Six Sigma and reliability science are concepts that originated within industry and are now finding a niche in health care. Six Sigma methodology was developed by Motorola, a company who went on to win the coveted Malcolm Baldridge Award for Quality in 1998 for its impact. Six Sigma, a strategy rooted in manufacturing, aims to eliminate variation in order to reduce the number of defective products to fewer than 3.4 per million units, or opportunities, or within six standard deviations of the mean. Given that in health care, quality problems occur much more frequently, at rates of 20–50%, or 200,000–500,000 per million, there has been interest in applying the methodology of Six Sigma to improve outcomes in service industries such as health care.[49]

Six Sigma is based on the premise that "variation is evil because a high level of variation means that customers will not get what they want – with all that that implies for retention, marketing efficiency, and revenue growth."[50] In order to improve defect free production, Six Sigma is a disciplined, data driven strategy, that uses the DMAIC Process (Define, measure, analyze, improve, control) to solve problems. There are reports of the process being used successfully to decrease

Table 9.3 Design concepts for improving reliability[58]

Level 1 reliability	Level 2 reliability	Level 3 reliability
• Basic standardization, e.g. CPGs • Memory aids such as checklists • Feedback mechanisms • Awareness raising and training	• Reminders • Differentiation (e.g. color coding) • Built-in decision aids and prompts • Desired actions as default choices • Redundancy • Leveraging existing habits and patterns • Agreement from staff to follow and learn from standardized processes	• Redesign after identifying failure modes

central line associated blood stream infections, and to increase compliance with hand hygiene.[51, 52]

Reliability can be defined as "failure-free operation over time," and failure rate, or unreliability, as "1 minus reliability."[53] Muething and Kotagal have given clinical examples of different levels of reliability.[54] A process such as improving the delivery of asthma care, may have a goal of 90% reliability, i.e. an error rate of 1 of 10 (Level 1 reliability). Strategies to prevent surgical site infections may target level 2 reliability, or 1 error or infection in 100 patients. A system to prevent adverse drug events in a hospital will aim toward error rates of 1 in 1,000 patients (99.9% reliability), which is level 3 reliability. Anesthesia in healthy patients is traditionally the only medical discipline to achieve a reliability level between 5 and 6,[55] and a recent report of applying the principles of reliability science to improve blood stream infections in an ICU was able to achieve Level 4 reliability, or <1 infection/1,000 line days.[56] The application of six sigma strategies to the administration of breast milk in the newborn intensive care unit reduced errors to 3.4 mistakes per one million opportunities.[57] Strategies to achieve the different levels of reliability are listed in Table 9.3. For further information the reader is referred to the IHI white paper.[58]

9.8   Standardization of Care as the Standard of Care?

Concerns have been raised that CPGs could be used to establish negligence in malpractice litigation.[8] A study in the USA found that in 17 of 259 (7%) malpractice claims did practice guidelines played a significant role, and this was more often to establish rather than to refute a claim of negligence.[59] Although a robust CPG may provide a benchmark for the standard of care, it has been claimed that they are not a substitute for expert testimony.[60, 61]

9.9 Conclusion

Facilitating standardization of care is an example of the role of informatics in promoting patient safety. The efficiency and effectiveness of this modality stands to be further increased in time by continued collaboration between experts in medical informatics and those in guideline and clinical standard development.[62, 59]

References

1. Kohn LT, Corrigan JM, Donaldson MS. *To Err Is Human: Building a Safer Health System.* Washington, DC: National Academy Press; 2000.
2. Vincent C. *Patient Safety.* Toronto: Elsevier Churchill Livingston; 2006.
3. Institute of Medicine. *Crossing the Quality Chasm.* Washington, DC: National Academy Press; 2000.
4. Bakken S, Cimino JJ, Hripcsak G. Promoting patient safety and enabling evidence-based practice through informatics. *Med Care* 2000;42:II49–II56.
5. Smith H. A model for validating an expert's opinion in medical negligence cases. *J Leg Med.* 2005;26:207–231.
6. Field MJ, Lohr KN eds. *Guidelines for Clinical Practice: From Developments to Use.* Washington, DC: Institute of Medicine, National Academy Press; 1992.
7. U.S. Department of Health and Human Services, Public Health Service, Agency for Health Care Policy and Research. *Depression Guideline Panel. Depression in Primary Care: Volume 1. Detection and Diagnosis. Clinical Practice Guideline 5.* Publication AHCPR 93-0550; 1993.
8. Andrews EJ, Redmond HP. A review of clinical guidelines. *Br J Surg.* 2004;100:956–964.
9. Woolf SH. Practice guidelines: a new reality in medicine. I. *Recent Dev Arch Intern Med.* 1990;150(9):1811–1818.
10. Homer CJ, Lannon CM, Harbaugh N, et al. Classifying recommendations for clinical practice guidelines. *Pediatrics.* 2004;114:874–877.
11. Grimshaw JM, Russell IT. Effect of clinical guidelines on medical practice: a systematic review of rigorous evaluations. *Lancet.* 1993;342:1317–1322.
12. Odwazny R, Hasler S, Abrams R, McNutt R. Organizational and cultural changes for providing safe patient care. *Q Manage Health Care.* 2005;14:132–143.
13. Cabana MD, Rand CS, Powe NR, et al. Why don't physicians follow clinical practice guidelines? A framework for improvement. *JAMA.* 1999;282:1458–1465.
14. Christakis DA, Rivara FP. Pediatricians' awareness of and attitudes about four clinical practice guidelines. *Pediatrics.* 1998;101(5):825–830.
15. Cohen AL, Rivara FP, Davis R, Christakis DA. Compliance with guidelines for the medical care of first urinary tract infections in infants: a population-based study. *Pediatrics.* 2005;115(6):1474–1478.
16. Glickman SW, Ou FS, DeLong ER, et al. Pay for performance, quality of care, and outcomes in acute myocardial infarction. *JAMA.* 2007;297(21):2373–2380.
17. Walter LC, Davidowitz NP, Heineken PA, Covinsky KE. Pitfalls of converting practice guidelines into quality measures. Lessons learned from a VA performance measure. *JAMA.* 2004;291:2466–2470.
18. The McDonnell Norms Group. Enhancing the use of clinical guidelines: the social norms perspective. *J Am Coll Surg.* 2006;202:826–836.
19. Chin HL, Wallace P. Embedding guidelines into direct physician order entry: simple methods, powerful results. *Proc AMIA Symp.* 1999;221–225.

20. Asaro PV, Sheldahl AL, Char DM. Embedded guideline information without patient specificity in a commercial emergency department computerized order-entry system. *Acad Emerg Med.* 2006;13:452–458.
21. Green G, Defoe EC Jr. What is a clinical algorithm? *Clin Pediatr (Phila).* 1978;17:457–463.
22. Margolis CZ. Uses of clinical algorithms. *JAMA.* 1983;249(5):627–632.
23. Margolis CZ, Warshawsky SS, Goldman L, Dagan O, Wirtschafter D, Pliskin JS. Computerized algorithms and pediatricians' management of common problems in a community clinic. *Acad Med.* 1992;67:282–284.
24. Fischer MA, Lilly CM, Churchill WW, Baden LR, Avorn J. An algorithmic computerized order entry approach to assist in the prescribing of new therapeutic agents. Case study of activated protein C at an academic medical center. *Drug Saf.* 2004;27:1253–1261.
25. Neidig JR, Megel ME, Koehler KM. The critical path: an evaluation of nursing case management in the NICU. *Nursing Manage.* 1992;11:45–52.
26. Chu S, Cesnik B. Improving clinical pathway design: lessons learned from a computerized prototype. *Int J Med Inform.* 1998;51:1–11.
27. The Joint Commission. Raising the bar with bundles: treating patients with an all-or-nothing standard. *Jt Comm Perspect Patient Saf.* 2006;6(4):5–6.
28. Department of Health, London. *Comprehensive Critical Care; A Review of Adult Critical Care Services;* 1999.
29. Institute for Healthcare Improvement. Bundle Up for Safety; 2004. Available at: http://www.ihi.org/IHI/Topics/CriticalCare/IntensiveCare/ImprovementStories/BundleUpforSafety.htm. Accessed December 20, 2008.
30. Resar R, Pronovost P, Haraden C, Simmonds T, Rainey T, Nolan T. Using a bundle approach to improve ventilator care processes and reduce ventilator-associated pneumonia. *Jt Comm J Qual Patient Saf.* 2005;31(5):243–248.
31. Fulbrook P, Mooney S. Care bundles in critical care: a practical approach to evidence-based practice. *Nurs Crit Care.* 2003;8(6):249–255.
32. Crunden E, Boyce C, Woodman H, Bray B. An evaluation of the impact of the ventilator care bundle. *Nurs Crit Care.* 2005;10(5):242–246.
33. Levy MM, Pronovost PJ, Dellinger RP, et al. Sepsis change bundles: converting guidelines into meaningful change in behavior and clinical outcome. *Crit Care Med.* 2004;32(11 Suppl):S595–S597.
34. Institute for Healthcare Improvement. Pursuing Perfection: Report from HealthPartners' Regions Hospital on Reducing Hospital-Acquired Infection: Ventilator-Associated Pneumonia and Catheter-Related Bloodstream Infection; 2004. Available at: http://www.ihi.org/IHI/Topics/CriticalCare/IntensiveCare/ImprovementStories/PursuingPerfectionReportfromHealthPartnersonReducingVAPCRBSI.htm. Accessed December 20, 2008.
35. Edson BS, Williams MC. 100,000 lives campaign and the application to children. *JSPN.* 2006;11:138–142.
36. Pediatric Affinity Group. How to Guide Pediatric Supplement: Central Line Associated Infection; 2002. Available at: http://www.childrenshospitals.net/AM/Template.cfm?Section=Homepage&Template=/CM/ContentDisplay.cfm&ContentFileID=2358. Accessed December 20, 2008.
37. Nolan T, Berwick DM. All-or-none measurement raises the bar on performance. *JAMA.* 2006;295(10):1168–1170.
38. Degani A. (1990) *Human Factors of Flight-Deck Checklists: The Normal Checklist.* Ames Research Center, National Aeronautics and Space Administration.
39. Horwitz LI, Kosiborod M, Lin Z, Krumholz HM. Changes in outcomes for internal medicine inpatients after work-hour regulations. *Ann Intern Med.* 2007;147(2):97–103.
40. Beckmann U, Gillies DM, Berenholtz SM, Wu AW, Pronovost P. Incidents relating to the intra-hospital transfer of critically ill patients: an analysis of the reports submitted to the Australian Incident Monitoring Study in Intensive Care. *Intensive Care Med.* 2004;30:8, 1579–1585.

41. Streitenberger K, Matlow A. *Check and Cross-Check: Using a Standardized Checklist to Reduce Adverse Events During Patient Transfer.* National Initiative for Child Health Quality (NICHQ) 4th Annual Meeting. San Diego, CA.
42. Berenholtz SM, Pronovost PJ, Lipsett PA, et al. Eliminating catheter-related bloodstream infections in the intensive care unit. *Crit Care Med.* 2004;32(10):2014–2020.
43. Wall RJ, Ely EW, Elasy TA, et al. Using real time process measurements to reduce catheter related bloodstream infections in the intensive care unit. *Qual Saf Health Care.* 2005;14(4):295–302.
44. Rall M, Dieckmann P. Safety culture and crisis resource management in airway management: general principles to enhance patient safety in critical airway situations. *Best Pract Res Clin Anaesthesiol.* 2005;19(4):539–557.
45. Lingard L, Espin S, Rubin B, et al. Getting teams to talk: development and pilot implementation of a checklist to promote interprofessional communication in the OR. *Qual Saf Health Care.* 2005;14(5):340–346.
46. Kingdon B, Newman K. Determining patient discharge criteria in an outpatient surgery setting. *AORN J.* 2006;83(4):898–904.
47. Hart EM, Owen H. Errors and omissions in anesthesia: a pilot study using a pilot's checklist. *Anesth Analg.* 2005;101(1):246–250.
48. Schwarz SK. Can items on an aviation-style checklist for preparation of cesarean delivery under general anesthesia present a threat for patient safety? *Anesth Analg.* 2006;102(3):970.
49. Chassin MR. Is health care ready for Six Sigma quality? *Milbank Q.* 1998;76(4):565–591.
50. George ML. *Lean Six Sigma: Combining Six Sigma Quality with Lean Speed.* New York: McGraw Hill.
51. Eldridge NE, Woods SS, Bonello RS, et al. Using the six sigma process to implement the Centers for Disease Control and Prevention Guideline for Hand Hygiene in four intensive care units. *J Gen Intern Med.* 2006;21(Suppl 2):S35–S42.
52. Frankel HL, Crede WB, Topal JE, Roumanis SA, Devlin MW, Foley AB. Use of corporate Six Sigma performance-improvement strategies to reduce incidence of catheter-related bloodstream infections in a surgical ICU. *J Am Coll Surg.* 2005;201(3):349–358.
53. Resar RK. Making noncatastrophic health care processes reliable: learning to walk before running in creating high-reliability organizations. *Health Serv Res.* 2006;41(4 Pt 2):1677–1689.
54. Muething SE, Kotagal U. Reliability of the health care delivery system. *J Pediatr.* 2005;146:581–582.
55. Amalberti R, Auroy Y, Berwick D, Barach P. Five system barriers to achieving ultrasafe health care. *Ann Intern Med.* 2005;142:756–764.
56. Render ML, Brungs S, Kotagal U, et al. Evidence-based practice to reduce central line infections. *Jt Comm J Qual Patient Saf.* 2006;32(5):253–260.
57. Drenckpohl D, Bowers L, Cooper H. Use of the six sigma methodology to reduce incidence of breast milk administration errors in the NICU. *Neonatal Netw.* 2007;26(3):161–166.
58. Nolan T, Resar R, Haraden C, Griffin FA. Improving the reliability of health care. Institute for Healthcare Improvement; 2004. Available at: http://www.ihi.org/NR/rdonlyres/7BD559B7-11A0-4BA5-ABDE-BF10003788F1/0/ReliabilityWhitePaper2004revJune06.pdf. Accessed December 20, 2008.
59. Hyams AL, Brandenburg JA, Lipsitz SR, Shapiro DW, Brennan TA. Practice guidelines and malpractice litigation: a two-way street. *Ann Int Med.* 1995;122:450–455.
60. McDonagh RJ, Lavis JN, Sharpe G. Clinical practice guidelines as explicit standards of care: medico-legal considerations. *Ann RCPSC.* 2002;35: 9–12.
61. Hurwitz B. How does evidence based guidance influence determinations of medical negligence? *BMJ.* 2004;329:1024–1028.
62. Biondich PG, Downs SM, Carroll AE, Shiffman RN, McDonald CJ. Collaboration between the medical informatics community and guideline authors: fostering HIT standard development that matters. *AMIA Annu Symp Proc.* 2006:36–40.

Chapter 10
Evidence-Based Medicine and Pediatrics

Donna M. D'Alessandro

Objectives

Upon completion of this chapter the reader will learn about:

- The definition and process of evidence-based medicine (EBM)
- Barriers and considerations when implementing EBM into practice
- Information technology in bringing evidence to the point-of-care
- Specific evidence-based resources for pediatric care

10.1 Introduction

The informed pediatrician, one who is aware of current medical research relevant to patient care, is evolving. Although many pediatricians are becoming better connected to current evidence, many barriers remain to its full incorporation into care. Information science and technology offer potential solutions to overcome these barriers to bring evidence to the point-of-care for effective decision making and for continuous professional development of pediatricians.

10.2 The Vision and Reality of Evidence-Based Medicine

Evidence-based medicine (EBM) is "the conscientious, explicit and judicious use of current best evidence in making decisions about the care of individual patients." EBM practice is active integration of individual clinical expertise with the best available external clinical evidence from systematic research.[1] The EBM movement originated, in part, with the publication of Dr. Archibald Cochrane's 1972 book, *Effectiveness and Efficiency: Random Reflections on Health Services*,[2] which was influential in creating the field. The term "evidenced-based medicine" to describe these concepts first appeared in 1992.[3]

C.U. Lehmann et al. (eds.), *Pediatric Informatics: Computer Applications in Child Health*, Health Informatics,
© Springer Science+Business Media, LLC 2011

The EBM process consists of collecting and summarizing research studies using an explicit review process to integrate evidence about prevention and therapy for a broad array of clinical problems.[4] EBM summaries "result in recommendations that are more consistent with the evidence than do [other] approaches" such as expert recommendations. Patients receiving efficacious therapy based on evidence, in the setting and context of routine care, have better outcomes.

Adoption and dissemination of EBM techniques and findings are enhanced by their availability in the form of clinical decision support tools at the point and time of care, through active physician engagement (interactive educational meetings, educational outreach visits) and through audit and feedback to providers from patient care indicators (see Case Study). Acceptance and use is further enhanced by local opinion leaders and champions and organizational support to improve quality, safety and to decrease costs through the provision of better care.[5]

The use of EBM in the course of clinical pediatric care is evolving. More pediatricians are connected to the Internet in their offices (95%), are using the Internet (50%), and an increasing number are using personal digital assistants (PDAs, 38%).[6] These tools, which provide easy access to information, have fundamentally changed pediatricians' expectations. Dissemination of important medical information from trusted sources (such as the American Academy of Pediatrics, the Centers for Disease Control and local health departments) is now be measured in hours instead of days to weeks (through e-mail alerts, Internet, and newsfeeds (RSS, really simple syndication) from trusted sources). Still, this vision has not been fully realized.

10.3   Practice Barriers

10.3.1   Time

Clinical workflow is busy and consequently important patient care questions arise but may go unanswered. Physicians' information needs may vary from 0.01–5.0 questions per patient encounter.[7, 8] On average, primary care physicians require 2–12 min to search textbooks, 2–6 min to search Internet resources and 20 min to do an average MEDLINE search.[9, 10]

10.3.2   Practical Internet Access

Although pediatricians may have office computers, this does not equal true accessibility to electronic resources such as clinical practice guidelines, journals, textbooks, and even consultants. Physical placement away from the point-of-care (such as the front office), slow connections and shared use may create functional and practical barriers to access. In one sample of pediatricians, only 33% said they accessed the Internet at work and the majority (44%) had slow (modem) connections.[6,8,11,12]

10.3.3 Understanding Clinical Information Needs

Primary care physicians' information needs have been well documented[7,13–23] in adult medicine, but pediatrician's information needs have been less well studied.[12, 19, 24, 25] The first primary study of pediatric clinical information needs in 2004[26] found that pediatricians articulated needs for clear definitions for medical conditions, physical findings and laboratory testing information. It also found that pediatricians may pursue clinical questions at a higher rate than other physicians.[8,26] Of particular importance to general pediatricians is the need for pharmacology (especially drug-dosing) and infectious disease information.[12,25]

10.3.4 Finding and Using Evidence Efficiently

To answer many questions, physicians may use convenient resources such as textbooks (which may be outdated) and colleagues (who may not have appropriate or current knowledge).[8,12,13,23,25] To use published evidence, a framework for asking clinical questions when searching primary literature has been suggested (PICO), in which a question is defined by:

- Patient population
- Intervention or exposure
- Comparison
- Outcome of interest

A pediatric example is: "In 3–5 year olds with recurrent otitis media, does insertion of pressure-equalizing tubes decrease the number of infections when compared to children treated with prophylactic antibiotics?"

It takes time and experience to formulate an effective question and to search the primary literature. A more time-efficient method is to use abstractions of evidence: clinical guidelines, systematic reviews, evidence-linked textbooks on a topic. However, unfamiliarity with specific knowledge resources within a domain and uncertainty of their accuracy may increase the time needed to find an appropriate resource. For example, general pediatricians usually use the AAP Red Book® as the authority on pediatric infectious diseases, but may not be as familiar with other infectious disease texts. While the use of abstracted EBM resources may be more efficient for clinicians, the costs associated with access (commercial information sources) may be prohibitive to small practices that are not affiliated with hospitals or academic centers.

10.4   Pragmatics

10.4.1   Educational and Quality Assurance

The evolution of formal continuing medical education (CME) throughout the last century originally separated physicians from practice in classroom settings. Educational content was (and often still is), passive, course-centered, and teacher-driven. This is not an efficient nor effective form of learning for clinicians,[27,28] and changes in continuing education have emphasized continuous professional development (CPD) where the educational content is active, physician-centered, and practice driven. Other areas of changing focus in continuing education include collaborative, interprofessional team training and professional communities of practice and learning.[29,30]

The American Board of Pediatrics (ABP), along with other members of the American Board of Medical Specialties (ABMS), now requires evidence of lifelong learning and self-assessment and satisfactory practice performance as two of the four parts of the maintenance of certification (MOC).[31] The American Academy of Pediatrics (AAP) provides online tools through its Pedialink© (http://www.pedialink.org) Website: educational modules, an activity finder, a CME hour tracking tool and a system for developing an individualized learning plan (ILP) for lifelong learning. ILPs are now required during residency training and may become an intrinsic part of CPD for practicing pediatricians in the future.[32] The AAP's eQIPP© (Educational in Quality Improvement for Pediatric Practice) program also supports CPD by providing pediatric practices with a structured clinical performance feedback process based on data collected from patient charts to identify opportunities for practice improvement based on performance compared to published evidence[31] (see Case Study). Structured feedback affects the individual pediatrician, and also the entire healthcare team by identifying areas for practice team education, organizational change and evaluation of outcomes.

10.4.2   Workflow and Organizational Issues

Ideally, physicians would like to streamline and combine their information use and maximize its benefits. They would like to have best evidence on hand (wherever they are) to answer all their clinical questions efficiently during patient encounters. They would like to be able to measure and document the effectiveness of their use of evidence in improving patient outcomes while concurrently receiving credit (both educational and reimbursement) for doing so. This ideal cannot be met easily, but there are (intertwined) steps that can move pediatricians along the continuum toward this ideal.

The physical placement of information access for easy use in clinician workflow is dependent on practice size (Chapters 16 and 17). In larger practices, assessment of workspace and workflow to identify optimum locations for computers, printers, and other devices becomes more complex. Sharing of computers and prioritization of staff access may affect clinician use of resources or may determine the type of access (handheld devices, cellular telephones). The more streamlined the access to information, the more likely they will be used.

10.4.3 Financial Issues

Cost is the major consideration and barrier for technology acquisition and maintenance. Solutions may include cooperation with other practices or entities (such as hospitals or nonprofit organizations) in cost sharing or volume discounts to decrease individual practice costs for information technology. Such sharing arrangements may also improve communications between groups (such as a hospital and pediatric practice or several practices) because of increased interoperability and familiarity due to same systems in different locations. Access to EBM resources may similarly be shared or granted through partnerships such as affiliations with other physicians and practices, education institutions, public health registries or clinical research projects, although such agreements should considered in the context of possible violations of federal antikickback laws and regulatory safe harbors prior to signing.[33]

The cost of EBM resource access may be reduced if open-source publication models of peer-reviewed journals gains wider acceptance in the medical community (Ex: Public Library of Science, PLoS, www.plos.org or BioMed Central, http://www.biomedcentral.com/). In open-source publishing, scientific manuscripts undergo traditional peer review, but payment for publication comes from authors or membership institutions (which pay fees to allow its employees to publish), resulting in free access to research studies. This public access policy is encouraged by the National Institutes of Health,[34] and some commercial publishers are allowing free online access to their journals after a specified period of time.

10.5 Assessing the Quality of Available Health Information

10.5.1 Rating the Quality of Published Evidence

Ratings to assess the quality of published evidence have been developed. The Centre for Evidence-Based Medicine[35] rates the validity of a research study on five levels of evidence:

1. Randomized clinical trials or meta-analysis of randomized control trials = best
2. Individual cohort trial or systematic review of cohort trials
3. Case control study or systematic review of case control studies

4. Case series or poor quality cohort/case control studies
5. Expert opinion = worst

Recommendations are based on consistency among research studies:

A. Consistent Level 1 studies = best
B. Consistent Level 1 studies or extrapolations from Level 1 studies
C. Consistent Level 4 studies or extrapolations from Level 2, 3 studies
D. Level 5, inconsistent or inconclusive studies = worst

This system or modifications are often used (e.g. National Cancer Institute's PDQ® Cancer Information Summaries, http://www.nci.nih.gov/cancertopics/pdq), but it can be cumbersome to remember particularly because of sublevels of the validity scale (Ex: a Level 1c). Some authors opt to make a summary statement (Ex: "data is based upon literature analysis and expert panel consensus," e.g. National Guideline Clearinghouse, http://www.guideline.gov). What is most important for clinicians to know is the type of evidence recommendations upon which they are based.

10.5.2   The Internet and Information Quality

The Internet was originally developed in 1969 as a means of improving communications among defense researchers (i.e. ARPANET). In the 1980s and 1990s software tools such as Gopher, WAIS, and the FTP Archive list[36] were used to organize online information. In 1992, the World Wide Web (or the Internet) was developed and revolutionized communication and information access. The Internet is a massive information resource and ~ one billion people (1/6 of the world's population) have used it. The Internet is estimated to have grown ~190% in the past 5 years.[37] There are no published data of the size of the pediatric Internet, but a monitored subset of it grew 135% in 2001–2002 (D'Alessandro DM, unpublished data).

The World Wide Web facilitated the creation, distribution, and linkage of EBM resources through digital libraries for answering questions and solving problems. The first Internet-based medical digital library was the Virtual Hospital® from the University of Iowa which was developed in 1992. The National Library of Medicine's digital library followed soon afterward in 1993. The pediatric component of the Virtual Hospital was reorganized into the Virtual Children's Hospital in 1997. An associated example of a pediatric digital library is GeneralPediatrics.com (http://www.generalpediatrics.com)[38] (see Specific Resources below).

Determination of the quality of health information on the Internet information has been studied.[39,40] Standards to denote integrity of online material include display of authorship, reference, sponsorship and/or ownership and currency (e.g. Health on the Net, www.hon.ch). Some Websites also use traditional peer-review where individuals or small groups review information prior to publication (e.g. Cochrane Collaboration, http://www.cochrane.org/). Other Websites use an accreditation model designed to judge works that change over time.[41] Another metric that has been used is bibliometric analysis of the Internet search engine results, using page rank and number of connections (hyperlinks) to other online documents as indicators of authority (higher rankings in the search engine results indicate higher authority and quality of information). These methodologies are being studied more and appear to have value in assessing quality of information.[42–45]

10.6   Bringing Evidence to the Point-of-Care

10.6.1   Incorporation of Evidence

Pediatricians have traditionally been trained that answers to clinical queries often lie in original research studies. With the Internet, improved searching strategies and knowledge of EBM, searching is easier, faster, and produces better results. A "5-S" (5 layer) model[4] of the evolution of evidence incorporation into care systems has been proposed. In it, evidence can be found in:

- *Studies*: Evidence begins as research published in the form of original journal articles. These may be found through MEDLINE (PubMed, http://www. pubmed.gov) or through commercial indexing services (Ex: EMBASE http:// www.embase.com, Highwire Press http://www.highwire.org). Google Scholar™ (http://scholar.google.com/) is a World Wide Web search engine that searches journal articles as well as "peer-reviewed papers, theses, books, abstracts, and articles, from academic publishers, professional societies, preprint repositories, universities, and other scholarly organizations."
- *Syntheses*: Summaries of research studies and other evidence are published as systematic reviews. These may be found through MEDLINE (systematic review subsets and PubMed Clinical Queries: http://www.ncbi.nlm.nih.gov/entrez/query/ static/clinical.shtml) or through the Cochrane Database of Systematic Reviews.
- *Synopses*: Brief descriptions of original articles and reviews using defined (and transparent) methods, which may provide enough information to base clinical actions. These are found in collections of focused articles that look at clinical problems and questions in a structured manner (Ex: a PICO question answered in a PICO format). Collections may be found at: the ACP Journal Club (http://www. acpjc.org/), Evidence-Based Medicine (http://ebm.bmjjournals.com/) and Essential Evidence Plus (formerly InfoPOEMs, http://www.essentialevidenceplus.com).
- *Summaries*: Published integration of best available evidence from previous layers (particularly syntheses) to provide evidence on management options for a given health problem. These may be found in evidence-based textbooks (Ex: Moyer VA, Elliott E, Davis RL, Gilbert R, Klassen T, Logan S, Mellis C, Williams L, eds. Evidence Based Pediatrics and Child Health, 2nd Edition, London, BMJ Books, 2004; Feldman W. Evidence-Based Pediatrics. Hamilton,

Ontario, BC Decker Inc, 2000) and published clinical practice guidelines (indexed in the National Guideline Collection http://www.guideline.gov).

- *Systems*: The full integration of best evidence to care of individual patients consists of incorporation of decision support into information tools such as electronic medical records (EMRs), electronic prescribing and computerized order entry. Important aspects of systems layer implementation of evidence are source transparency (the basis of decision support rules on previous layers) and currency (based on new research), as well as protocols, procedures (critical paths) and information sources that reflect current evidence.

10.6.2   Evidence Resources for Patient Care

An annotated bibliography of available online EBM resources is included in Table 10.1.

GeneralPediatrics.com is an online user-centered, problem-based pediatric digital library based on the common pediatric problems discovered through a literature-based needs assessment. This digital library provides access to current, easily accessible, authoritative pediatric information. One study showed that computer-based resources, including GeneralPediatrics.com, were as effective as other more traditional information resources, e.g. consulting people, journals, textbooks, etc., but computer-based information resources were much more time efficient.[36,46] Since this study, others have documented that pediatricians are spending more and more of their time using computer-based resources.[6]

10.6.3   Evidence Resources for Continuous Professional Development

A major challenge for practitioners is to keep updated on clinical research. Technology can help to manage information overload and to guide CPD effectively and efficiently. However, it depends in part on self-knowledge of information preferences and their association to personal learning.

- "What's new" pages on (pediatric) information Web sites can summarize updates and new journal articles of interest. Pediatric updates are available through the American Academy of Pediatrics Websites (as well as through journal Web sites and pediatric portals). "Bookmarks" can be reviewed on demand, with e-mail alerts notifying users of updates.[47]
- News aggregators provide digest versions of new information using RSS (Really Simple Syndication) and e-mail technologies (where information from multiple sources is sent to one e-mail box for easy review). The federal government offers free health-related RSS feeds,[48] including one that allows notification of customized MEDLINE searches.

Table 10.1 Annotated list of EBM resources

Name	Sponsor	Description	Cost	Notes
GeneralPediatrics.com	University of Iowa	General pediatric portal for evidence-based information	Free	Curated WWW resource (See text for description)
				http://www.generalpediatrics.com
AAP Red Book	American Academy of Pediatrics (AAP)	Pediatric infectious disease authority	Free with AAP membership, varies	Print, CD-ROM, Online, Handheld versions, updated every 3 years
				http://www.aapredbook.org
AAP Policy Statements	AAP	Pediatric policy and technical statements	Free	Published in Pediatrics, updated every 3 years
				http://www.aappolicy.org
AAP Clinical Practice Guidelines (CPG)	AAP	CPG subset of AAP Policy Statements	Free	Published in Pediatricsl
				http://aappolicy.aappublications.org/ practice_guidelines/index.dt
National Guideline Clearinghouse	Agency for Healthcare Research and Quality (AHRQ)	Comprehensive database of EBM CPGs	Free	From original sources
				http://www.guideline.gov
Online Mendelian Inheritance in Man (OMIM)	National Library of Medicine (NLM) and the Johns Hopkins University	Comprehensive and collaborative database of human genes and genetic disorders	Free	Continually updated
				http://www.ncbi.nlm.nih.gov/sites/ entrez?db=omim

(continued)

Table 10.1 (continued)

Name	Sponsor	Description	Cost	Notes
PubMed	NLM	Online database of over 17 million citations from MEDLINE with links to full text articles and other resources.	Free (links to full-text articles may have charges).	Continually updated, uses a controlled vocabulary for indexing and retrieval (MeSH). Links to related articles, configurable interface (including e-mail and RSS alerts) http://www.pubmed.gov
Highwire Press	Stanford University	Online repository over 1,000 high impact, peer-reviewed journals, with links to full text articles	Free (Index access is free, but journal links may have charges)	Configurable for searching, browsing, e-mail alerts and purchasing subscriptions http://www.highwire.org
Cochrane Reviews	The Cochrane Collaboration	Collection of systematic reviews, pediatric reviews are limited to neonatology	Free abstracts, cost for full documents	Configurable for searching, browsing, and abstract reading http://www.cochrane.org/reviews/
Essential Evidence Plus (formerly Patient Oriented Evidence that Matters (InfoPOEMs)	Wiley Interscience	Part of essential evidence plus information commercial product, provides EB summaries on topics of interest to family physicians	Subscription	Configurable for searching, browsing, handheld computing and e-mail alerts http://www.essentialevidenceplus.com/
Google Scholar	Google	Searches scholarly peer-reviewed literature across many disciplines and sources	Free, currently in beta production	Primarily search, but can be configured for mobile computing http://scholar.google.com/

- Podcasting is a popular way of distributing video or audio programs for use on mobile devices (e.g. Apple iPod® or cell phones). Subscribers can be automatically alerted to updates when new content is available for download.[49] Podcasts are being used by many universities, professional societies, non-profit organizations and government agencies are using to provide CME, news bulletins and other updates.
- Handheld computers, personal digital assistants (PDAs) and cell phones are combining online and information technologies which now include complete textbooks, medical calculators, and journal subscriptions. Increasingly digital information is being made available in formats for mobile computing. Examples include: the AAP Red Book® and mobilePDR™. A good source for handheld evidence resources for pediatricians is Pediatrics On Hand (http://www.pediatricsonhand.com).[50]

10.7 EBM and the Future

10.7.1 Communities of Practice

Translation of research into practice and the development of evidence requires communication and interaction of researchers, clinicians, and tools that disseminate knowledge. Information technology facilitates these connections by allowing users to overcome time and space limitations. In addition to some of the functions discussed, IT has empowered the growth of communities of practice in pediatrics (and other fields). A community of practice is defined as a "group of people who share the same concern or passion for something they do and learn how to do it better as they interact regularly."[30]

One pediatric community is in pediatric critical care. PedsCCM: The Pediatric Critical Care Website (http://pedsccm.wustl.edu) has been in existence for 10 years and is a multidisciplinary information source which includes clinical resources, usable bibliographies, and critically appraised journal reviews contributed by its members. Another pediatric community is in pediatric education. PediatricEducation.org© (www.pediatriceducation.org) is a chronologically-organized, case-based pediatric digital library and learning collaboratory supporting pediatricians by answering common questions and supporting inquiry into related topics. Currently, there are over 200 cases covering all age ranges and specialties.[51] Future enhancements will include implementation of CME and expansion of the learning community of practice.

10.7.2 The Special Needs of Incorporating Evidence into Pediatric Practice

When considering the impact of evidence-based care on pediatric outcomes of children:

- Children are not little adults. Children have specialized healthcare needs and evidence that is used to provide medical care for them must be pediatric-specific.
- Children receive their health care from many different types of providers (beyond pediatricians): physician assistants, nurses, family medicine physicians and emergency medicine physicians (the largest percentage from nurses and family medicine physicians). Children's health concerns comprise only ~30% of the scope of practice of these healthcare providers, whose information needs, resources, and communities of practice are distinct from pediatricians.

Therefore, facilitated access to current EBM about children's health is important for all pediatric healthcare providers (including pediatricians), especially those for whom pediatrics is not the main focus of their clinical practice. This will become more important as electronic information systems become more prevalent.

10.8 Case Study: An Example of Evidence Based Resources in Practice

A 9 month-old infant boy is being seen in a general pediatrician's office in June, prior to traveling to Ecuador because of a family death. The parents are experienced international travelers and the boy has accompanied them on long trips within the continental US, but this is his first trip abroad. On examination, he is a healthy male. The family wants to know which immunizations he will require prior to travel.

The pediatrician, Dr. Cook, knows of the problem-oriented pediatric digital library GeneralPediatrics.com, and during the patient's visit searches the professional's information page and chooses the Centers for Disease Control (CDC) and Prevention Traveler Health (Yellow Book) Website. Dr. Cook searches by region and country to find current information on infectious diseases in Ecuador. She locates and reviews information on potential exposure risks, including Hepatitis A, Hepatitis B, Rabies, Typhoid, and Malaria. Using the patient's electronic medical record (EMR), she confirms the recommended immunizations he has already received and which are contraindicated due to his young age. From the CDC Traveler Health Website, the pediatrician learns that measles and malaria are currently not of concern in Quito and another large city the patient would be visiting.

Dr. Cook shares this information with the parents who verify using an online CDC map that they will not be traveling to an area at risk for Yellow Fever. Dr. Cook prints the CDC-based information for the family about decreasing exposure risks including animal exposures, the use of insect repellent and the clean water and reviews general information about traveling abroad with infants. Using the EMR's prescription writing software, she also transmits a prescription directly to the pharmacy for World Health Organization oral rehydration solution (ORS) packets for the family to pick up and gives provides printed instructions on their proper use and instructions on when to seek medical attention when abroad.

After the visit, the discussion about traveler's diarrhea reminds Dr. Cook to check on a question she has about the uptake of rotavirus vaccine in her patient population. She asks her office manager to query the practice's EMR database about uptake of the rotavirus vaccine for her eligible patients and finds it to be low. Searching the CDC site for better patient education materials about the vaccine, she receives 30 minutes of continuing medical education electronically for reviewing the vaccine research trial data and vaccine information and begins a program to improve rotavirus immunization rates using her online practice management quality tool.

References

1. Center for Evidence-Based Medicine. Glossary of terms in evidence-based medicine; 2005. Available at: http://www.cebm.net/glossary.asp. Accessed December 20, 2008.
2. Cochrane AL. *Effectiveness and Efficiency. Random Reflections on Health Services* (reprinted 1999 by the Royal Society of Medicine, London). London: Nuffield Provincial Hospitals Trust; 1972.
3. Guyatt G, Cairns J, Churchill D, et al. for the Evidence-Based Medicine Working Group Evidence-based medicine. A new approach to teaching the practice of medicine. *JAMA.* 1992;268:2420–2425.
4. Haynes RB. Of studies, syntheses, synopses, summaries, and systems: the "5S" evolution of information services for evidence-based healthcare decisions. *Evid Based Med.* 2006;11(6):162–164.
5. Guyatt G, Rennie D. *Users' Guide to the Medical Literature. A Manual for Evidence-Based Clinical Practice.* Chicago, IL: American Medical Association; 2002: 216–218.
6. American Academy of Pediatrics. Periodic Survey of Fellows. Use of Computers and Other Technologies Executive Summary; 2003. Available at: http://www.aap.org/research/periodic-survey/ps51exs.htm. Accessed December 20, 2008.
7. Gorman P. Information needs of physicians. *J Am Soc Inform Sci.* 1995;46:729–738.
8. Coumou HCH, Meijman J. How do primary care physicians seek answers to clinical questions? A literature review. *J Med Libr Assoc.* 2006;94(1):55–60.
9. Gorman PN, Helfand M. Information seeking in primary care: how physician choose which clinical questions to pursue and which to leave unanswered. *Med Decis Mak.* 1995;15:113–119.
10. Alper BS, Stevermer JJ, White DS, Ewigmann BG. Answering family physicians' clinical questions using electronic medical databases. *J Fam Pract.* 2001;50(1):960–965.
11. Green ML, Ruff TR. Why do residents fail to answer their clinical questions? A qualitative study of barriers to practicing evidence-based medicine. *Acad Med.* 2005;80(2):176–182.
12. Kim GR, Bartlett EL Jr, Lehmann HP. Information resource preferences by general pediatricians in office settings: a qualitative study. *BMC Med Inform Decis Mak.* 2005;5:34. Available at: http://www.biomedcentral.com/1472–6947/5/34. Accessed December 20, 2008.
13. Woolf SH, Benson DA. The medical information needs of internists and pediatricians at an academic medical center. *Bull Med Libr Assoc.* 1989;77:372–380.
14. Timpka T, Ekstrom M, Bjurulf P. Information needs and information seeking behavior in primary health care. *Scan J Prim Health Care.* 1989;7:105–109.
15. Osheroff JA, Forsythe DE, Buchanan BG, et al. Physicians' information needs: analysis of questions posed during clinical teaching. *Ann Intern Med.* 1991;114:576–581.
16. Forsythe DE, Buchanan BG, Osheroff JA, Miller RA. Expanding the concept of medical information: an observational study of physician's information needs. *Comput Biomed Res.* 1992;25:181–200.

17. Ely JW, Burch RJ, Vinson DC. The information needs of family physicians: case-specific clinical questions. *J Fam Prac*. 1992;35:265–269.
18. Dee C, Blazek R. Information needs of the rural physician: a descriptive study. *Bull Med Libr Assoc*. 1993;81:259–264.
19. Ely JW, Osheroff JA, Ebell MH, Bergus R, Levy BT, Chambliss ML, Evans ER. Analysis of questions asked by family doctors regarding patient care. *BMJ*. 1999;219:358–361.
20. Phillips, SA, Zorn M. Assessing consumer health information needs in a community hospital. *Bull Med Libr Assoc*. 1994;82:288–293.
21. Gorman PN. Information needs in primary care: a survey of rural and nonrural primary care physicians. *Medinfo*. 2001;10(pt.1):338–342.
22. Smith R. What clinical information do doctors needs? *BMJ*. 1996;313(7064):1062–1068.
23. Andrews JE, Pearce KA, Ireson C, Love MM. Information-seeking behaviors of practitioners in a primary care practice-based research network (PBRN). *J Med Libr Assoc*. 2005;93(2):206–212.
24. Ely JW, Osheroff JA, Gorman PN, et al. A taxonomy of generic clinical questions: classification study. *BMJ*. 2000;321:429–432.
25. D'Alessandro DM, Kreiter CD, Peterson MW, Kingsley P, Johnson-West J. An analysis of patient care question of asked by pediatricians at an academic medical center. *Amb Pediatrics*. 2004;4;18–23.
26. D'Alessandro DM, Kreiter C, Peterson MW. An evaluation of information-seeking behaviors of general pediatricians. *Pediatrics*. 2004;113:64–69.
27. American College of Physicians, American Society of Internal Medicine. The Effort to Build Better CME. ACP-SIM Observer; 1999. Available at: http://www.acponline.org/journals/news/nov99/bettercme.htm. Accessed December 20, 2008.
28. Davis D, O'Brien MA, Freemantle N, Wolf FM, Mazmanian P, Taylor-Vaisey A. Impact of formal continuing medical education: do conferences, workshops, rounds, and other traditional continuing education activities change physician behavior or health care outcomes? *JAMA*. 1999;282(9):867–874.
29. McLoud TC, Bisset GS, Bresolin L. RSNA teaching and learning conference: summary and findings. *Radiographics*. 2006;26:529–542.
30. Wenger E. Communities of Practice: A Brief Introduction; 2004. Available at: http://www.ewenger.com/theory/index.htm. Accessed December 20, 2008.
31. American Board of Pediatrics Website; 2008. Available at: http://www.abp.org. Accessed December 20, 2008.
32. American Academy of Pediatrics. Pedialink Frequently Asked Questions; 2008. Available at: http://www.pedialink.org/faqs-view.cfm. Accessed December 20, 2008.
33. Office of Inspector General. Department of Health and Human Services. Federal Anti-kickback Law and Regulatory Safe Harbors; 1999. Available at: http://oig.hhs.gov/fraud/docs/safeharborregulations/safefs.htm. Accessed December 20, 2008.
34. Office of Extramural Research National Institutes of Health. NIH Public Access Policy; 2008. Available at: http://publicaccess.nih.gov. Accessed December 20, 2008.
35. Centre for Evidence-Based Medicine. Levels of Evidence. Levels of Evidence and Grandes of Recommendation; 2001. Available at: http://www.cebm.net/levels_of_evidence.asp. Accessed December 20, 2008.
36. Wikipedia. History of the Internet; 2008, last modification. Available: http://en.wikipedia.org/wiki/Internet_history. Accessed December 20, 2008.
37. Miniwatts Marketing Group. World Internet Statistics; 2008. Available at: http://www.internetworldstats.com/stats.htm. Accessed December 20, 2008.
38. D'Alessandro DM, Kingsley P. Creating a pediatric digital library for pediatric health care providers and families: using literature and data to define common pediatric problems. *J Am Med Inform Assoc*. 2002;9(2):161–170.
39. Bernstam EV, Shelton DM, Walji M, Meric-Bernstam F. Instruments to assess the quality of health information on the world wide web: what can our patients actually use?. *Int J Med Inform*. 2005;74(1):13–19.

40. Health on the Net Foundation. HON Code of Conduct (HONcode) for Medical and Health Web Sites; 2006. Available at: http://www.hon.ch/HONcode/Conduct.html. Accessed May 4, 2006.
41. Argos Limited Area Search of the Ancient and Medieval Internet. Available at: http://web. archive.org/web/20000815085931/http://argos.evansville.edu/about.htm. Accessed December 20, 2008.
42. Hernandez-Borges AA, Macias-Cervi P, Gaspar-Guardado MA, Torres-Alvarez de Arcaya ML, Ruiz-Rabaza A, Jimenez-Sosa A. Can examination of WWW usage statistics and other indirect quality indicators distinguish the relative quality of medical web sites?. *J Med Internet Res*. 1999;1(1):E1.
43. Hernandez-Borges AA, Macias-Cervi P, Gaspar-Guardado A, Torres-Alvarez De Arcaya ML, Ruiz-Rabaza A, Jimenez-Sosa A. User preference as quality markers of paediatric web sites. *Med Inform Internet Med*. 2003;28(3):183–194.
44. Griffiths KM, Christensen H. Website quality indicators for consumers. *J Med Internet Res*. 2005;e55.
45. Berstam EV, Herskovic JR, Aphinyanaphongs Y, Aliferis CF, Sriram MG, Hersh WR. Using citation data to improve retrieval from MEDLINE. *J Am Med Inform Assoc*. 2006;13:96–105.
46. Magrabi F, Coiera EW, Westbrook JI, Gosling S, Vickland V. General practitioners' use of online evidence during consultations. *Int J Med Inform*. 2005;74(1):1–12.
47. ATS Consulting AS. WatchThatPage.com; 2005. Available at: http://www.watchthatpage. com. Accessed December 20, 2008.
48. US General Services Administration. FirstGov.gov: Health RSS Feeds; 2008. Available at: http://www.firstgov.gov/Topics/Reference_Shelf/Libraries/RSS_Library/Health.shtml. Accessed December 20, 2008.
49. Wikipedia. Podcast; 2008, last update. Available at: http://en.wikipedia.org/wiki/Podcasting. Accessed December 20, 2008.
50. Children's National Medical Center. Pediatrics on Hand; 2008. Available at: http://www. childrensnational.org/pdas. Accessed December 20, 2008.
51. D'Alessandro DM, D'Alessandro MP. *Formative Evaluation of a Chronologically-Organized, Case-Based Digital Library Delivering an Unstructured Pediatric Curriculum*. Pediatric Academic Societies Meeting. San Francisco, CA; 4/29/2006.

Chapter 11
Clinical Practice Guidelines: Supporting Decisions, Optimizing Care

Richard N. Shiffman

Objectives

- To distinguish clinical practice guidelines from other quality improvement tools
- To outline the production of and barriers to guidelines
- To provide an overview of guideline implementation and a pediatric example

11.1 Introduction: Why Guidelines are Important

Clinical practice guidelines (CPGs) are repositories of high quality medical knowledge. During the past decade and a half, as techniques for distilling clinical knowledge from basic research have improved, data may be gathered efficiently and transformed in a timely basis into useful summaries of the best available evidence. CPGs are the subject of considerable interest in clinical medicine and informatics. Clinicians look to guidelines for credible assistance in resolving problems they face in daily practice.

Informaticians view guidelines as a mechanism to overcome the "knowledge acquisition bottleneck," i.e., the extraction of knowledge from experts in a format that can be processed by computers. Other problems in CPG dissemination include selection of the "best" guideline on a particular topic when "competing" documents for management of common conditions are developed[1] and the high cost of CPG development (US guidelines cost on average $100,000–200,000[2] and require periodic updating).

11.2 What is a Guideline? How Guidelines Differs from Other Quality Improvement Tools

In 1992, the Institute of Medicine[3] created the most commonly quoted definition for a guideline: a "systematically developed statement to assist practitioner and patient decisions about appropriate health care for specific clinical circumstances."

C.U. Lehmann et al. (eds.), *Pediatric Informatics: Computer Applications in Child Health,* Health Informatics,
© Springer Science+Business Media, LLC 2011

Synonyms include *practice standards, protocols, practice parameters, algorithms, care plans*, and *critical pathways*. Each term represents a minor variation which fulfills the elements of the IOM definition.

Guidelines may also serve as criteria for *medical review, performance measures* and *reimbursement*, although these are generally applied after care has been provided to assess its quality. In these cases, their use does not fit the criterion of assisted decision-making that would allow them to meet the definition of practice guidelines.

11.3   The Guideline Lifecycle

The guideline lifecycle is a series of stages from conception to revision.[4]

- The lifecycle begins with the ***perception of a need to standardize processes***. This perception may be based on recognition of variations in care delivery, of the need to clarify the evidence base supporting a topic or an expectation of cost savings.
- Once the need for a guideline is recognized and resources are assembled, ***authoring*** begins. Authoring is translation of published evidence and expert consensus into formal policy statements. Ideally, a multidisciplinary group of stakeholders and experts define a set of questions that the guideline addresses. Following an exhaustive literature search and a filtering process to select well-performed and relevant studies that address the clinical questions, guideline authors develop a draft document that defines appropriate diagnosis and management, based on synthesis of evidence and weighing of anticipated benefits, risks, harms, and costs. Several drafts are prepared and critiqued until consensus is reached. The penultimate draft is then circulated to nonparticipant stakeholders for critical review and revision if necessary and finally sanctioned by the sponsoring organization.
- In ***dissemination***, the guideline is circulated to its intended audience in a non-targeted manner. Guidelines are published in professional journals, sent directly to stakeholders who may be interested in the topic and/or made available online via sponsoring organizations. The Agency for Healthcare Research and Quality maintains the National Guidelines Clearinghouse on a website (www.guidelines.gov) that archives and indexes almost 2,000 practice guidelines.
- Guideline ***implementation*** is the assimilation of recommendations into clinical care processes, through operationalization in specific clinical settings to improve local outcomes of care. Guideline implementation into information systems requires ***encoding*** to make them computer-executable.
- Guideline ***maintenance*** by representatives of the authoring organization focuses on revision of recommendations based on changes in the evidence base. Most organizations specify a time period after which each guideline must be reviewed, revised if necessary or retired.

11.4   Selection of Guideline Topics

Because guideline development is resource-intensive, organizations that develop guidelines often apply explicit criteria to prioritize the topics they address. A number of parameters are regularly considered:

- The prevalence of a health problem
- The degree of variability that exists in current practice in managing a problem
- The health burden (e.g., mortality, morbidity) endured by those suffering from a problem
- The economic burden of a problem (including its prevention, diagnosis, treatment, and management)
- The potential improvement of health outcomes
- The availability of scientific evidence upon which recommendations will be based
- The ethical, legal, and social impact of a guideline

Although efforts have been made to weight these criteria using a standardized formula, the results have been, on the whole, unsatisfactory. Therefore, topic selection, in many cases, is based on a less formal consensus process.

11.5   Assessment of Guideline Quality

Over the last 15 years, ad hoc standards for "high-quality" guidelines have emerged from several sources. In 1990, the Institute of Medicine described characteristics of valid and usable guidelines. In 1999, Shaneyfelt created a set of 25 quality criteria, the Guidelines Quality Assessment Questionnaire (GQAQ)[5] that contains ten items to evaluate the process of guideline development and format, ten items to evaluate evidence identification and synthesis, and five items to evaluate formulation of recommendations. When a large number of guidelines were tested according to these criteria, most guidelines failed almost half of them.

In 2002, a Conference on Guideline Standardization (COGS) at Yale[6] brought together guideline authors, disseminators, and implementers to define information that should be incorporated in CPGs to assure their validity and usability. The resulting COGS checklist is best applied while guidelines are being created to assure inclusion of critical elements. In 2001, a large international collaborative effort created an Appraisal of Guidelines Research and Evaluation (AGREE) instrument[7] that offers a systematic framework for appraisal of guideline quality. AGREE is best applied once a guideline has been published.

However, none of the aforementioned quality appraisal tools focuses on implementation issues. In 2005, the Guideline Implementability Appraisal (GLIA)[8] was released. This tool addresses each recommendation of a guideline as a unit of implementation and focuses potential problems that might be anticipated. The two most critical dimensions assessed by GLIA are a recommendation's *decidability* (the precise conditions under which the recommendation is to be performed) and its *executability* (the specific action to perform under the defined conditions). Both criteria must be satisfied for a guideline recommendation to be implementable.

11.6 Barriers to Guideline Implementation

11.6.1 Extrinsic and Intrinsic Factors

A framework[9] for understanding failure in guideline implementation concentrates on factors *extrinsic* to the guideline itself including:

- Lack of awareness that there is a guideline on this topic and lack of familiarity with its content due to general information overload
- Lack of agreement with the general concept of guidelines
- Disagreement with the recommendations in a specific guideline
- Lack of motivation to adhere to the recommendations
- Lack of outcome expectancy, i.e., a belief that following the guideline will not lead to a desirable outcome
- Lack of self-efficacy, i.e., belief that the clinician is unable to perform the recommendation as prescribed
- Environmental factors limiting clinicians' ability to carry out the recommendations, such as lack of time, resources, reimbursement, malpractice litigation fears, or other organizational constraints

These factors complement *intrinsic* guideline factors such as vague language that undermines decidability and executability, limitations in validity, poor formatting, inflexibility, and nonmeasurable outcomes (which are identified by the GLIA tool).

11.6.2 Clinician Behavior

Publication of guidelines alone does not guarantee clinician behavior change, and as with guideline authoring, a generalized approach to the creation of guideline implementation systems has been lacking. Most systems that have been reported implement recommendations for only a single domain or a narrow range of domains.

Guideline knowledge is most likely to be applied when advice is tailored to specific patients and is available during a patient encounter. Use of computer-based decision support systems can lead to improvements in the provision of preventive care, appropriate drug dosing and general clinical management of patients. Intrinsic factors favoring clinician acceptance of guidelines also include clarity of recommendations, evidence-base, source integrity, especially if they have the imprimatur of a professional organization and promotion as improving quality of care.[10]

In general, passive educational methods – such as publication, lectures, and grand rounds presentations – improve awareness but do not change behavior. Individual audit and feedback (with "report cards") involving local opinion leaders and educated consumers have met with variable success[11,12]. Effective modalities include reminders[13] (when used sparingly), individual outreach ("academic detailing"),[14] interactive educational programs, interventions that focus directly on recognized barriers and combined strategies.

11.6.3   Lack of Standard Implementation Systems

Although computerized systems can be effective in implementing guidelines in clinical practice, creating computer-mediated implementation systems has proven to be onerous and not uniformly successful. Challenges include: lack of explicit definitions, focus on errors of omission rather than errors of commission, not accounting for other factors (such as comorbid conditions, concurrent treatments, timing of interventions and follow-up). One suggestion has been for all guideline recommendations to be written in a simple if-then-else format with all parameters strictly defined using routinely collected clinical data. Nonetheless, this recommendation has not gained acceptance in the US.[15]

Informaticians have long struggled with transforming knowledge contained in clinical practice guidelines into systems that reliably influence clinician behavior. Implementers currently create computer-based decision support systems from published guidelines by applying poorly specified, largely tacit knowledge acquisition processes to a wide variety of knowledge representations. This approach often results in inconsistent encoding of guideline knowledge and potential inaccuracy of the advice that is provided. In addition guideline recommendations regularly fail to address a topic comprehensively, leaving users to design their own solutions for situations that are not covered.[16]

11.7   Approaches to Guideline Implementation

11.7.1   Knowledge Representation

Recent publications comparing features of guideline implementation systems have focused on representing guideline knowledge. Projects that represent executable guideline knowledge (Asbru, EON, GLIF, GUIDE, PRODIGY, and PROforma)[17] vary in their intended scope, the way that decisions are applied and the ways that clinical goals are represented and utilized. In projects where authoring has been included (PRODIGY, ZYNX), it has been performed by dedicated multidisciplinary teams that fit their analyses of the medical literature into templates that facilitate implementation.

In guideline implementation projects, knowledge acquisition can be identified as model-centric or document-centered.[18] In a model-centric approach,[19] a knowledge engineer reads and assimilates the guideline narrative, formulates an internalized conceptual model and converts the model to a fully operational (i.e., computable) representation (Table 11.1). Translation is implicit and mediated by the engineer

Table 11.1 Choices for guideline knowledge representation
A comparison of several prominent guideline-modeling approaches. Note that authoring of guidelines is rarely a focus and that several systems have not been implemented in health care settings

Project (encoding)	Authoring	Implementations
Arden (HL7) – a standardized format for encoding logic; encoding tools exist; there are difficulties encoding complex guideline logic[17]	–	Sharable Medical Logic Modules (MLMs); in use in several commercial EHR environments
EON (Stanford)/SAGE (SAGE Consortium); encoding with Protégé/SAGE workbench, which requires some expertise in knowledge engineering [18]	–	EON, ATHENA, T-Helper systems based on Protege; SAGE implementations not yet evaluated in practice setting
GLARE (U. Piemonte Orientale, IT)[19]	–	Graphical guideline execution tool; In use in bladder ca, reflux esophagitis, CHF
GASTON (Eindhoven, NL); encoding with Protege [20]	–	DSS implemented in critical care, family practice, psychiatry, cardiology; limited interface with existing IT systems
GLIF (Intermed Collaboratory); encoding tools exist but inconsistent encoding has been demonstrated [21]	–	GLEE Execution engine, GELLO Exp/Query language; diabetes foot care guideline
GUIDE (Pavia); workflow-aware encoding using Petri nets[27]	–	In use for stroke, breast cancer, CHF
HGML (UMDNJ) has an XML markup tool for encoding recommendation logic only[28]	–	Applications are "under development" but not currently deployed
PROforma (Cancer Research UK) uses JAVA-based, commercially available AREZZO tool for encoding[29]	–	Commercial product used in HIV (Retrogram), cancer care, (ARNO) renal anemia management (ORAMA)
ZYNX; MLMs[30]	Recommendations are created following a meta-analysis by a dedicated authoring team using templates	EKM-web-based rule sets and orders for advice on >100 topics for inpatient management; implementation advice available; commercial product
GEM (Yale University) GEM Cutter transforms published guideline into XML format[26]	In use by two US national specialty societies in guideline authoring activities; GEM-Q, GEM-COGS, GEM-Arden tools available	Implementations in chronic asthma management, glaucoma diagnosis and management, smoking cessation counseling

"who is responsible for the initial 'text-to-model leap'." Ultimately, the relationship of the model to the original document may be only "indirect" or "tangential." This "top-down" approach has been used in EON, Asgaard, GLIF, and PRODIGY activities. In document-centric knowledge acquisition,[20] the original text of a guideline is systematically marked up with semantically meaningful tags and maintained as a structured document in XML. Using this "bottom-up" approach, text content "evolves" into an operational format and the interpreting expert is constrained by the explicit content of the guideline.

The implicit nature of the model-centered approach leaves its output subject to the domain expertise and skills of the knowledge engineer to a greater degree than does the document-centered approach. As a result, the accuracy of the output is open to question, with considerable variability in systems engineered by different members of their team from the same clinical guidelines. Recommendations differ for the same patient when conceptualized by different knowledge engineers. In addition, many model-centered knowledge representations have little or no capability to encode content that does not directly relate to recommendation logic, such as objectives, rationales for creating the guideline, the intended audience, the setting for recommendations, the quality of the evidence supporting a recommendation, and the guideline authors' view of the strength of the recommendation (all of which are important for successful implementation).

The document-centered approach grounds the transformation process explicitly in the guideline publication, thereby enhancing auditability and perhaps diminishing erroneous encoding. When a guideline is fully marked up (i.e., beyond the recommendation logic), additional capabilities become apparent. Feedback can be provided to guideline authors regarding validity, usability, and adherence to recognized authoring standards. Likewise, those charged with selecting guidelines for use within a particular healthcare organization can use such information to help compare guidelines to meet local needs.

11.7.2   An Example of Document-Centric Knowledge Acquisition: Guideline Elements Model (GEM)[12]

The Guideline Elements Model (GEM) represents clinical practice guideline knowledge in electronic form. GEM is a hierarchy of over 100 concepts that describe the content of clinical practice guideline documents. It was conceived in extensible markup language (XML) to allow encoding without programming skill. GEM has expressiveness to convey the complexities and nuances of clinical medicine while retaining informational equivalence to the original guideline and flexibility to deal with a wide variety of guideline topics and multiple levels of abstraction. GEM allows encoded guidelines to be comprehensive, comprehensible to domain experts, reusable, and sharable among institutions.

The GEM implementation model begins with selection of a guideline, followed by markup and creation of a GEM document and detailed specification of the relevant knowledge (atomization, de-abstraction, disambiguation, verification of completeness, addition of explanation and building of executable code).[31] The GEM model then focuses on workflow integration.[32] GEM users specify origins of decision variables and insertions of actions into clinical workflow, define action-types, select associated implementation strategies, choose interface components and ultimately create a specification that can be instantiated by local information technology teams.

11.7.3 Pediatric Guidelines: The Role of the American Academy of Pediatrics

The American Academy of Pediatrics (AAP) has been a leader in the development and implementation of evidence-based guidelines for child health. The earliest example of a specialty-society guideline is its Report of the Committee on Infectious Diseases, also known as the AAP Red Book (first published in the 1930s, and currently available in print, CD-ROM, online, and handheld formats).[33] Since the early 1990s, the AAP has regularly convened multispeciality panels to review evidence and provide guidelines and technical reports on the management of common pediatric problems (including urinary tract infection, febrile seizures, head trauma, attention deficit and hyperactivity disorder, gastroenteritis, otitis media with effusion, developmental dysplasia of the hip, and bronchiolitis.[34]

In recognition of the importance of practice guideline implementation strategies, the AAP recently formed the Partnership for Policy Implementation (PPI), which includes pediatric informaticians with special interest in guideline-based decision support and expertise in pediatric quality improvement. The PPI works with AAP guideline (and policy) authoring committees to assure that the developed recommendations will be implementable in practice settings.

The AAP Steering Committee on Quality Improvement and Management (SCOQIM)[35] has oversight over AAP guideline development. A scheme for classifying pediatric guideline recommendation strength based on evidence quality and consideration of the benefits, risks, harms, and costs associated with implementation has been published. Transparency of guidelines (the degree to which their purpose and development are made clear to users) is emphasized.

To participate fruitfully in guideline development, committee members must understand the guideline authoring process and have skill in critical appraisal of the scientific literature.

11.8 Case Study: Decision Support for Pediatric Chronic Asthma

A multidisciplinary team at Yale University has developed and implemented a decision support system for chronic asthma management in children based on National Heart Lung and Blood Institute (NHLBI) guidelines. The Pediatric Primary Care

Center at Yale New Haven Hospital functions as a resident continuity clinic and uses the Centricity (GE Medical Systems, Fairfield, CT) ambulatory electronic health record system.

Following a careful parsing of the guidelines, supplemented with input from Pediatric Respiratory Medicine experts, a set of data collection templates and forms that provide guideline-based advice were designed and refined. An example of system operation is:

A pediatric patient (Willy Wheeze) with identified chronic asthma comes for an appointment for health maintenance. His mother notes that he recently experienced his first asthma exacerbation that required a trip to the Emergency Room. The primary care pediatrician (Dr. Jones) clicks a button that adds the asthma management forms to the electronic health record health maintenance templates that are presented for the visit. The asthma forms prompt Dr. Jones to ask about the frequency of wheezing, cough, chest tightness, etc. As Dr. Jones records Willy's mother' responses, a rule-based template calculates, per the NHLBI guidelines, the severity level of Willy's asthma. The frequency of Willy's symptoms indicates his asthma severity is mild persistent.

Dr. Jones next inquires about Willy's level of asthma control, based on answers to questions about missed school and emergency department visits. Results of pulmonary function testing (PFTs) are also recorded. The decision support system, using data from the history and PFTs, indicates that Willy's control is suboptimal. A third panel of questions prompts questions about asthma triggers and activities the family has put into place to diminish Willy's exposure.

The system summarizes findings and returns that Willy's asthma is mild persistent and suboptimally controlled. Dr. Jones considers the assessments, considers overriding the suggestions and notes her reasoning in modifying or accepting the assessments. The system recommends a series of appropriate interventions based on the guideline, including rescue and controller medications. The system also notes that inhaler propellants will be changing in the near future and will require modification and refresher training for patients. Dr. Jones selects appropriate medications from a list and gets additional information on options offered by an onscreen "Info-button." Dr. Jones clicks on her selections, which are automatically added to Willy's EHR medication list as prescriptions are prepared for electronic transfer to the pharmacy. An individualized asthma action plan according to NHLBI guidelines is automatically prepared and printed to which Dr. Jones can add additional information.

References

1. Bosson JL, Labarere J. Determining indications for care common to competing guidelines by using classification tree analysis: application to the prevention of venous thromboembolism in medical inpatients. *Med Decis Mak.* 2006;26(1):63–75.
2. Burgers JS, Grol R, Klazinga NS, Makela M, Zaat J. Towards evidence-based clinical practice: an international survey of 18 clinical guideline programs. *Int J Qual Health Care.* 2003;15(1):31–45.

3. Institute of Medicine. *Clinical Practice Guidelines: Directions for a New Program*. Field MJ, Lohr KN, eds. Washington, DC: National Academy Press.
4. Peleg M, Boxwala AA, Tu S, et al. The InterMed approach to sharable computer-interpretable guidelines: a review. *J Am Med Inform Assoc*. 2004;11(1):1–10.
5. Shaneyfelt TM M-SM, Rothwangl J. Are guidelines following guidelines? The methodological quality of clinical practice guidelines in the peer-reviewed medical literature. *JAMA*. 1999;281:1900–1905.
6. Shiffman RN, Shekelle P, Overhage JM, Slutsky J, Grimshaw J, Deshpande AM. Standardized reporting of clinical practice guidelines: a proposal from the Conference on Guideline Standardization. *Ann Intern Med*. 2003;139(6):493–498.
7. AGREE Collaboration. Development and validation of an international appraisal instrument for assessing the quality of clinical practice guidelines: the AGREE project. *Qual Saf Health Care*. 2003;12(1):18–23.
8. Shiffman RN, Dixon J, Brandt C, et al. The GuideLine Implementability Appraisal (GLIA): development of an instrument to identify obstacles to guideline implementation. *BMC Med Inform Decis Mak*. 2005;27(5):23.
9. Cabana MD, Rand CS, Powe NR, et al. Why don't physicians follow clinical practice guidelines? A framework for improvement. *JAMA*. 1999;282(15):1458–1465.
10. Grilli R, Magrini N, Penna A, Mura G, Liberati A. Practice guidelines developed by specialty societies: the need for a critical appraisal. *Lancet*. 2000;355:103–106.
11. Matthews JC, Johnson ML, Koelling TM. The impact of patient-specific quality-of-care report cards on guideline adherence in heart failure. *Am Heart J*. 2007;154(6):1174–1183.
12. Jimbo M, Nease DE Jr, Ruffin MT 4th, Rana GK. Information technology and cancer prevention. *CA Cancer J Clin*. 2006;56(1):26–36.
13. Johnson KB, Feldman MJ. Medical informatics and pediatrics. Decision-support systems. *Arch Pediatr Adolesc Med*. 1995;149(12):1371–1380.
14. O'Brien MA, Rogers S, Jamtvedt G, et al. Educational outreach visits: effects on professional practice and health care outcomes. *Cochrane Database Syst Rev*. 2007;17;(4):CD000409.
15. Tierney WM, Overhage JM, Takesue BY, et al. Computerizing guidelines to improve care and patient outcomes: the example of heart failure. *J Am Med Inform Assoc*. 1995;2:316–322.
16. Institute of Medicine.. *Setting Priorities for Clinical Practice Guidelines*. Field MJ, ed. Washington, DC: National Academy Press; 1995.
17. de Clercq PA, Blom JA, Korsten HH, Hasman A. Approaches for creating computer-interpretable guidelines that facilitate decision support. *Artif Intell Med*. 2004;31(1):1–27.
18. Svátek V, Ruzicka M. Step-by-step mark-up of medical guideline documents. *Int J Med Inform*. 2003;70(2–3):329–335.
19. Peleg M, Tu S, Bury J, et al. Comparing computer-interpretable guideline models: a case-study approach. *J Am Med Inform Assoc*. 2003;10(1):52–68.
20. Shiffman RN, Michel G, Essaihi A, Thornquist E. Bridging the guideline implementation gap: a systematic, document-centered approach to guideline implementation. *J Am Med Inform Assoc*. 2004;11(5):418–426.
21. OpenClinical. OpenClinical: Knowledge Management for Health Care Website; 2008. Available at: http://www.openclinical.org. Accessed June 5, 2008.
22. Kim S, Haug PJ, Rocha RA, Choi I. Modeling the arden syntax for medical decisions in XML. *Int J Med Inform*. 2008;77(10):650–656.
23. Musen MA, Tu SW, Das AK, Shahar Y. EON: a component-based approach to automation of protocol-directed therapy. *J Am Med Inform Assoc*. 1996;3(6):367–388.
24. Terenziani P, Montani S, Bottrighi A, Torchio M, Molino G, Correndo G. The GLARE approach to clinical guidelines: main features. *Stud Health Technol Inform*. 2004;101:162–166.
25. De Clercq PA, Blom JA, Hasman A, Korsten HH. GASTON: an architecture for the acquisition and execution of clinical guideline-application tasks. *Med Inform Internet Med*. 2000;25(4):247–263.
26. Patel VL, Allen VG, Arocha JF, Shortliffe EH. Representing clinical guidelines in GLIF: individual and collaborative expertise. *J Am Med Inform Assoc*. 1998;5(5):467–483.

27. Ciccarese P, Caffi E, Boiocchi L, Quaglini S, Stefanelli M. A guideline management system. *Medinfo*. 2004;2004:28–32.
28. Hagerty CG, Chang J, Pickens DS, Kulikowski CA, Sonnenberg FA. Semi-automated encoding of guidelines. *Medinfo*. 2004:1625.
29. Sutton DR, Taylor P, Earle K. Evaluation of PROforma as a language for implementing medical guidelines in a practical context. *BMC Med Inform Decis Mak*. 2006;6:20.
30. Zynx Health; 2008. Available at: http://www.zynx.com. Accessed June 8, 2008.
31. Shiffman RN, Michel G, Essaihi A, Thornquist E. Bridging the guideline implementation gap: a systematic, document-centered approach to guideline implementation. *J Am Med Inform Assoc*. 2004;11(5):418–426.
32. Yale University. Guideline Elements Model Website; 2008. Available at: http://gem.med.yale.edu/default.htm. Accessed June 5, 2008.
33. American Academy of Pediatrics. AAP Red Book Online; 2008. Available at: http://aapredbook.aappublications.org/. Accessed June 5, 2008.
34. American Academy of Pediatrics. AAP Policy Website; 2008. Available at: http://aappolicy.aappublications.org/. Accessed June 5, 2008.
35. American Academy of Pediatrics. Steering Committee on Quality Improvement and Management Steering Committee on Quality Improvement and Management Website; 2008. Available at: http://www.aap.org/visit/scoqim.htm. Accessed June 5, 2008.

Chapter 12
Diagnostic Decision Support

Mitchell J. Feldman

Objectives

- To describe the history and previous work in the field of medical diagnostic decision support, including Bayes' Law, on which much of this work is based
- To illustrate three currently available systems, DXplain, GIDEON, and Isabel
- To consider how diagnostic decision support could be useful in practice

12.1 Introduction

In 1763, the Reverend Thomas Bayes published "a method by which we might judge concerning the probability that an event has to happen, in given circumstances, upon supposition that we know nothing concerning it but that, under the same circumstances, it has happened a certain number of times, and failed a certain other number of times."[1] This is Bayes' Law, which in 1959, was applied to medical diagnosis[2] to form the basis of diagnostic decision support.[3, 4] Because almost all computer-based medical diagnostic decision support systems (MDDSS) use some application of Bayes' Law, it is instructive to review basic principles.

12.2 Testing: Sensitivity and Specificity

Medical decision making is predicated on an explicit or implicit use of sensitivity, specificity, and prevalence:

- The **sensitivity** of a test is the probability that a test for a disease will be positive in a patient with the disease. A highly sensitive test will be positive in most cases in patients with the disease. In a test of low sensitivity, many patients with the disease will test negative.
- The **specificity** of a test is the probability that the test will be negative in a patient without the disease. A highly specific test will be negative in most cases

C.U. Lehmann et al. (eds.), *Pediatric Informatics: Computer Applications in Child Health*, Health Informatics,
© Springer Science+Business Media, LLC 2011

in patients without the disease. In a test of low specificity, many patients without the disease will test positive.

- The **prevalence** of a disease is the frequency with which it is found in a population.

Symptoms, signs and tests of high sensitivity are useful for ruling out a diagnosis because a negative result suggests exclusion (low false negative rate). Those with high specificity are useful for confirming a diagnosis because a positive result suggests inclusion (low false positive rate). Clinicians initially use highly sensitive symptoms, signs, and tests to screen for disease. Following screening, clinicians will then use specific symptoms, signs, and tests to confirm the final diagnosis.

For diagnoses of high impact (morbidity, mortality, or significance), symptoms, signs, and tests of both high sensitivity and specificity are needed. For diagnoses of high impact but of low prevalence, high sensitivity is more important than specificity.

Newborn metabolic screening tests for congenital hypothyroidism are highly sensitive, resulting in few missed (false negative) cases, with a lower specificity that results in a small number of erroneously identified healthy (false positive) cases. High sensitivity is crucial because early treatment is essential to prevent impairment, whereas misidentification of a healthy newborn is corrected by confirmatory testing (of higher specificity). "Gold standard" tests (highest positive predictive value (See next section)) are used to confirm and prevent harm from unnecessary interventions.

12.3 Diagnosis: Prevalence and Positive Predictive Value

How do clinicians diagnose? Several methods are likely incorporated, depending on the complexity of the case. Pattern recognition is helpful in simple cases. Deduction is useful in complex cases where a set of individual hypotheses about a diagnosis is investigated, and the set is revised based on new information.[5] Knowledge of the **prevalence** of clinical findings and likely diseases both in the general population and in the patient's demographic is helpful in arriving at a correct diagnosis, especially with common conditions. Knowledge of the probability of a particular disease occurring in a patient with a given finding (**positive predictive value**, or **PPV**) is of great importance. A clinician tacitly combining these processes is applying Bayes' Law.[6]

In a medical context, Bayes' Law asks:

*Given the prevalence of a disease and the probabilities of a particular finding (or test result) in patients with and without that disease, what is the probability that given this finding in a patient, that the patient has the disease (What is the **positive predictive value (PPV)** of the finding or positive test result)?*

In mathematical terms:

*The **positive predictive value (PPV)** of a test or finding with respect to a disease (the probability that a patient with a positive test or finding has the disease (P(D|F)):*

$$PPV = P(D|F) = \frac{P(F|D) \times P(D)}{P(F|D) \times P(D) + P(F|-D) \times P(-D)}$$

(where P() = "probability of," | = "given," F = finding, D = Disease, and –D = absence of Disease)

$$= \frac{(\text{sensitivity of finding or test for the disease}) \times (\text{prevalence of disease})}{(\text{sensitivity} \times \text{prevalence}) + (1 - \text{specificity}) \times (1 - \text{prevalence})}$$

An illustration that demonstrates the importance of prevalence is the calculation of avian influenza (AI, "bird flu") risk when compared with the calculation of a very common disease, the "common cold." AI is rare, with 385 human cases reported by June 2008 and 34 cases in 2008 thru July 2.[7] Using an estimate of the world population of 6,707,380,479,[8] AI prevalence in humans is approximately 5.1×10^{-9}. If disease (D) = avian influenza and the finding (F) is "cough," the probability of a patient having AI, given that cough is present AND that 20% of patients without AI have cough (P(F|–D) = 0.2; specificity (1–P(F|–D) = 80%), and that the sensitivity of cough in patients with AI (P(F|D)) is 90%, then:

$$\left.\begin{array}{l}\text{The PPV of cough}\\\text{for Avian influenza}\end{array}\right\} = \frac{0.9 \times 5.1 \times 10^{-9}}{(0.9 \times 5.1 \times 10^{-9}) + 0.2 \times (1 - 5.1 \times 10^{-9})}$$

$$= \frac{4.6 \times 10^{-9}}{\sim 0.2}$$

$$= 2.3 \times 10^{-8}$$

Therefore, cough alone is not predictive of the diagnosis of avian influenza.

This contrasts markedly with the example of a nonspecific upper respiratory infection (URI). If the sensitivity of the presence of "cough" is 60% in patients with URI (sensitivity = P(F|D) = 0.6), the prevalence of URI in the population is 10% (P(D) = 0.1) and if 10% of patients without URI have cough (P(F|–D) = 0.1; specificity = 90%), then the PPV of cough alone for URI is 0.4 or 40%, given our assumptions. This has face validity, with the other 60% of diseases presenting with cough alone including allergic rhinitis, bronchitis, pneumonia, asthma, sinusitis, pertussis, and others (including avian influenza!).

12.4   Decisions: Influences and Information Support

Diagnostic thinking is influenced by several factors:

- **Total and recent experience**: A rare disease seen recently may come more easily to mind than a highly prevalent disease that has never been encountered
- **Heuristics** (rules of thumb): Algorithms or decision rules
- **Parsimony** (Ockham's razor): The explanation of findings in as few diagnoses as possible[9]
- **Prevalence**: Experienced pediatric clinicians teach that having two common diagnoses is much more likely than having a single very rare disease[10]

The art of medicine may really be the implicit combination of estimates of prevalence, positive and negative predictive values, sensitivity and specificity, monetary and invasiveness costs of further testing as well as degrees of severity of illness and opportunity costs of not diagnosing or treating. Bayes' Law incorporates some of these elements, but it is likely that clinicians do not formally use these calculations in their daily work[3] This is just as well, since pure Bayesian theory requires two assumptions that rarely apply: (a) mutual exclusivity of diseases (each patient may have only one disease that explains the given findings) and (b) conditional independence of findings (e.g. using patient data about both a red throat and a sore throat may not produce the correct calculations since they are likely connected).

Despite these limitations, computer-based diagnostic decision support that uses probabilistic data may be helpful to guide clinicians. Computers can sort and store data on thousands of diseases and clinical findings. Programs can provide reminders such as unconsidered differential diagnoses. Others have stated that physicians usually do not retain more than five simultaneous diagnostic hypotheses, and never consider more than seven.[10] Thus computers may help augment the clinician's thinking.

Would MDDSS be useful in practice? In an observational study of 103 family doctors, researchers recorded 1,101 questions that arose during clinical care, of which 24% were potentially answerable by MDDSS. The questions were typically of the forms:

"What is the cause of symptom X or physical finding Y, or test finding Z?"

"Could this patient have disease or condition Q?"[11]

Early MDDSS, using a "Greek Oracle" model (the "all-knowing" computer delivers "the answer" after patient information is entered), have been used for diagnosing congenital heart disease,[12] abdominal pain[13] and general medical problems.[14] The model has evolved to include the idea that physicians will always have more complete knowledge of the patient than can be entered into a system for consideration. While computers excel at storing and sorting data, human knowledge and reasoning are not easily duplicated.[15] These systems are likely to be most useful early in the diagnostic process, when definitive data are not yet available.

Recent MDDSS have had the more modest and attainable goal of providing diagnostic reminders. In a series of 100 cases involving diagnostic errors, cognitive factors played a role in 74 of the cases, with the most common factor (39 instances) being premature closure: "the failure to continue considering reasonable alternatives after an initial diagnosis was reached."[16] While it is usually more likely for two common diseases to be present than a single very rare one, it is impossible to know a priori when Ockham's razor will apply or when a single rare disease is the more likely explanation. Therefore, most MDDSS provide a list that includes both common and rare diseases.

The characterization of clinical decision support systems can be based on five attributes:

• The intended function
• The mode by which the system offers advice (passive or active)
• The consultation style (consulting or critiquing)

- The underlying decision-making process (how the program works; its algorithms and logic)
- Factors related to human–computer interaction[17]

Three MDDSS systems: DXplain, GIDEON, and Isabel are reviewed, with each system characterized according to this scheme along with more detailed description.

12.5   Examples of MDDSS

12.5.1   DXplain

- Intended function
  - Diagnostic decision support in general internal medicine, its subspecialties and pediatrics
- Mode by which advice is offered
  - Passive: User accesses system when needed
- Consultation style
  - Consulting model
- Underlying decision-making process
  - Heuristic modification of approximation to sequential Bayesian calculation
- Human–computer interaction
  - Easy to use web-based interface

DXplain is a Web-enabled MDDSS with information on over 2,300 disease states and more than 4,800 clinical findings. Under development since 1984 in the Laboratory of Computer Science (LCS) at the Massachusetts General Hospital (MGH),[18] DXplain provides clinicians access to a medical diagnosis knowledge base (KB) of relationships between clinical findings (history, physical exam and laboratory test data) and diagnoses. The KB includes diagnoses from general internal medicine, its subspecialties, pediatrics, surgery, and gynecology. The system provides two modes:

- Case analysis mode: A user can enter a set of clinical findings and the system will return a list of plausible diagnoses.
- Electronic textbook mode: A user can retrieve a differential diagnosis for any of the 4,800 findings, or a description of any of the 2,300 diseases, with clinical finding associations and an indication of how frequently each finding is seen in the disease. A separate section displays diagnostically helpful findings, with links to current abstracts through PUBMED.[19]

Research has shown that physicians use only a small number of features of MDDSS,[20] therefore simple and streamlined interfaces enhance usability. DXplain's developers designed the system to be easy to use without prior training. Users can enter clinical findings in narrative form, and the system's extensive synonym matching, misspelling tolerance, and broad recognition of medical terminology allow for tolerant mapping to the system's controlled medical vocabulary. Another important design goal was the system's ability to explain its reasoning. A user can obtain "Evidence for Dx" for any of the diseases shown on DXplain's list (see Figs. 12.1 and 12.2).[21] The system will then display the entered findings that support the diagnosis, as well as other important findings associated with the diagnosis.

DXplain's structure and heuristics were influenced by previous work (Internist-I and QMR.[14]) in which the functional unit is the "disease profile." In DXplain, each disease profile contains an average of 53 clinical findings (10 to 100 +). Each finding is related to one or more diseases by two parameters:

- Term Frequency (TF) indicates how often a finding is seen in a disease and is analogous to sensitivity.
- Evoking Strength (ES) answers the question "Given this finding, how strongly should I consider that disease?" and is analogous to positive predictive value (PPV).
- Term Importance (TI), is disease independent, and indicates the significance of a particular clinical finding, ranging from 1 (unimportant) to 5 (must be explained (e.g. "coma")).

There are approximately 244,000 (2 × 53 × 2,300) data points describing disease-finding relationships in the KB.[22]

Factors that contribute to scoring diseases in DXplain include heuristic approximations of PPV, prevalence, TI, and sensitivity.[18] Pediatric ages (such as a child or infant) will exclude adult diseases (e.g. Alzheimer Disease), and some diseases (hypothyroidism, gastroesophageal reflux disease) may contain separate profiles

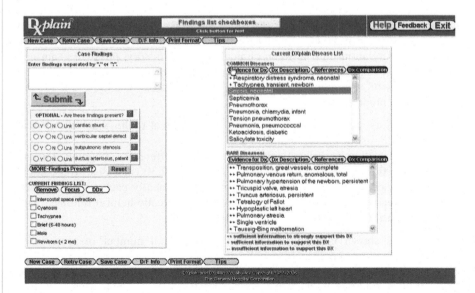

Fig. 12.1 DXplain: Case Analysis of a newborn with cyanosis, tachypnea, and retractions

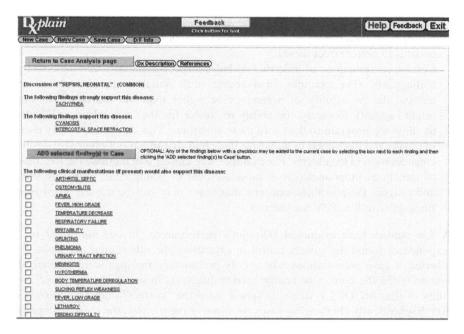

Fig. 12.2 DXplain: Evidence for Disease: Neonatal Sepsis

for adult and pediatric forms. Users enter an average of four non-demographic findings per case. Additional findings are often entered from the system's prompts called "Findings present?". After an initial analysis, the system asks the user if findings with high TF or ES are present or absent. Findings with high TF for a given disease that are absent help to rule out that disease; findings with high ES that are present raise the support for that disease.

The system is available via the World Wide Web. Advantages over prior distribution methods (e.g. PC–based versions) include the ability to update the system easily and to collect feedback from users. Such feedback has proven to be a very useful resource for the DXplain editors to correct knowledge base errors and deficiencies and to improve the program. In the last five years, over 11,000 users have accessed the application each year.[22]

In 2006, Epocrates Sx, which uses a subset of the DXplain KB, was developed jointly by the LCS and Epocrates. The program allows users to enter clinical findings on a handheld computer. It then displays an index of plausible diagnoses, which are hyperlinked to the Epocrates Dx product, which is based on the 5 Minute Clinical Consult textbook.[23]

Limitations of the system include:

• Prevalence values that are not regionally adjusted (though in some diseases, geographic prevalence is listed as a clinical finding, e.g. "North American, Southwestern" in "Coccidioidomycosis").

- Incorrect or missing data from the KB are possible sources of error (user feedback and quality assurance measures by the developers allow for continuing updates to help correct these).
- Certain combinations of independent but nonspecific findings can underweight a diagnosis. (For example, in a young adult female with amenorrhea and nausea, the probability of pregnancy is higher than the individual findings might suggest). Recently, the ability to cluster findings was added to DXplain to allow the program to deal with these situations. This can be especially useful in raising the likelihood of a disease in a child that might not otherwise deserve consideration in the elderly. For example, one cluster will increase the likelihood of infectious mononucleosis in an adolescent or young adult with sore throat and fatigue. Despite these clusters, diagnoses may still be missed when many findings with low PPV are entered.

A few studies have evaluated DXplain's performance. In one study, 29 of 34 respondents found the system useful in expanding the differential diagnosis.[24] In a series of case presentations where only preliminary findings were entered, the system listed the correct or nearly correct diagnosis in seven of ten cases.[25] In a study of four MDDSS systems, DXplain listed the "correct" diagnosis in 69% of 105 diagnostically challenging cases (in some of these cases, the correct diagnosis was not contained in DXplain's KB), 75% when adjusted to cases (96) whose diagnoses were contained in the KB. DXplain suggested an average of two or more additional diagnoses per case that expert physicians found relevant but did not consider.[26] In a study of the system at a teaching hospital, 80% of residents using the system stated it was useful, 94% stated the system was easy to use and over 70% stated the system provided them with diagnoses they would not have otherwise considered.[27]

12.5.2 GIDEON

- Intended function
  - Diagnostic decision support limited to infectious diseases
- Mode by which advice is offered
  - Passive: User accesses system when needed
- Consultation style
  - Consulting model
- Underlying decision-making process
  - Bayesian matrix
- Human–computer interaction
  - Streamlined intuitive modular interface

GIDEON (Global Infectious Diseases and Epidemiology Network) is an MDDSS that contains data on 337 infectious diseases and 231 countries, available via CD and via the World Wide Web. The system is comprised of four modules: Diagnosis, Epidemiology, Therapy, and Microbiology:

- *Diagnosis module*: This consists of an interface where users may input any combination of 217 signs, symptoms, laboratory findings, and demographics, using a checkbox exploding hierarchical tree interface (Fig. 12.3). The system returns a ranked differential diagnosis calculated using Bayes' rule. The user can drill down to further information on a disease by "clicking" on the listed diagnosis (including an approximation of the P(F|D) for each finding). The user can also click on "Why Not" to see why specific diagnoses have been omitted and display findings which exclude the diagnosis. GIDEON has the ability to differentiate prevalence regionally. For example, in a child with diarrhea and abdominal pain in Haiti, Shigella is the more likely diagnosis, whereas in the United States, it is Campylobacter (See Figs. 12.3 and 12.4).[28] GIDEON is limited to one of the 337 infectious diseases in its KB.
- *Epidemiology module*: This is a compendium of epidemiologic information about each of the 337 diseases, including agent names, synonyms, phenotype, reservoir, vector, incubation period, diagnostic tests, clinical hints, vaccines (when available), typical adult and pediatric therapy including dosing, geographic distribution including historical (for some diseases dating back to 1917) annual incidence, images, and expanded clinical information. This module is also accessible from the ranked list in the Diagnosis Module.

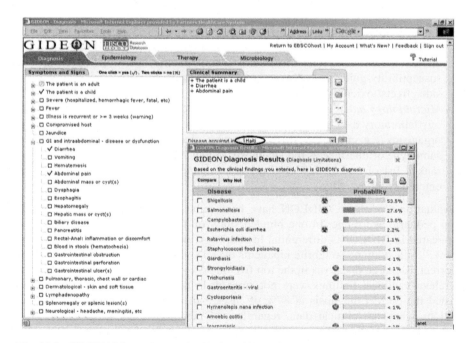

Fig. 12.3 GIDEON Diagnosis module: Haitian child with diarrhea and abdominal pain

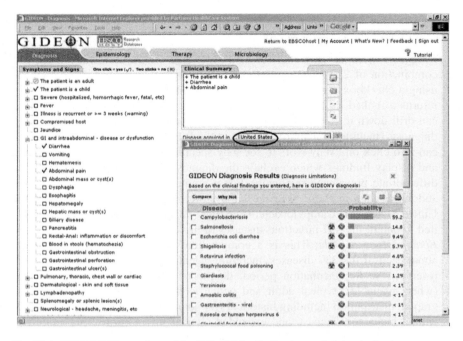

Fig. 12.4 GIDEON Diagnosis module: U.S. child with diarrhea and abdominal pain

- *Therapy module*: Contains information on 269 drugs and 65 vaccines. Therapeutic information includes: mechanism of action, adult, and pediatric dosage, half life and excretion, side effects, interactions, trade names, microbial spectrum and susceptibility guidelines. A user can filter therapies by pathogen susceptibility, side effects/toxicities and drug interactions.
- *Microbiology module*: This is an interface for accessing specifics on microbiology laboratory data. A user can enter laboratory test-specific information about organisms (e.g. catalase positive or negative, glucose fermenter or not) using the same type of interface as the Diagnosis Module. The system returns a Bayesian ranked list of any of the 1,147 possible organisms within the KB that fit the entered criteria.[29, 30]

Evaluation studies on GIDEON have been published, although they are not in the pediatric age range. In one blinded study of 495 cases, the correct diagnosis appeared in GIDEON's differential list 94.7% of the time, and was ranked first in 75%.[31] In a study of 86 febrile inpatients over 18 years of age, GIDEON listed the correct discharge diagnosis in the top five on 36% of cases; this rose to 69% when irrelevant clinical findings were not entered. In the same study, junior residents listed the correct diagnosis in 87% of cases.[32] In a study of 50 inpatient consultations where all clinical data, regardless of perceived clinical relevance, were entered, the infectious disease consulting team's diagnosis was among GIDEON's top five diagnoses 22% of the time. In this study, the consulting team's top diagnosis matched the patient's discharge diagnosis in 92% of cases. The authors note that in 73% of cases where GIDEON's top diagnosis did not match the discharge diagnosis, the final diagnosis was not contained in GIDEON's KB, which was attributed to unusual infections seen primarily in quaternary care hospitals such as those complicated by invasive lines or surgical hardware.[33]

12.5.3   Isabel

- Intended function
  - Diagnostic decision support in pediatrics, internal medicine and their subspecialities
- Mode by which advice is offered
  - Passive: User accesses system when needed
- Consultation style
  - Consulting model
- Underlying decision-making process
  - Proprietary pattern recognition software indexing of pediatric and internal medicine texts. Case findings are matched to the textbook index and relevant diagnoses are displayed.
- Human–computer interaction
  - Web-based reminder system based on user text entry

Isabel is a Web-based diagnostic reminder system, with the goal of reducing diagnostic and decision errors.[34] The system, available since 2002, initially covered pediatrics and in 2005 was expanded to include adult medicine. The pediatric content derives from two texts on general pediatrics, one on neonatology and one on toxicology. A proprietary pattern recognition program extracts concepts from these texts.[35]

Whereas search engines are optimized for keyword searching and retrieval, the pattern recognition program used in Isabel provides search results optimized for meaning and context. It is described as "using non-linear adaptive digital signal processing techniques to find patterns that naturally occur in text based on the frequency of terms that correspond to concepts" and as using Bayesian inference and a principle of information theory (the less frequently a word or phrase occurs, the more information it conveys) to arrive at the probability that a particular document pertains to a specific subject. Bayesian calculations categorize the context of the content, and information theory is used to infer its significance.[36] After the pattern recognition program extracts concepts from the textbook's documents, they are linked to diagnoses. According to the developer, synonyms for document terms are identified and prevalence values for diagnoses are assigned and are adjusted regionally[37].

Isabel's underlying knowledge base (KB) contains textbook information and proprietary concept extractions on 3,500 diagnoses. The user inputs clinical findings into a textbox interface. The program then searches the KB text and it matches documents whose concepts are most similar to the concepts matching the findings entered by the user. Diagnostic possibilities are displayed, grouped by body system or etiology.[38] Diagnoses are linked to original material from pediatric texts. Limitations of the system include:

- Lack of recognition of negative findings and of certain abbreviations (Ex: PTT, PPD).
- Omission of clinical findings if textbook descriptions are incomplete or if there is a mismatch between the terminology used by the author and the user. This limitation is minimized by the use of synonyms and by indexing larger numbers of textbooks. Initially, the developers did not rank order the diagnostic lists (to reinforce Isabel's function as a reminder system[35]), but have since added a "degree of match view" to provide a goodness of fit measure between each matched diagnosis and the entered terms.

Several studies have evaluated Isabel's performance. In one study of inpatients, 91% of expected diagnoses (in 90 of 99 hypothetical cases) were listed by Isabel. In the second stage of this study, the final diagnosis from the discharge summary was listed by Isabel in 95% (83 of 87) of real cases for which the Isabel KB contained the diagnosis.[35] A second study using the same dataset with two pediatricians working together to determine a gold standard (one to four diagnoses per case), showed Isabel listing all gold standard diagnoses in 73% of cases, and in an additional 15% of cases, Isabel listed at least half of gold standard diagnoses.[38] A retrospective evaluation of records from 200 pediatric intensive care unit patients in an Indian hospital showed Isabel listing the final diagnosis (from discharge summary, death certificate, or autopsy report) 80.5% of the time.[39] In a prospective study analyzing 161 patients admitted to five pediatric intensive care units in the United Kingdom and the United States where the diagnosis was not known at admission, and where a discharge diagnosis was available, the admitting team's differential contained the ultimate discharge diagnosis in 89.4% of cases whereas Isabel listed the final diagnosis in 92.5%.[40]

12.6   Challenges to Developers and Users of MDDSS

12.6.1   Evaluating MDDSS

In none of these evaluations was the program used as it would likely be used in actual clinical practice. In all cases, MDDSS output was compared directly with the discharge diagnosis (and the gold standard for discharge diagnosis often was not specified, e.g. pathology etc.), or a list of diagnoses developed by clinicians independent of the system. In actual practice, providers using the MDDSS would more likely filter advice by considering diagnostic reminders, and may or may not alter working differential diagnoses. One study[41] of medical students, residents, and faculty listing differential diagnoses for cases based on actual patients before and after using MDDSS showed a small but significant increase in both the number of correct diagnoses and the plausibility of the other diagnoses listed (as determined by a plausibility score assigned by consensus of the study's clinical coinvestigators). The effect was greater for medical students than residents and greater for residents than faculty, suggesting a role for these systems in education. This study used two other systems, QMR and Iliad, both of which are no longer available, as the MDDSS.

A validated composite score that holds promise for evaluating the usefulness of MDDSS[42] weighs the quality of differential diagnoses and management plans (including further testing and treatment) on a user's lists generated both before and after use of the MDDSS. The score rewards both relevance and comprehensiveness of differential diagnosis and management plans. The reliability and validity of this measure is based on data from 71 subjects on six simulated cases, however it is not clear how the MDDSS affected the subjects' before and after results.

12.6.2   Developing MDDSS: Scope, Vocabularies, Level of Detail

MDDSS developers face several challenges in regard to medical vocabularies. The classification and nomenclature of diseases and findings are not always clear (in the context of decision-making). Scope decisions, which diseases and findings to include (and exclude), can be controversial. Many MDDSS programs have specific names for entities such as "Pneumococcal Pneumonia" and "Mycoplasma pneumonia," in their disease vocabularies and will list all pneumonias in their differential lists when pertinent clinical findings are entered, even if the data available do not yet support a specific type of pneumonia. This approach confers advantages to both the developers and the users. Using specific disease names prevents such systems from needing several hierarchical layers of disease vocabulary and the corresponding knowledge relating more specific diseases to higher level disease processes. Also, the end-level diagnostic reminders displayed may be more useful in helping the clinician build a differential diagnosis than would be a higher level term. "Lumpers" and "splitters" have a fertile field for discourse in the area of MDDSS. For example, in designing a diagnostic reminder system for general pediatrics, it may not be initially clear if a diagnosis list should include "ADHD" alone or "ADHD inattentive type," "ADHD hyperactive type" and "ADHD combined type."

12.6.3   Using MDDSS: Education

The Liaison Committee on Medical Education[43] lists two educational objectives that are relevant to teaching diagnostic skills to medical students:

- ED-28: "Evaluation of problem solving, clinical reasoning, and communication skills"

- ED-12: "Practical opportunities for the direct application of…critical analysis of data…[and] computer-based exercises where students either collect or utilize data to test and/or verify hypotheses or to address questions about biomedical principles and/or phenomena… the ability to collect, analyze, and interpret data"

An Association of American Medical Colleges Report in 1998 also recommended certain relevant competencies for medical students, including the ability to "identify and locate, when possible, the crucial pieces of missing clinical information, and determine when it is appropriate to act on incomplete information" and to "make critical use of decision support, demonstrating knowledge of the available sources of decision support which range from textbooks to diagnostic expert systems to advisories issued from a computer-based patient record."[44] Because many MDDSS allow a student to observe how a change in clinical data can incrementally affect diagnostic considerations, such systems can be helpful as adjuncts to teaching concepts of medical decision making. Students can learn, interactively, which clinical data strongly raise consideration of particular diagnoses (high PPV clinical findings). Many medical school faculty and students already use MDDSS programs.

12.7   Case Study: A Teenager with Rabies[45]

As an illustrative example (not intended to be a comprehensive analysis or detailed comparison of the three systems), a published case of rabies in a teenager where the history of a bat bite is omitted is used to compare the three MDDS systems described. This was the first reported case of a patient who survived rabies that had not been treated by either vaccine or postexposure prophylaxis. Once the history of a bat bite was revealed, the diagnosis was straightforward, but without that critical history, the diagnosis can be challenging and MDDSSs could be useful.

Non-demographic findings in the initial presentation from the published case report were extracted, omitting the history of the bat bite. There were 17 non-demographic findings that were entered into each system as allowed. For DXplain, 14 of 17 findings were enterable (using its controlled vocabulary); for GIDEON, 4 of 17 findings were enterable; and for Isabel (since it accepts narrative text entries rather than a controlled vocabulary) all 17 findings were entered. In addition, the case was run a second time in Isabel using the entire textual description as published in the report.

For DXplain: Rabies was not in the 50 top diagnoses displayed (see Fig. 12.5). Many of the entered findings had low PPV for rabies resulting in a low score (see Fig. 12.6). Most suggested diagnoses were CNS lesions or other noninfectious neurologic conditions though encephalitis, an infectious disease concept related to rabies, does appear on DXplain's list. Given that this patient has fever, a user may want DXplain to focus more on infectious etiologies. The "FOCUS" feature (see Fig. 12.7) eliminates diagnoses that do not contain "fever," and causes rabies to appear as a Rare Diagnosis. The "Disease Description" function (see Figs. 12.8–12.10) allows the user to see the findings in DXplain's KB for any disease.[21]

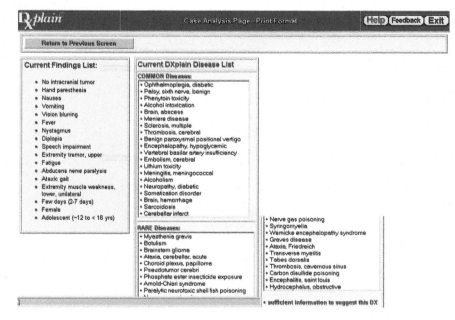

Fig. 12.5 DXplain Case Analysis: case study

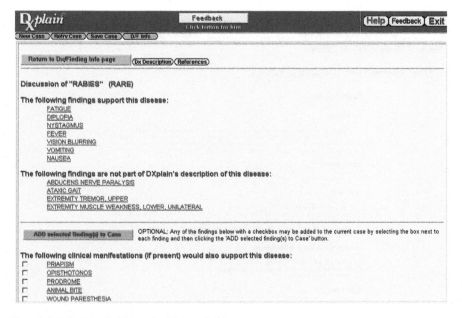

Fig. 12.6 DXplain: Evidence for Disease Rabies

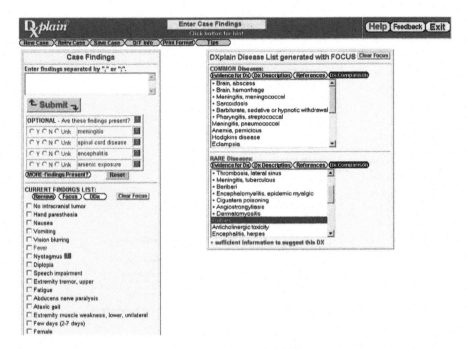

Fig. 12.7 DXplain: Case Analysis with FOCUS on "fever"; diseases shown only if they include fever

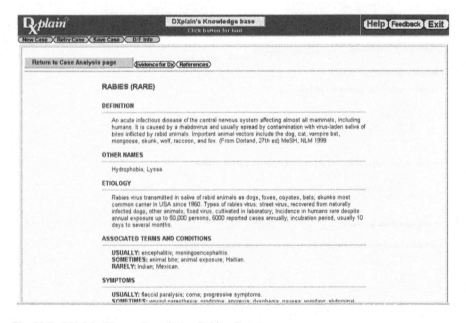

Fig. 12.8 DXplain Disease Description Rabies, Part 1

SOMETIMES: wound paresthesia; prodrome; anorexia; dysphagia; nausea; vomiting; abdominal pain; diplopia; vision blurring, vision impairment; headache; malaise; consciousness disturbance; vertigo; numbness; hallucination; insomnia; anxiety; auditory hallucination; visual hallucination; sleep disturbance; irritability; dyspnea; apnea; few days (2-7 days); diarrhea; joint stiffness; dysuria; oliguria; bladder atonia; photophobia; sore throat; throat constriction; communication impairment; delirium; dementia; hyperacusis; hyperesthesia; paresthesia; sensory disorder; cough; choking sensation; wound burning sensation; wound pain.
RARELY: priapism; lethargy; fatigue.
ADDITIONAL NOTES: Painful contraction of pharyngeal muscles, initially precipitated by attempt to drink; drooling.
MAKE DIAGNOSIS LESS LIKELY: very brief (< 6 hours).

PHYSICAL FINDINGS

USUALLY: drooling; salivation increase; agitation.
SOMETIMES: opisthotonos; muscle spasm; lacrimation; fever, low grade; dysarthria; nystagmus; hyperreflexia; depression; despondency; unresponsiveness; pulse weakness; tachycardia; hypotension; meningismus; pharyngeal inflammation; aphonia; fever; seizure; Babinski sign positive; emotional instability; mania; personality change; hyperventilation; hypoventilation.
RARELY: fever, recurrent; fever, high grade; optic neuritis.

LABORATORY FINDINGS

USUALLY: serum creatine phosphokinase elevated; serum creatine phosphokinase MM fraction elevated.
SOMETIMES: leukocytes increased; cerebral spinal fluid protein increased, slight; cerebral spinal fluid protein increased; glycosuria; pyuria; proteinuria; cerebral spinal fluid protein increased, marked.
ADDITIONAL NOTES: Culture of virus from saliva, brain at autopsy, possibly CSF.

DIAGNOSTICALLY HELPFUL

ALWAYS CONSIDER DIAGNOSIS: wound paresthesia.
VERY STRONGLY SUPPORTS: drooling.
STRONGLY SUPPORTS: encephalitis; flaccid paralysis; opisthotonos; prodrome; salivation increase; priapism; animal bite.

COURSE

Prognosis: rapidly fatal in humans; recovery doubtful.

PATHOLOGY

Fig. 12.9 DXplain Disease Description Rabies, part 2

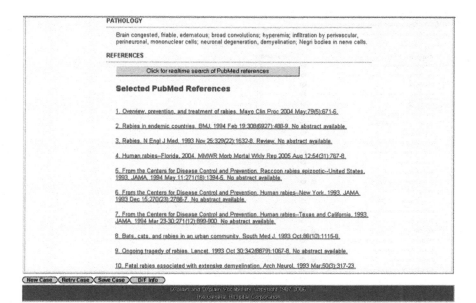

Fig. 12.10 DXplain Disease Description Rabies, part 3

For GIDEON: Rabies appears in the fifth position with a probability of 6.8% (worldwide: without specifying a geographic location) and in the 11th position with a probability of less than 1% (within the United States) (see Figs. 12.11–12.13). Figure 12.14 shows the findings in GIDEON's KB for rabies. GIDEON's tailored

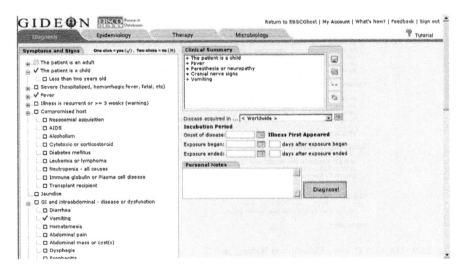

Fig. 12.11 GIDEON Diagnosis module: case study

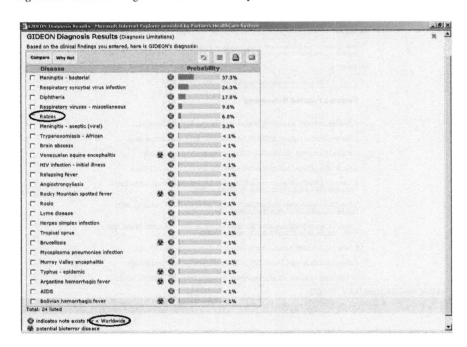

Fig. 12.12 GIDEON Diagnosis module: diagnosis results, worldwide

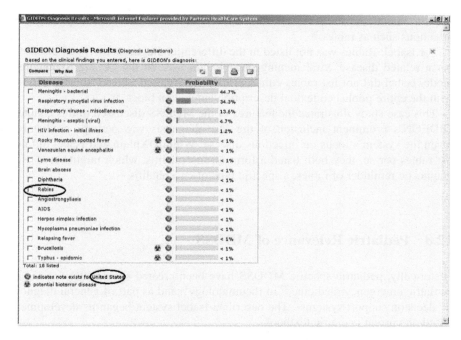

Fig. 12.13 GIDEON Diagnosis module: diagnosis results, U.S

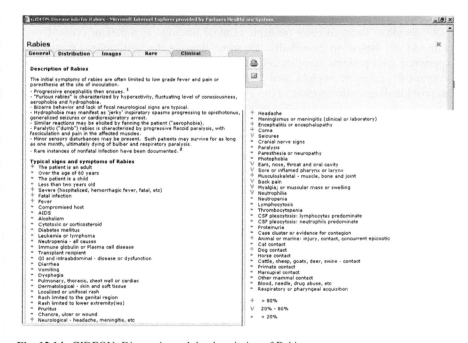

Fig. 12.14 GIDEON: Diagnosis module; description of Rabies

KB on infectious diseases makes it appropriate and useful to help diagnose infections such as rabies.[28]

For Isabel: Rabies was not listed in the differential diagnosis of 10–15 diseases, but a related disease, viral meningoencephalitis was. In the "Using Synonyms" mode, Isabel did not list rabies either with the 17 findings entered individually or with the entire published textual description entered en block.[46]

This case study illustrates the features of the MDDSS discussed in this chapter. GIDEON's prominent inclusion of the case diagnosis was perhaps predictable given the system's focus on infectious disease. While DXplain and Isabel did not list rabies per se, they both listed a form of encephalitis, which might serve as a diagnostic reminder of rabies, a specific type of encephalitis.

12.8   Pediatric Relevance of MDDSS

Historically, pediatric-specific MDDSS have been created specifically for use in pediatric emergency medicine,[47] in rheumatology[48] and as part of general diagnostic decision support systems.[4] The described Isabel system began its development based on current pediatric textbooks.

Major pediatric textbooks are each over 2,500 pages in length, organized largely by disease process, which require users to be familiar with the diagnoses contained within them. There are also differential diagnosis handbooks in pediatrics[49] (and other fields) that guide users through algorithms based on individual findings. MDDSSs allow users to enter multiple clinical findings as a patient presents with them and are based on essentially the same data as the textbooks, i.e. clinician experience with patients summarized in the medical literature, but it is their ability to organize, aggregate, weight, and display this information in a useful format that can provide diagnostic support to the clinician, enhancing the care process.

12.9   Conclusion: Current Clinical Relevance of MDDSS

How are MDDSS useful in current clinical practice?

- **Expand a differential diagnosis**
  - ○ MDDSS can provide differential diagnoses of a single clinical finding or of a set of findings and can add unconsidered diagnoses
- **Educate clinicians about specific diagnoses**
  - ○ MDDSS can provide links to disease-specific information from differential diagnosis lists
- **Guide diagnosis in specialty domains**
  - ○ MDDSS may be helpful in domains, such as GIDEON in infectious diseases to guide further testing and therapy

Will physicians modify their behavior in response to computer-based suggestions? One study by McDonald 30 years ago showed that physicians responded to more than twice as many (from 22% to 51%) clinical events such as lab abnormalities or medication side effects after seeing computer-based reminders than when not seeing them.[50] While this study did not look at the specific area of diagnosis, it does show that computer-based suggestions can alter behavior.

MDDSS are unlikely to be used on a widespread basis until they are integrated to match clinicians' thinking and workflow, as closely as possible:

- **Work silently**
  - A background agent, with natural language processing capabilities that silently extracts clinical findings from the medical record (without the need for clinicians to re-enter findings) and automatically activate the MDDSS, is needed.
- **Work intelligently**
  - Such an agent would need sufficient natural language capabilities: (a) to map clinician-entered narrative text accurately and effectively into a controlled vocabulary that can be used in decision logic ("cough" as an abnormal respiratory symptom), (b) to capture and convey nuances such as negation (the explicit absence of "cough"), quantity (not much "cough," "coughs" half the night, hardly ever "coughs") and quality (mild "cough," deep hacking "cough") and (c) to interpret nonstandard descriptions and unanticipated semantic variations (staccato or tic "cough").
- **Work independently**
  - The nonintrusive ideal is an agent that requires few (or no) direct interactions between the system and the clinician to maintain workflow.

Achieving the optimal balance between clarifying user intent and minimizing workflow disruption is a major challenge for system developers. Despite this, as practices approach the tipping point for widespread EMR adoption, we will soon have the opportunity to integrate decision support to facilitate and improve patient care.

Further information about DXplain, GIDEON, and Isabel is available at the programs' respective websites:

www.dxplain.org
www.gideononline.com
www.isabelhealthcare.com

Author Disclosure Statement:
Dr. Feldman works at the Massachusetts General Hospital's Lab of Computer Science, where DXplain was developed.

References

1. Bayes T Rev. An Essay towards solving a Problem in the Doctrine of Chances. *Philos Trans R Soc Lon.* 1763;53:370–418.
2. Ledley RS, Lusted LB. Reasoning foundations of medical diagnosis. *Science.* 1959;130:9–21.
3. Miller RA. Medical diagnostic decision support systems-past, present, and future: a threaded bibliography and brief commentary. *J Am Med Inform Assoc.* 1994;1:8–27.

4. Johnson KB, Feldman MJ. Medical informatics and pediatrics. Decision-support systems. *Arch Pediatr Adolesc Med.* 1995;149(12):1371–1380.
5. Elstein AS, Schwarz A. Clinical problem solving and diagnostic decision making: selective review of the cognitive literature. *BMJ.* 2002;324(7339):729–732.
6. Sox HC. The evaluation of diagnostic tests: principles, problems and new developments. *Annu Rev Med.* 1996;47:463–471.
7. World Health Organization. Cumulative Number of Confirmed Human Cases of Avian Influenza A/(H5N1) Reported to WHO; 2008. Available at: http://www.who.int/csr/disease/avian_influenza/country/en/. Accessed December 20, 2008.
8. US Census Bureau. U.S. and World Population Clocks; 2008. Available at: http://www.census.gov/main/www/popclock.html. Accessed December 20, 2008.
9. Wikipedia. Occam's Razor; 2008. Available at: http://en.wikipedia.org/wiki/Occam's_razor. Accessed December 20, 2008.
10. Oski FA, Oski JA. The diagnostic process. In: McMillan J et al., ed. *Oski's Pediatrics: Principles & Practice.* Philadelphia, PA: Lippincott; 2006:43–44.
11. Ely JW, Osheroff JA, EBell MH, et al. Analysis of questions asked by family doctors regarding patient care. *BMJ.* 1999;319:358–361.
12. Warner HR et al. A mathematical approach to medical diagnosis. Application to congenital heart disease. *JAMA.* 1961;177(3):75–81.
13. deDombal F et al. Computer-aided diagnosis of acute abdominal pain. *BMJl.* 1972;2:9–13.
14. Miller RA, Pople HE, Myers JD. INTERNIST-1, an experimental computer-based diagnostic consultant for general internal medicine. *N Engl J Med.* 1982;307:468–476.
15. Miller RA, Masarie FE Jr. The demise of the 'Greek Oracle' model for medical diagnostic systems. *Method Inform Med.* 1990;29:1–2.
16. Graber ML, Franklin N, Gordon R. Diagnostic error in Internal Medicine. *Arch Intern Med.* 2005;165:1493–1499.
17. Musen MA, Shahar Y, Shortliffe EH. Clinical decision support systems. In: Shortliffe EH et al., ed. *Medical Informatics: Computers Applications in Health Care and Biomedicine.* New York: Springer; 2001:583.
18. Barnett GO, Cimino JJ, Hupp JA, Hoffer EP. DXplain. An evolving diagnostic decision-support system. *JAMA.* 1987;258(1):67–74.
19. National Library of Medicine. PubMed. Available at: http://www.pubmed.gov. Accessed May 29, 2008.
20. Berner ES, Maisiak RS. Physician use of interactive functions in diagnostic decision support systems. *AMIA Annu Symp Proc.* 1997. Available at: http://www.pubmedcentral.nih.gov/picrender.fcgi?artid=2233322&blobtype=pdf. Accessed December 20, 2008.
21. DXplain; 2008. Available at: http://dxplain.org. Accessed December 20, 2008.
22. Hoffer EP, Feldman MJ, Kim RJ, Famiglietti KT, Barnett GO. DXplain: patterns of use of a mature expert system. *AMIA Annu Symp Proc.* 2005: 321–325.
23. ePocrates. Epocrates Collaborates with Massachusetts General Hospital to Offer Unique Decision Support Tool; 2006. Available at: http://www.epocrates.com/company/news/10239.html. Accessed December 20, 2008.
24. Barnett GO, Cimino JJ, Hupp JA, Hoffer EP. DXplain: experience with knowledge acquisition and program evaluation. *Proceedings of the Eleventh Annual Symposium on Computer Applications in Medical Care.* New York: IEEE Computer Society Press; 1987:150–154.
25. Feldman M, Barnett GO. Pediatric computer-based diagnostic decision support. *Scientific program, Section on Computers and Other Technologies, American Academy of Pediatrics.* New Orleans, LA: American Academy of Pediatrics; 1991.
26. Berner ES, Webster GD, Shugerman AA, et al. Performance of four computer-based diagnostic systems. *New Engl J Med.* 1994;330:1792–1796.
27. Bauer BA, Lee M, Bergstrom L, et al. Internal medicine resident satisfaction with a diagnostic decision support system (DXplain) introduced on a teaching hospital service. *Proc/AMIA Annu Symp.* 2002:31–35.

28. Global Infectious Disease and Epidemiology Network (GIDEON); 2008. Available at: http://www.gideononline.com. Accessed December 20, 2008.
29. Global Infectious Disease and Epidemiology Network. The GIDEON Product: Content, Users, Accuracy, Requirements; 2008. Available at: http://www.gideononline.com/product.htm#Content. Accessed December 20, 2008.
30. Edberg SC. Global infectious diseases and epidemiology network (GIDEON): a world wide Web-based program for diagnosis and informatics in infectious diseases. *Clin Infect Dis.* 2005;40(1):123–126.
31. Berger SA. GIDEON: a computer program for diagnosis, simulation, and informatics in the fields of geographic medicine and emerging diseases. *Emerg Infect Dis.* 2001; 7(3 Suppl):550.
32. Ross JJ, Shapiro DS. Evaluation of the computer program GIDEON (Global Infectious Disease and Epidemiology Network) for the diagnosis of fever in patients admitted to a medical service. *Clin Infect Dis.* 1998;26(3):766–767.
33. Luo RF, Bartlett JG. Use of the computer program GIDEON at an inpatient infectious diseases consultation service. *Clin Infect Dis.* 2006;42(1):157–158.
34. Britto J. ISABEL at the helm. A web-based diagnosis system speeds clinical decisions for pediatric physicians. *Health Manag Technol.* 2004;25(7):28–29.
35. Ramnarayan P, Tomlinson A, Rao A, Coren M, Winrow A, Britto J. ISABEL: a web-based differential diagnostic aid for paediatrics: results from an initial performance evaluation. *Arch Dis Child.* 2003;88:408–413.
36. Autonomy Corporation. Frequently Asked Questions: What does Autonomy do? at: http://www.autonomy.com/content/Autonomy/FAQ/. Accessed December 20, 2008.
37. Britto J. (2005) Personal Communication,
38. Ramnarayan P, Tomlinson A, Kulkarni G, Rao A, Britto J. (2004) A novel diagnostic aid (ISABEL): development and preliminary evaluation of clinical performance. Medinfo. 2004; 11(pt 2):1091-5.
39. Bavdekar SB. Pawar M. (2005) Evaluation of an Internet delivered pediatric diagnosis support system (ISABEL) in a tertiary care center in India. Indian Pediatrics. 42(11):1086-91.
40. Thomas NJ, Ramnarayan P, Bell MJ et al. (2008) An international assessment of a web-based diagnostic tool in critically ill children. Technology and Health Care. 16:103-110.
41. Friedman CP, Elstein AS, Wolf FM et al. (1999) Enhancement of clinicians' diagnostic reasoning by computer-based consultation: a multisite study of 2 systems. JAMA. 282:1851-1856.
42. Ramnarayan P, Kapoor RR, Coren M et al. (2003) Measuring the impact of diagnostic decision support on the quality of clinical decision making: development of a reliable and valid composite score. Journal of the American Medical Informatics Association 10(6):563-572.
43 Liaison Committee on Medical Education. (2008) Functions and Structure of a Medical School, Standards for Accreditation of Medical Education Programs Leading to the M.D. Degree. URL: http://www.lcme.org/functions2008jun.pdf [last accessed 20 December 2008].
44. [No authors listed] (1999) Contemporary issues in medicine--medical informatics and population health: report II of the Medical School Objectives Project. Acad Med. 74(2):130-41.
45. Willoughby RE Jr. Tieves KS. Hoffman GM. Ghanayem NS. Amlie-Lefond CM. Schwabe MJ. Chusid MJ. Rupprecht CE. (2005) Survival after treatment of rabies with induction of coma.New England Journal of Medicine. 352(24):2508-14.
46. Isabel Healthcare. (2008). Isabel Website. URL: http://www.isabelhealthcare.com [last accessed 20 December 2008].
47. Simon JE. (1992) Computerized diagnostic referencing in pediatric emergency medicine. Pediatr Clin North Am. 39(5):1165-74.
48. Athreya BH, Cheh ML, Kingsland LC 3rd. (1998) Computer-assisted diagnosis of pediatric rheumatic diseases. Pediatrics. 102(4):e48.
49. Berman S. (2003) Pediatric Decision Making. 4th ed. Mosby.
50. McDonald CJ. (1976) Protocol-based computer reminders: The quality of care and the nonperfectability of man. New England Journal of Medicine 295:1351-1355.

Chapter 13
Managing Pediatric Knowledge Resources in Practice

Prudence W. Dalrymple, Bernard A. Cohen and John S. Clark

Objectives

- To guide clinicians in aligning information needs and resources in practice
- To list a practical inventory of information resources available to pediatricians

13.1 Introduction

Information and communication technology (ICT) provides busy clinicians with access to timely health information: e-mail updates, online educational programs, podcasts etc. to the point of overload. The abundance of information has increased user expectations about the availability of timely and useful medical information, but has perhaps reduced user objectivity in distinguishing evidence from opinion and advertisement as messages from different sources: professional associations, patient groups, pharmaceutical companies, news agencies and policymakers are all cast along the same channels in similar formats.

An ongoing problem for working clinicians is how to manage available information resources to provide the best care for patients while staying informed and current without becoming overwhelmed. Beyond the technical aspects of how to approach this problem (how to choose and use tools and resources) are considerations of which resources are free and which should be purchased (or leased).

13.2 A Cognitive Model of Clinical Information Use

Choosing "best" information sources requires understanding of how clinicians need them in practice. During clinical encounters, they discover and prioritize questions, many of which may be easily answered, some which may be ignored, some which may trigger further queries (history, exam, laboratory test), and others which require selecting and consulting appropriate resources.

13.2.1 The Clinical Encounter

In a clinical encounter between a practitioner and patient and family, data about the patient's medical needs (clinical problems and diagnoses requiring resolution, therapy and education) are elicited, collected and documented by the physician (from history and physical examination) to formulate hypotheses and problem lists (based on clinical knowledge and expertise). Interventions (diagnostic testing and/or therapy) are guided by the clinician's application of medical knowledge (decisions based on the training and experience).[1]

Within the clinical encounter, the clinician uses formal and informal knowledge (Table 13.1) dynamically to make diagnostic and therapeutic decisions and may have information needs during any part of the encounter. In many cases, informal knowledge or resources ("tribal knowledge,"[3] consultation with a colleague) are used, but frequently, formal sources of medical knowledge (textbooks, journal articles, databases) and patient data (medical records) are needed to fill an individual clinician's data or knowledge gaps.

It is not sufficient to have access to information resources. Clinicians must also have familiarity with tools and when (and how) to use them. Many practicing clinicians have favorite and familiar resources that are kept at hand,[4] but need guidance when those resources fail them in answering a question.

13.2.2 Recognizing and Prioritizing Information Needs

The first step in using information resources is recognition of an "information gap" in personal knowledge ("what I don't know") that prevents effective problem solving. Unrecognized personal information gaps may go unresolved[5] or may be addressed by clinical decision support (guided choices and knowledge-based prompts) and/or by educational programs. Once an information need is recognized, other factors such as the urgency of patient need and the expectation that an answer will be found may affect prioritization of consulting information resources.[6]

Table 13.1 Types and formality of medical information[2]

	General medical knowledge	Patient-specific data
Informal	• Stereotypes about types of patients or practitioners • Undocumented information about side-effects of particular drugs or procedures	• Knowledge about particular patients • Practitioners' shared impressions about causality of local phenomena
Formal	• Information contained in texts and national databases • Causal models and general procedures accepted throughout medicine	• Information in medical records and hospital information systems

The timing of information needs in clinical workflow[7] may cause delays or lapses in asking questions that require resource use.

13.2.3 Formulating Questions, Matching and Navigating Information Resources

Once an information need is recognized and prioritized, the next step is formulating a clinically answerable question[2] and selecting resources most likely to provide useful answers. Frequently asked questions (such as drug dosages for specific indications) may be answered more directly by a drug formulary rather than a comprehensive pharmacology textbook. Questions about initial care for a specific condition (estimating prognosis, deciding on a treatment plan, counseling and educating families) may be better answered by a general than a specialty text. Anticipated questions may be answered by a just-in-time "Infobutton"[8] to a knowledge source such as MEDLINE abstracts to help support decisions.

13.3 Linking Information Needs to Resources

Selecting the "best" resource is becoming progressively difficult because of the growing number of available information products. Becoming familiar with what is available, what is useful and what is cost-effective is challenging. Frequently, the most important (and first) resource consulted is a phone call to an established network of professional colleagues.

What follows is a brief catalog of online information resources according to the types of information needs clinicians may bring to them. These include resources that match medical knowledge to questions about:

- Clinical findings
- Clinical constellations
- General information on diseases
- Information on pediatric specialties
- Information for families

13.3.1 Clinical Findings

Clinical findings include history, physical examination and laboratory test results that clinicians use to arrive at a diagnosis. Electronic resources can assist the clinician by: (1) providing audio samples and photographs of auditory and visual data and (2) linking findings to differential diagnoses.

For pediatricians, a common visual information need is identification of normal and abnormal skin findings and their linkage to disease states ("What is this rash?"). Practitioners may capture and store visual data on skin samples using digital cameras, which can be forwarded electronically to remote experts for tele-consultation. Alternatively, online image repositories may be helpful for additional discussions on unusual or interesting cases.

- **Dermatlas** (www.dermatlas.org) is a free, collaborative, open access repository (from Johns Hopkins University School of Medicine) of over 10,000 images contributed by more than 400 physicians worldwide. Clinicians may enter clinical observations in text format, and then retrieve skin images that correspond to their observations, thus helping to confirm a diagnosis and pointing to additional resources for treatment and prognosis. Dermatlas has a differential diagnosis feature that links visual findings to aid the diagnostic process. It also links diagnoses to medical literature references (via PubMed) and other information resources.
- **VisualDx** (www.logicalimages.com/prodVDxProven.htm) is a subscription-based online (or standalone) service (from Logical Images/Thomson Healthcare) that provides clinical images and reference text to guide clinicians in making diagnoses. Originally developed for dermatology, this tool is being extended to other domains, including oral health. For skin lesions, users may use a specially developed dermatology lexicon to enter lesion types, such as "lump or bump," "scabs" or "raised lesions" to augment a search based on historical findings (exposures, previous diseases or travel).

A common auditory information need is the distinction of functional and pathologic heart murmurs. Despite advanced technology for diagnosing structural heart disease, auscultation is still the primary diagnostic examination, and auditory identification of heart sounds and linkage to structural lesions is an important pediatric skill. A library of heart sounds plays a similar role to the visual image repositories.

- **CARD** (www.murmurlab.com/card6) is an online library of digitized heart sounds (from Johns Hopkins University School of Medicine) collected from pediatric patients who have undergone echocardiography. To date, the database contains over 5,000 individual recordings from over 900 patients, representing a variety of normal and abnormal heart murmurs. The application allows adjustments in heart rates and frequencies and graphic rendering of sounds, providing an optimal learning and reference environment that can both educate and help determine whether to refer for additional work-up. It is available free of charge.[9]

13.3.2   Clinical Constellations

A diagnosis is often made not on the basis of a single finding (except for pathognomonic associations), but on a co-occurrence of several findings in one patient. Constellations of findings (history, examination, laboratory test results) associated with diseases or syndromes, based on statistical knowledge of the presence of these combinations in diagnosed patients, are part of the knowledge that clinicians develop with exposure and experience.

Information resources that support clinical decisions associate clinical findings to diseases by using: (1) logical inference based on epidemiologic prevalence of findings and diseases or (2) bibliometric linkages. Discussion of the former appears elsewhere in this book, and this discussion will be restricted to the latter.

Bibliometric linkages measure the frequency with which a conceptual entity (finding, disease or other term) is associated with another entity within a set of documents, such as the chapters in a book or articles within a journal. Bibliometric linkages do NOT reflect epidemiologic frequencies, but may be important conceptually. For example, many reports, about a single case of a rare disease may associate it with a specific finding. The strength of this approach depends on the relevance of the set of documents, the query, the linkage rules ("search engine") and the user/clinician's expertise in interpreting the results. Two tools discussed here are Isabel, designed to assist diagnosis by increasing recall of diagnostic possibilities, and the familiar search engine Google.

- **Isabel** (www.isabel.org.uk/) is a subscription-based online/mobile-accessible resource that may be integrated into an electronic medical record (from Isabel Health Care) that provides links to a pediatric knowledge base in response to clinical features entered using natural language. The system, using a proprietary natural language tool/engine, searches the knowledge base for similar terms and related concepts (diseases) to create differential diagnoses. It is not an expert system and does not prioritize diagnoses, but rather expands the list of relevant diagnoses to consider.[10]
- **Google** (www.Google.com/) is a popular Web search engine that uses a mathematical algorithm called "PageRank"[11] as a measure of authority of a given World Wide Webpage in response to an entered query. In addition, Google has created access to scholarly journals that are incorporated into general searches (Google scholar: http://scholar.google.com/) across many journals and disciplines (including medicine) (see Case Study).

13.3.3 General Information on Diseases

Often, all a clinician needs or wants is a quick overview/review of a disease to make a clinical decision or to update his/her personal knowledge. This type of information (disease manifestations, history, diagnosis, etc.) usually does not change drastically over time and may be found in standard textbooks (print or electronic). Many publishers now provide time-limited subscription to online, CD-ROM and PDA versions of traditional textbooks with search features and automated update capabilities. Web-based textbooks are often bundled as part of a collection of books and standard journals in a particular specialty (such as general pediatrics). Most collections have electronic enhancements that allow simultaneous searching across multiple textbooks.

Access to such resources may be provided through libraries of hospitals as a service to physicians on medical or house staff. For clinicians with affiliation with academic medical centers, remote access from community practices may also be available through virtual private networks and secure connections. Ongoing costs of subscription are borne by these institutions (which may be considerably higher than for single subscribers) who monitor their usage closely.

Commercial packages that include online versions of traditional pediatric texts as well as a variety of other resources are:

- **MD Consult** (http://www.mdconsult.com, Elsevier) provides online and mobile access to several dozen textbooks, including **Nelson's Pediatrics**, **Harriet Lane Handbook** and the **Pediatric Clinics of North America** in a fully searchable format in addition to access to journals, drug information, medical synopses, guidelines and patient education materials. It may be used on a PDA and is available through personal or institutional subscription.
- **Stat!Ref** (http://www.statref.com, Teton Data System) provides an online gateway to health resources, including the evidence-based Physician Information and Education Resource (PIER) created by the American College of Physicians and **Rudolph's Pediatrics** as well as tools such as calculators and decision trees. It is available in a variety of formats through personal or institutional subscription.
- **Books @Ovid** (http://www.ovid.com/site/products/books_landing.jsp, Wolters Kluwer Health) provides a large number of electronic texts including a pediatric collection that includes **Oski's Pediatrics, 5-Minute Pediatric Consult** and subspecialty texts (in orthopedics, oncology and adolescent health). It is available through personal, pay per view or institutional subscription.
- **UpToDate** (http://www.uptodate.com/physicians/pediatrics_primary.asp, UpToDate) provides disease-oriented physician-written summaries with a section focused on pediatrics endorsed by the American Academy of Pediatrics that can be used to earn CME credit. It provides succinct summaries that can be readily used for patient care. It is available via Web, PDA or CD-ROM. Subscriptions are priced for personal use, for a single workstation updated every 4 months via CD-ROM, or for a single institution (on-site only).
- **Pediatric Care Online** (http://www.pediatriccareonline.org/pco/ub, Unbound Medicine and the American Academy of Pediatrics) is an online resource linked with the AAP textbook Primary Pediatric Care with open-source applications for use in patient care. It is scheduled for release in 2008.

Free online resources are also available (some requiring registration):

- **E-Medicine** (http://www.emedicine.com, WebMD) contains numerous current articles and offers continuing education credits.
- **MerckMedicus** (http://www.merckmedicus.com, Merck) is an online portal that is free to licensed healthcare professionals (registration required). It provides access to books and journals (through MDConsult), as well as diagnostic and therapeutic tools such as **DxPlain** (epidemiologic-based decision support)

and **TheraDoc** (drug dosing), patient education materials, slides and continuing education. It also provides access to an online version of the **Merck Manual** as well as a mobile version of resources.

13.3.4   Information on Pediatric Specialties

13.3.4.1   Infectious Diseases

Infectious diseases, their diagnosis and management, are a frequent focus of pediatric practice. Practitioners often depend on consultation with local experts and a few key resources:

- The **American Academy of Pediatrics Red Book** (aapredbook.aappublications.org/, The American Academy of Pediatrics) is the internationally recognized authority on pediatric infectious diseases, available for subscription/purchase in a number of formats: print, CD-ROM, PDA and online. Electronic versions provide multimedia sections on physical manifestations of disease, care management guidelines and patient information sheets.
- The **Johns Hopkins Division of Infectious Diseases Antibiotic Guide** (http://www.hopkins-abxguide.org/, Johns Hopkins University School of Medicine) provides information about diagnosis, pathogens, and antibiotics to treat specific disease entities. Not limited to pediatrics and more academic in tone, the Hopkins guide is free and available in both online and mobile versions.
- The **Centers for Disease Control and Prevention Yellow Book** (http://www.cdc.gov/travel/yb/, The Centers for Disease Control and Prevention) is the international reference on health care for international travelers. This online resource is also available (at cost) in print and allows creation of customizable reports for patients with actionable vaccination recommendations.

13.3.4.2   Genetics and Genomics

Genetic information plays an increasingly important role in personalizing medical care. Pediatricians and families will need to know more about the impact of genetic information on diagnosis and treatment[12] presently and in the future. There are a number of free resources available to help clinicians, parents, and prospective parents.

- **Genetics Home Reference** (http://ghr.nlm.nih.gov, National Library of Medicine) is a searchable online resource designed for health consumers that provides free, nontechnical overviews of genetics and genetic conditions with links to other NLM resources (PubMed, MedlinePlus, ClinicalTrials.gov and the Online Mendelian Inheritance in Man) and directories to genetic counselors by geographic area.

- **Online Mendelian Inheritance in Man (OMIM)** (http://www.ncbi.nlm.nih. gov/entrez/query.fcgi?db=OMIM, National Center for Biomedical Information (NCBI) and Johns Hopkins University) is an online catalog of human genes and genetic disorders. The database contains clinical data (findings, diagnostic tests and therapies) with linkages to PubMed, gene sequence records and other related resources in the NCBI database. There are a number of searching options, and because the database is specialized to genetics information, the retrieval can be comprehensive without being overwhelming.
- **GeneTests** (http://www.genetests.org, University of Washington, Seattle; funded by the National Library of Medicine) provides a number of up-to-date reports from national experts on clinical information on genetic syndromes (GeneReviews), US specialty clinics that provide genetic expertise and services, laboratories and availability of clinical testing for diseases in the database, research testing and testing trends over time.

13.3.4.3 Drug Information

Many electronic sources of formulary data, dosing information and contraindications exist, particularly for handheld devices that incorporate decision support (calculators, interaction guides).[13, 14]

- **Epocrates** (http://www.epocrates.com/, Epocrates, Inc) provides an updatable database on pediatric and adult drug information in online and handheld formats. The basic versions are free with additional services for subscription (dictionary, coding tools, diagnostic/therapeutic aids).
- **Lexi-Drugs** (http://www.lexi.com/, Lexi-Comp, Inc) provides a pediatric suite of tools for desktop and handheld computers, including a pediatric/neonatal specific drug database, interaction tools, toxicology information, calculators and a point-of-care textbook.
- **Thomson/Micromedex Healthcare Series** (http://www.micromedex.com, Thomson/Micromedex) is a suite of detailed databases on diseases, drugs and toxicology accessible through an integrated interface for online and handheld use in clinical settings (such as emergency departments). **Clinical Xpert** is the general handheld version and **Neofax** is an online/handheld reference with decision support tools for neonatal care.
- **Harriet Lane Handbook** (available through MDConsult, Elsevier and Johns Hopkins) is the familiar pediatric resource, now available in print, online, desktop and handheld versions. Computer versions provide calculators, but the print version may still be the most usable.

Online government resources of note that contain drug information include:

- **MEDLINEplus** (http://www.medlineplus.gov, National Library of Medicine) contains a consumer-oriented database of medication information sheets.
- **Food and Drug Administration Office of Pediatric Therapeutics** (http:// www.fda.gov/oc/opt/default.htm) is the source for regulatory information and

news on pediatric drug safety and research. A free e-mail alerting service is available.

- **Toxicology Data Network (including the Hazardous Substances Data Base)** (http://toxnet.nlm.nih.gov/cgi-bin/sis/htmlgen?HSDB, National Library of Medicine) is a reference database of peer-reviewed toxicology information that may be used in conjunction with local poison centers for information on toxins, their effects, diagnosis and treatment.
- **National Institute on Drug Abuse** (http://www.nida.nih.gov, National Institutes of Health) Website contains extensive data, news and resources on substance abuse for practitioners, researchers and patients.
- **National Network of Libraries of Medicine (US) and National Network of Libraries for Health in Canada** (http://nnlm.gov/, National Library of Medicine, http://cisti-icist.nrc-cnrc.gc.ca/main_e.html, National Research Council Canada) These resources can assist practitioners even in remote areas to stay abreast of new developments and obtain access to resources. Residents of the United States, can contact a Regional Medical Library at 1-800-338-7657, Monday–Friday 8:30 AM–5:30 PM EST; they will provide information on how to contact libraries in the local area. Residents of Canada may contact the Canada Institute for Scientific and Technical Information (CISTI) at 1-800-668-1222.

13.3.4.4 Research Questions

The approach to evidence-based medicine is discussed in Chapter 10. Several core resources (beyond those discussed here) are available to help clinicians find published research on specific health topics:

- **AAP Policy Statements** (http://www.aappolicy.org, American Academy of Pediatrics) contains policy statements and technical reports published and endorsed by the AAP that are updated every 3 years.
- **MEDLINE/PubMed** (http://www.pubmed.gov, National Library of Medicine) provides free online search of 15 million citations from 5,000 medical and research journals. Interface tools allow users to limit searches to age groups, publication types (systematic reviews, case studies) and therapy/diagnosis/etiology/prognosis. Free interfaces for mobile computing (http://www.nlm.nih.gov/mobile/) are available.
- **Morbidity and Mortality Weekly Report** (http://www.cdc.gov/mmwr/, Centers for Disease Control and Prevention) is available for free online, as e-mail alerts, newsreader feeds and podcasts.
- **National Center for Health Statistics** (http://www.cdc.gov/nchs/) and **CDC WONDER** (http://wonder.cdc.gov/) (both from the Centers for Disease Control and Prevention) provide direct access to health statistical data from federal collaborative studies including the National Health and Nutrition Examination Survey (NHANES).

13.3.5 *Information for Families*

Reliability, accessibility and usability of health information for families are three areas of concern in recommending resources. In addition, issues of language, literacy and culture must be considered in content and format of such resources. There is a growing body of literature on these aspects of patient-provider communication, especially as US demographics change over time. As such, resources are also changing to meet these evolving patient needs. Two examples are:

- **MedlinePlus** (http://www.medlineplus.gov, National Library of Medicine) provides current and readable health information in English and Spanish on diseases, therapies and drug information in Web pages and patient information sheets. When possible, linkages to local resources are provided.
- **Patient Education Online** (http://patiented.aap.org/index.aspx, American Academy of Pediatrics) is a subscription service for pediatricians that provides current English or Spanish patient information sheets produced by the AAP for download, that may be printed in the office for families, and may also be used as a practice marketing tool. A big advantage of the online format is paper reduction.
- **HealthVault Search** (http://www.healthvault.com, Microsoft Corporation) is a consumer-targeted search engine to a number of vetted sources of health information as part of a personal health information management system where users may create accounts for storing and using health information.

13.4 Conclusion

The increasing availability of electronic medical information for patient care, education and research provide great opportunities for practicing pediatricians to be more efficient, productive and better communicators and learners. Integration of general medical knowledge resources with patient-specific applications (such as electronic health records) will continue to evolve, but knowing what resources will be useful to practitioners in specific clinical environments is essential to get the best return on investment in electronic resources.

13.5 Case Study: Using the World Wide Web and Google for Health

The Google World Wide Web search engine (See "Clinical Constellations" earlier in this chapter) uses a mathematical algorithm called "PageRank"[11] as a measure of authority of a given Webpage in response to an entered query. While most clinicians are not likely to depend solely on Google for diagnosing patients, they may use it to expand a query (such as patient findings) to find a subset of documents (Webpages) where partial answers may be found and conceptual navigation may be easier. With sufficient guidance, clinicians can continue their information seeking. The inclusion of links to medical journal citations (from PubMed and from journal Websites) via Google Scholar may lead clinicians to original articles, may provide insights into patient perceptions and problems with specific disease processes[15] and information about specific providers. Interestingly, in a recent informal, but published experiment, Google returned correct diagnoses in response to 15 of 26 queries,[16, 17] however, this use is fraught with bias that is strongly dependent on the use of language, terminology and topic of search. An even more interesting use of the WWW uses its characteristic as an open system (one in which new information is constantly entering) as a surveillance tool for global disease alerts[18] using news reports and a querying/filtering/visualization tool for online display.[19]

References

1. Johns RJ, Fortuin NJ. Clinical information and clinical problem solving. In: Harvey AM, Johns RJ, McKusick VA, Owens AH, Ross RS, eds. *The Principles and Practice of Medicine.* 22nd ed. Norwalk, CT: Appleton & Lange; 1998:1–4.
2. Forsythe DE, Buchanan BG, Osheroff JA, Miller RA. Expanding the concept of medical information: an observational study of physicians' information needs. *Comput Biomed Res.* 1992;25(2):181–200.
3. Tribal knowledge. SixSigma; 2008. Available at: http://www.isixsigma.com/dictionary/Tribal_Knowledge-488.htm. Accessed December 17, 2007.
4. Zipf GK. *Human Behavior and the Principle of Least Effort; an Introduction to Human Ecology.* Cambridge, MA: Addison-Wesley; 1949:8–18.
5. Ely JW, Osheroff JA, Ebell MH, et al. Analysis of questions asked by family doctors regarding patient care. *BMJ.* 1999;319(7206):358–361.
6. Gorman PN, Helfand M. Information seeking in primary care: how physicians choose which clinical questions to pursue and which to leave unanswered. *Med Decis Making.* 1995;15(2):113–119.
7. Westbrook JI, Gosling AS, Coiera E. Do clinicians use online evidence to support patient care? A study of 55,000 clinicians. *J Am Med Inform Assoc.* 2004;11(2):113–120.
8. Cimino JJ, Li J, Bakken S, Patel VL. Theoretical, empirical and practical approaches to resolving the unmet information needs of clinical information system users. *Proc AMIA Symp.* 2002: 170–174.
9. Thompson WR, Hayek CS, Tuchinda C., Telford JK, Lombardo JS. Use of automated cardiac auscultation for detection of pathologic heart murmurs in children and young adults. *Pediatr Cardiol.* 2001;22:373–379.
10. Ramnarayan P, Roberts GC, Coren M, et al. Assessment of the potential impact of a reminder system on the reduction of diagnostic errors: a quasi-experimental study. *BMC Med Inform Decis Making.* 2006;6:22.
11. Brin S, Page L. The anatomy of a large-scale hypertextual Web search engine. *From Proceedings of the seventh international conference on World Wide Web.* 1998;7:107–117.
12. Andrews LB et al. *Assessing Genetic Risks: Implications for Health and Social Policy.* Institute of Medicine. Washington, DC: National Academy Press; 1994.
13. Knollmann BC, Smyth BJ, Garnett CE, et al. Personal digital assistant-based drug reference software as tools to improve rational prescribing: benchmark criteria and performance. *Clin Pharmacol Ther.* 2005;78(1):7–18.

14. Galt KA, Rule AM, Houghton B, Young DO, Remington G. Personal digital assistant-based drug information sources: potential to improve medication safety. *J Med Libr Assoc.* 2005;93(2):229–236.
15. Mehta SA. What can physicians learn from the blogs of patients with uveitis? *Ocul Immunol Inflamm.* 2007;15(6):421–423.
16. Tang H, Ng JH. Googling for a diagnosis–use of Google as a diagnostic aid:internet based study. *BMJ.* 2006;333(7579):1143–1145.
17. Twisselmann B. Use of Google as a diagnostic aid: summary of other responses. *BMJ.* 2006;333(7581):1270–1271.
18. Freifeld CC, Mandl KD, Reis BY, Brownstein JS. HealthMap: global infectious disease monitoring through automated classification and visualization of Internet media reports. *J Am Med Inform Assoc.* 2008;15(2):150–157.
19. Children's Hospital Informatics Program. Healthmap. Harvard-MIT Division of Health Sciences & Technology; 2008. Available at: http://www.healthmap.org. Accessed January 2, 2008.

Chapter 14
Supporting Continuing Pediatric Education and Assessment

Peter S. Greene, Valerie Smothers and Toby Vandemark

Objectives

By the end of this chapter, the reader will be able to:

- Describe the role of technology standards in supporting continuing medical education and maintenance of certification of pediatricians
- Identify the organizations involved in developing and applying technology standards for healthcare education and competence assessment

14.1 Introduction

Numerous organizations are involved in the continuing education and assessment of pediatricians, yet the information flow among them is often inefficient or nonexistent. Professional societies, academic medical centers and other Continuing Medical Education (CME) providers support continuing professional development (CPD). Certification boards, such as the American Board of Pediatrics (ABP), are commissions that set standards for assessment, certification and periodic recertification of physicians' competence to deliver high quality care within a medical or surgical specialty.[1] Licensing boards are organizations charged with protecting the public that determine jurisdictional and legal requirements physicians must meet to practice medicine.[2]

Each of these organizations is dependent on data managed by the others. Licensing boards require data on approved CME activities, specialty certifications and other state licenses in order to grant medical licenses. Certification boards also require CME data, as well as practice improvement and other professional activities and licensure/certification data from other boards. Umbrella organizations, such as the Federation of State Medical Boards (FSMB) and the American Board of Medical Specialties (ABMS) collect disciplinary action and certification data respectively from their member boards for sharing with other organizations,[3, 4] such as hospital credentialing committees. The combined effort for this interorganizational data

C.U. Lehmann et al. (eds.), *Pediatric Informatics: Computer Applications in Child Health,* Health Informatics,
© Springer Science+Business Media, LLC 2011

exchange is redundant and will become progressively worse as accountability and reporting requirements increase.

Information technology (IT) standards for healthcare education and competence assessment provide an efficient way to exchange important professional development and credentialing data among these organizations. We will describe IT standards that support the education, assessment and maintenance of certification of physicians and how they are implemented to support the evolving CPD of pediatricians.

14.2 Standards in Healthcare Education and Assessment

IT standards and specifications relevant to healthcare education and competence assessment have been created for use by organizations that create, manage and track CME activities and data. The MedBiquitous Consortium, an American National Standards Institute (ANSI) accredited standards development organization (SDO), has created a number of specifications for exchanging structured (electronic) data about CME and certification.[5]

MedBiquitous standards can be divided into four categories:

- Standards for tracking and evaluating professional education and certification activities
- Standards for discovering relevant education and information resources
- Standards for exchanging healthcare education content
- Standards for coordinating and tracking of competence assessment data

14.2.1 Standards for Tracking and Evaluating Professional Education and Certification Activities

14.2.1.1 Activity Report

The Activity Report provides a common format for an individual's professional education and certification accomplishments. With this draft standard, education and certification activities can be tracked across organizations. Organizations using the Activity Reports can collect CME and certification data to create individual e-portfolio systems that allow physicians to track their own professional activities.

14.2.1.2 Medical Education Metrics (MEMS)

MEMS provide a consistent format and data structure for representing aggregate evaluation data for a given learning activity. With this draft standard, healthcare educators can exchange evaluation data with accrediting bodies to simplify evaluation of an activity's reach and efficacy.

14.2.2 Standards for Discovering Relevant Education and Information

14.2.2.1 Healthcare Learning Object Metadata (Healthcare LOM)

Healthcare LOM, a customization of a Learning Object Metadata standard (from the Institute of Electrical and Electronics Engineers (IEEE)), provides a consistent way of describing healthcare educational content and activities, including CME activities. This description enables searching across multiple repositories to bring the most relevant learning resources to practitioners as they need them. Ultimately, point-of-care systems may educate and empower practitioners to improve clinical outcomes. Healthcare LOM is designed to support education for many health professionals as well as patients and caregivers.

14.2.3 Standards for Exchanging Healthcare Educational Content

14.2.3.1 SCORM for Healthcare

Based on the Advanced Distributed Learning Initiative's Shareable Content Object Reference Model (SCORM) for interoperable online learning, SCORM for Healthcare incorporates Healthcare LOM to enable interoperability of healthcare online learning. SCORM provides a consistent way to describe, package and run healthcare e-learning content and lets developers easily transfer e-learning content across learning management systems. Because SCORM uses a modular approach to content development, e-learning components can be disaggregated and reused in multiple courses and contexts, saving development costs and time. Healthcare-specific extensions in Healthcare LOM facilitate discovery of SCORM conformant content for both learners and developers.

14.2.3.2 Virtual Patients

Virtual Patients are interactive computer programs that simulate clinical scenarios for education and training. MedBiquitous Virtual Patient standards will allow interoperability to reduce costs and enhance the quality of education and assessment. The components include patient data, learning activities and multimedia resources to define and create rich learning experiences.

14.2.4   Standard for Coordinating and Tracking Competence Assessment Data

14.2.4.1   Healthcare Professional Profile

The Professional Profile simplifies the exchange of member or healthcare professional name, address, contact, education, training, certification, licensure, disciplinary action, academic appointment, occupation, and membership information by providing a common data format. With this building block, certifying, assessment, and licensing boards can better exchange competence assessment data and coordinate their activities.

14.3   Educational and Assessment Standards for Pediatric CPD

14.3.1   Maintenance of Certification

The American Board of Medical Specialties (ABMS) is the US regulatory organization that establishes quality standards for physician certification. It consists of 24 specialty member boards (including the American Board of Pediatrics (ABP), which is charged with credentialing and certification of general and specialty pediatricians solely and in conjunction with other specialty boards).

In 1998, the ABMS and its member boards, including the ABP, adopted a plan to develop and implement Maintenance of Certification (MOC) processes for ongoing certification of physician specialists to ensure that physicians maintain the competencies necessary to provide quality patient care in their area of certification. Maintenance of Certification consists of four parts:

- Evidence of professional standing, such as a license to practice medicine
- Evidence of a commitment to lifelong learning and self assessment to guide learning
- Evidence of cognitive expertise based on exam performance
- Evidence of evaluation of performance in practice[6]

IT standards for healthcare education and competence assessment are currently being developed and used to track certification data, to reconcile physician identity records across organizations and to coordinate education and assessment activities. As part of its transition to MOC, the ABP must track information about pediatrician certification activities for primary (general or specialty) and secondary (specialty) certificates they may hold.

Other organizations may deliver self-assessments and quality improvement activities that the ABP may accept to fulfill MOC requirements and licensure. The ABP is working with the American Academy of Pediatrics (AAP), a developer or pediatric educational and assessment activities, to define what activities are acceptable and eligible to fulfill MOC requirements for pediatricians. Once a process to establish this eligibility was in place, there was a need for a standard method by which activity completion could be communicated between the two organizations.

14.3.2 Case Study: Developing Data Links Between Two Pediatric Organizations

14.3.2.1 Problem

The American Academy of Pediatrics (AAP) and the American Board of Pediatrics (ABP) needed to create a standard by which electronic data about activities completed by AAP members could be transmitted to the ABP for use in MOC. The AAP and ABP use different computer platforms, languages and databases and therefore needed a common denominator to encode and share this data.

14.3.2.2 Requirements

In addition to being able to enable data sharing between the ABP and AAP, the ABP had an additional requirement for the standard to be flexible enough to handle data from any other organization that provided activities that met MOC criteria. Data fields for educational activities that needed to be shared with ABP include: sponsoring organization information, activity name, start and end dates of the activity, completion status, number of credits earned for the activity as well as data for the participant. In addition, ABP and AAP shared many members, requiring a matching process between the two organizations.

14.3.2.3 Design and Implementation

To accomplish this task, the ABP and the AAP agreed to use the MedBiquitous Healthcare Professional Profile that allowed matching of ABP diplomates with AAP members. The two organizations decided jointly what data points would be required to match physician identities across databases. A combination of fields, including Social Security Number, date of birth, first name, middle name, last name and address were used to perform an initial match, yielding 85% exact identification on all fields, with most of the rest successfully matched. The few that did not match may have been boarded pediatricians who were never members of the AAP. Once identities were matched, the MedBiquitous Activity Report was (developed and) used to transfer data on specific activities between the two organizations.

The two organizations employed a Web Services model to implement this transfer, in which each was able to export data in a format (eXtensible Markup

Language, XML) that allowed comparisons (the Healthcare Professional Profile), to encode and transmit data (the Activity Report) and to ensure security. The Web Service used by the ABP (WebSphere) employed 128-bit encryption, tokens and domain information to ensure the authenticity of the sender of the data. Keys held by each organization are also employed to further guarantee the integrity and safety of sender and receiver of data.

The ABP also allows reciprocity of MOC activities with other ABMS boards, specifically the American Board of Internal Medicine (ABIM), for pediatricians also certified as internists. For example, a pediatrician may complete a self-assessment activity offered by ABIM and use that activity to meet the self-assessment requirement for MOC in internal medicine AND pediatrics rather than having to complete two activities. The ABP is planning on using the MedBiquitous Activity Report to exchange data with the ABIM regarding these activities. The Activity Report is also being examined for data exchange between ABP and other boards for MOC activities where the pediatricians must participate in activities sponsored by those boards.

References

1. American Board of Pediatrics. Board Certification; 2008. Available at: http://www.abp.org/abpinfo/abouttheabp.htm. Accessed December 21, 2008.
2. Federation of State Medical Boards. About State Medical Boards; 2008. Available at: http://www.fsmb.org/smb_overview.html. Accessed December 21, 2008.
3. Federation of State Medical Boards. Federation Physician Data Center; 2008. Available at: http://www.fsmb.org/m_fpdc.html. Accessed December 21, 2008.
4. American Board of Medical Specialties. Board Certification Verification Resources; 2008. Available at: http://www.abms.org/Products_and_Publications/Certification_Verification. Accessed December 21, 2008.
5. MedBiquitous Consortium. Medbiquitous Website; 2008. Available at: http://www.medbiq.org. Accessed December 21, 2008.
6. American Board of Medical Specialties. ABMS Maintenance of Certification; 2008. Available at: http://www.abms.org/Maintenance_of_Certification/ABMS_MOC.aspx. Accessed December 21, 2008.

Additional Suggested Readings

Pasini N. The Who, What, Why, and How of E-learning Standards. The Medbiquitous E-Learning Discourse (MELD); 2006. Available at: http://meld.medbiq.org/primers/e-learning_standards_pasini.htm. Accessed April 6, 2009.
Smothers V, Clarke M, Van Dyck C. MedBiquitous and journal publishers: scholarly content and online medical communities. *Learn Publ.* 2006;19(2):125–132.

Part IV
Informatics and Pediatric Ambulatory Practice

Chapter 15
Pediatric Care Coordination: The Business Case for a Medical Home

Donald E. Lighter

Objectives

- To outline the needs of children, especially children and youth with special health care needs (CYSHCN) and an architecture for a clinical record to meet those needs
- To make a business case for adoption of an electronic health record for pediatrics, especially for CYSHCN
- To illustrate by way of a financial ledger the set-up, use and maintenance of an electronic health record for a pediatric practice and its positive impact on the quality of care

15.1 Introduction: The Medical Home

Children and Youth with Special Health Care Needs (CYSHCN) have complex health care issues that require multiple providers, as well as numerous procedures and medications that potentially can interact with each other to endanger health and safety (Chapter 5). The American Academy of Pediatrics created the Medical Home program in 1992 in a policy statement that defined the concept and recommended an infrastructure for children with conditions that fit the special needs criteria. That policy statement was updated in 2002[1] to include several enhancements (with emphasis on the concept of the Medical Home for ALL children) and specifying the following list of services provided:

1. Family centered care
2. Unbiased and clear information
3. Primary care, in the broadest definition
4. Assurance that care for acute and chronic conditions is continuously available
5. Continuity of care, including transitions to other providers
6. Appropriate and timely referrals to pediatric medical and surgical specialists
7. Interaction with early intervention programs
8. Care coordination

C.U. Lehmann et al. (eds.), *Pediatric Informatics: Computer Applications in Child Health*, Health Informatics,
© Springer Science + Business Media, LLC 2011

9. A centralized record with all information needed for comprehensive care
10. Developmentally appropriate, culturally competent health assessments and counseling

Of particular importance, the ninth service reads specifically as follows:

Maintenance of an accessible, comprehensive, central record that contains all pertinent information about the child, preserving confidentiality.

The need for information to facilitate care coordination is not only logical, but is a central factor in implementation of effective care management since the inception of the concept.[2] Only by having the complete picture of an individual's clinical status can cogent decisions be made about health care interventions. As pediatric electronic health records (EHRs) are deployed throughout the industry, recognition of the specific needs of children, particularly Children and Youth with Special Health Care Needs, must be central to the design of the record.

15.2   Architecture of the Clinical Record for CYSHCN

Most of the data elements for CYSHCN are similar to those required for all other children, but there are a number of important additional features that become important for these children, including:

• Storage and retrieval of consultant reports, not only by consultant, but also by consultant type (neurology, urology, etc.), dates of interventions/evaluations, types of interventions (e.g., CT scan, initiation of drug therapy)
• Appointment types and dates by consultant name or specialty
• Diagnostic or therapeutic interventions by procedure or type of procedure (e.g., radiology, surgical, etc.)
• Parental involvement in care, based on evaluations from all providers
• Child's functional level (assessed by outcome instruments like the Pediatric Evaluation of Disability Inventory, Gross Motor Function Classification System, etc.)
• Medication list and potential drug interactions

Case managers for CYSHCN require considerably more information than professionals who manage children with less complex conditions. For example, a child with cerebral palsy may be taking medications for seizures, osteopenia, gastroesophageal reflux, as well as receiving high calorie alimentation feedings for failure to grow. This combination of drugs and nutrients can produce abnormal drug levels, diminishing therapeutic effect or causing adverse drug reactions. Care managers must understand not only the scope of the child's therapeutic regimen, but also the potential interactions between all these factors.

Primary care pediatricians are often hesitant to provide Medical Home care coordination for uninsured or underinsured CYSHCN[3] partly because of the difficulty in assembling all of the information needed to adequately manage all of their needs. The paper chart world makes gathering all of the necessary information nearly impossible, or at least a daunting and time consuming task. Even when the paper chart contains all of the information, finding the necessary data and then correlating it with the child's current clinical status remains difficult at best. On the other hand, finding, sorting, and collating information in an electronic record can be much more expedient and certainly more accurate that relying on the traditional paper chart search methods. Thus, an electronic chart can make finding and organizing chart data much more achievable.[4-6]

Like all record keeping systems, however, getting data into the electronic chart is the key to having information available for clinical use. Direct access to consultant reports, lab and x-ray reports, as well as details of school performance and therapy interventions, is a critical component of coordinating complex care regimens and ensuring quality and safety. EHR systems for CYSHCN must be accessible for data entry by all of the child's consultants, as well as from laboratories, radiology departments and the many types of therapists who provide services for these children. Information in the chart must be available, if the child is to receive the best possible care, with access adequately secured, through biometric identification methods or through smartcards that authenticate and track all users of the record.

Informed care managers enable children to achieve a quality of care that exceeds that of those who are left to fend for themselves in the complicated health care environment. Through effective use and analysis of clinical information, these professionals can achieve the goal of the AAP's Medical Home Project, i.e. the highest quality care available for children and youth with special needs.[7-9]

15.3 Business Case for the EHR

If health care consists of multiple processes, and the delivery of care by physicians and other providers uses those processes to create diagnostic and therapeutic approaches for patients, then virtually every health care decision has economic implications. As every process has inputs and expected outcomes, so each process has expected costs and revenues. Some processes generate only costs, while others involve both costs and revenues. For example, when a child is evaluated by a pediatrician in the office, the process of care involves costs (physician time, overhead, capital costs for property and equipment) and revenues (payment for services). As with any business, the goal is to generate more revenues than costs, and so a variety of approaches are deployed to reduce costs and maximize revenues.

Maximization of revenues for CYSHCN can occur in only a few ways:

- Proper coding to ensure maximum reimbursement by third party payers
- Complete documentation to justify code levels
- Performance of lab tests, imaging studies, and special services (e.g., therapy) that can be billed to patients or third parties
- Sales of equipment or special devices for use by the child or parent

Most practices have a number of ways to reduce costs, however, including

- Staffing reductions
- Purchase lower cost supplies and perishables (e.g., vaccines)
- Automation of business processes
- Automation of clinical processes
- Improved efficiency (eliminating steps in processes that do not add value)
- Reduced costs for malpractice insurance due to improved documentation

The EHR provides a way of ensuring that several of these approaches are implemented effectively. For example, many EHRs now provide support for proper coding, with prompts that help practitioners understand the reasons for specific coding levels. After an encounter has been entered into the system, the program makes a recommendation for an Evaluation and Management (E&M) code that best fits the documentation that has been entered. If the clinician thinks that the visit should be coded differently, e.g., with a higher paying code, the system can provide the reasons for selection of the suggested code and recommendations for improving the documentation to justify a different code. Optimization of the E&M code in this way can ensure appropriate payment for services, as well as avoid legal problems and fines related to incorrect billing.[10]

The EHR can reduce risk and improve financial performance in other ways, as well. Although most EHR installations do not reduce staffing needs, in many cases staff can be reassigned to patient care duties that reduce costs and risks or generate revenue. Costs incurred for staff members finding charts, chasing down lab and x-ray results, or writing in paper charts can often be reallocated to pay staff members to provide billable services like telephone calls, blood drawing, office lab tests, and similar services. Thus, staff costs that originally were expended for non-revenue producing activities can be transferred to the revenue producing column of the ledger.

Implementation of an EHR should always include analysis of the processes of care to identify non-value added steps and improve efficiency. Automation of any process naturally changes the workflow and new work patterns must be developed as part of the transformation of a medical practice. This work redesign effort sometimes requires help from outside the practice. Almost invariably, effective automation can improve efficiency and reduce costs, but installing a computerized solution in a flawed process will always lead to frustration and increased costs, as well as risks to patient safety and effective care.[11]

Thus, the business case can be made for automating medical records through the following cost reduction and revenue producing enhancements:

- Reallocation of staff efforts to revenue producing activities
- Improved process of care to eliminate costly, non-value added processes
- Improved documentation for justifying appropriate coding

One final point about improving costs may be germane to some EHR users. Since documentation of the visit is generally improved for most practitioners, malpractice risk may actually be reduced at the same time that billing efficiency is enhanced. Some insurers provide discounts for physicians who use these electronic systems, since the amount of information that is recorded at each visit generally increases significantly. Thus, in the event of an untoward event that leads to litigation, the amount of information (particularly pertinent negatives) available to defense attorneys might make the difference for successfully defending the suit. For this reason, some insurers have reduced premiums for physicians using EHRs.[12,13]

Effective automation has the long term effect of enhancing revenues and reducing costs to actually produce a return on the investment made in computers and software. These results have been demonstrated in businesses from car repair to robotics manufacturing, and health care delivery is no exception. The multitude of methods by which revenues are increased and costs reduced should be considered in these calculations to create a business case to justify the expenditures and understand the return on investment.[14-16]

15.4 Business Case Study

Let's evaluate a typical business analysis of an EHR implementation in a pediatric practice, starting with the following assumptions:

- Five provider practice, three pediatricians, and two pediatric nurse practitioners
  - Currently dictate records, with two transcriptionists who comprise 1.5 FTEs
- Two receptionists who manage entry of the superbills into the billing system and creation of follow up appointments
- Three office nurses, two medical assistants whose functions include:
  - Finding and verifying lab and imaging results
  - Conducting office lab tests
  - Patient education and distribution of educational literature
  - Check patients into the "clinic area," do brief history, vital signs
  - Check all transcriptions for typographic errors and grammar
- An office manager who makes sure everything gets done and that collections are healthy

The worksheet in Table 15.1a provides a cost breakdown of the current practice situation. The practice is operating at a break-even level, with little or no profit from year to year. Medical assistants work at a level of two FTEs, and nurses at 3 FTEs, and a substantial amount of their work relates tracking and evaluating lab results, as well as proofreading transcriptions.

Assumptions for the pro forma include the following (Table 15.1b):

The practice decides to automate its medical record, and purchases a system with the following characteristics:

- Direct data entry of progress notes, histories, and physicals using templates
- Interface with the practice's hospital reference lab and x-ray department to receive reports in batches

Table 15.1a Pediatric practice abbreviated profit and loss statement before automation

	Income	Expenses
Provider services – outpatient	$ 1,100,000.00	
Provider services – inpatient	$ 385,000.00	
Office laboratory services	$ 480,000.00	
Total revenues	$ 1,965,000.00	
Salaries – providers		$ 550,000.00
Salaries – nurses		$ 105,000.00
Salaries – medical assistants		$ 36,000.00
Salaries – receptionists		$ 30,000.00
Salaries – transcriptionists		$ 37,500.00
Salaries (subtotal)		$ 758,500.00
Benefits		$ 242,720.00
Overhead charges		$ 884,250.00
Medical malpractice		$ 81,000.00
Total expenses		$ 1,966,470.00
Net Income	$ (1,470.00)	

Table 15.1b Assumptions for the pro forma

Item	Cost
Provider salaries	$140,000 per year
Nurse practitioner salaries	$65,000 per year
Nurse salaries	$35,000 per year
Medical assistant salaries	$18,000 per year
Receptionist salaries	$15,000 per year
Transcriptionist salary (1.5 FTE)	$25,000 per year
Benefit costs	32% of salaries
Medical malpractice – MDs	$19,000 per year
Medical malpractice – NPs	$12,000 per year
Overhead charges	45% of gross revenue

- Auto checking of notes for spelling and grammar errors using a medical dictionary
- Billing recommendations based on the structured note entered by the clinician
- Compliant with malpractice insurer's requirements for a 10% premium credit

The medical record system costs $175,000, which the practice pays by taking $35,000 from financial reserves and finances the remaining $140,000 at 5.5% interest for 48 months. The assumptions made for the calculations take into account the expected decline in productivity during the first year after implementation, as well as a number of other practice costs related to the new system:

- The time spent by the nurses and medical assistants in managing the paper chart are consumed with other duties, such as increasing reimbursable lab volumes done in the office by 10%.

- The level of transcription required decreases by half, since the structured notes can be entered by practitioners at the time of visit, which reduces the amount of dictation substantially.
- Providers will suffer a 25% decline in productivity, measured by the number of patients seen, during the first 6 months after implementation of the new system. That decline is reflected in the gross revenues generated by each provider.
- The practice will see an immediate 10% credit on malpractice premiums.
- Conversion of the paper records to the electronic system (Conversion costs) will total $25,000. This amount includes scanning required information for current patients into the electronic system.

The projections for the first 6 months post-implementation reveal a significant loss, primarily due to lowered productivity in the outpatient department (Table 15.2). Adjustments to income relate to the improved laboratory revenues, but some costs can be improved, as well, through savings on malpractice insurance and

Table 15.2 Pro forma statement – first 6 months post-implementation

Item	Cost	
System cost	$175,000.00	
Amount financed	$140,000.00	
Interest rate	5.5%	
Finance period	48 months	
Monthly payment	$8,338.20	
Increased lab volume	10%	
Transcription decrease	50%	
Productivity decrease	25%	
Medical malpractice credit	10%	
	Income	Expenses
Provider services – outpatient	$412,500.00	
Provider services – inpatient	$192,500.00	
Office laboratory services	$264,000.00	
Total revenues	$869,000.00	
Salaries – providers		$275,000.00
Salaries – nurses		$52,500.00
Salaries – medical assistants		$18,000.00
Salaries – receptionists		$15,000.00
Salaries – transcriptionists		$18,750.00
Salaries (subtotal)		$121,360.00
Benefits		$242,720.00
Overhead charges		$304,150.00
Medical Malpractice		$33,150.00
Loan payments		$50,029.18
Conversion costs		$25,000.00
Total expenses		$912,939.18
Net income	$(43,939.18)	

transcription costs. In spite of these improvements, however, the practice can expect to show a loss in the near term after implementation.

With assumptions

As practitioners become more skilled in use of the system and the practice begins to adjust financially to the new system, a number of improvements can be expected, as shown in Table 15.3. Providers can be expected to return to previous productivity levels during the second 6 months (Recovery in service rates 100%), and lab volume should continue to increase as nurses and medical assistants have more time to devote to doing lab tests that normally would have been sent to the reference lab because of lack of time to do the tests in the office. Additionally, medical assistants and nurses should start finding slack time available, for which the practice manager might want to begin making work time adjustments as noted in the assumptions (15% decrease in medical assistant time, 5% decrease in nurse time). The return to normal productivity, combined with modest decreases in nursing and medical assistant costs and elimination of the conversion costs, lead to a profit for the practice, which offsets the loss in the first 6 months post-implementation.

Assumptions

Thus, the financial case for the EHR can be made with the assumptions that the implementation will be expeditious, staff and providers cooperate with the

Table 15.3 Pro forma statement – second 6 months post-implementation

Item		
Recovery in service rates	100%	
Increased lab volume	10%	
Decreased medical assistant time	15%	
Decreased nurse time	5%	
	Income	Expenses
Provider services – outpatient	$440,000.00	
Provider services – inpatient	$192,500.00	
Office laboratory services	$290,400.00	
Total revenues	$922,900.00	
Salaries – providers		$275,000.00
Salaries – nurses		$49,875.00
Salaries – medical assistants		$15,300.00
Salaries – receptionists		$15,000.00
Salaries – transcriptionists		$18,750.00
Salaries (subtotal)		$373,925.00
Benefits		$119,656.00
Overhead charges		$276,870.00
Medical malpractice		$33,150.00
Loan payments		$50,029.18
Total expenses		$853,630.18
Net income	$69,269.82	

conversion, and productivity changes follow the usual pattern after a new system is installed. Within a year post-implementation, a practice can be not only back to normal rates of productivity, but in many cases can exceed previous levels through better allocation of resources to generate revenue.

15.5 Improved Quality of Care

A number of organizations have advocated automation of the medical record to improve the quality of care. The Leapfrog Group,[17] the Institute for Healthcare Improvement,[18] and the federal government[19] now promote widespread adoption of electronic records as one way to improve health care quality. Some ways in which this approach can promote better quality care include:

- Ready access to a complete medical record to improve data-based decision making
- Decreased redundancy of laboratory and x-ray tests that could be potentially harmful
- Better documentation and legibility of entries
- Enhanced detection of drug interactions and adverse reactions
- Improved ability to measure and analyze clinical data
- More rapid access to reference and supporting data for patient care

When the medical record is unavailable, practitioners have little recourse but to discern diagnostic and therapeutic histories from patients, who often have indistinct memories of past medical treatments. The clinician is left in the difficult position of trying to design a diagnostic and treatment regimen with incomplete information, leading to errors such as drug interactions or allergic reactions, repetition of potentially uncomfortable or harmful tests, and patient dissatisfaction. Additionally, standardized data entry can improve documentation and availability of information for decision support.[20,21]

Quality management hinges on measurement: "You can't manage what you can't measure." Measurement of clinical processes has relied on two basic sources of data: (1) transaction data from coded insurance company transactions and (2) paper chart audits performed by skilled reviewers. The transaction data come from coded forms submitted by providers to insurance companies for reimbursement. These data are flawed in a number of ways for measurement of clinical processes. First, the codes are not descriptive of the richness of a clinical encounter, since they only provide information regarding the diagnosis assigned and procedures performed during the patient visit. Many other issues often arise during an interaction between a provider and patient, and the codes used for an insurance claim rarely capture those elements, particularly for children with special health needs. Thus, a great deal of information does not make it into an insurance claim system.

Secondly, the data submitted on an insurance claim form are designed to optimize reimbursement for services rendered, rather than provide information relating to quality of care. As such, the codes will not contain important clinical parameters, such as lab test results or the results of imaging exams. Without such information, the outcomes related to particular procedures or interventions are difficult to assess, and so clinical quality cannot be determined.

Finally, numerous errors occur because of different coding approaches. Evaluation and management (E&M) codes have become increasingly complex, with multiple levels of codes used to define provider services using several factors leading to a high potential for errors. In fact, E&M coding error rates have remained relatively high, in spite of several years of provider experience with the system.[22] Thus, the use of insurance claims data for quality management of children with complex needs can be fraught with problems.

On the other hand, the gold standard for quality data collection, skilled review of patient paper charts, has attendant shortcomings. In most cases, a skilled reviewer, often a nurse or other relatively expensive, well-trained health professional uses a data collection tool or form to extract information from provider charts for later entry into an electronic data management system. The process of chart review is usually straightforward, but often tedious and subject to a number of potential flaws. Foremost, this method of data collection is the most expensive, since reviewer salaries are often quite high. Most of these types of studies target specific issues and are generally reserved for the most critical problems facing an organization. Additionally, the process involves identifying and pulling patient charts, which disrupts office routine and usually leads to costs incurred by the provider, as well. Several other problems arise during these reviews, such as errors in interpretation of entries in the record, unclear operational definitions, entry errors into the data management system, and inability to read chart entries. All of these issues support the need for an electronic method of capturing data at the point of care.

Perhaps one of the greatest advantages of an electronic health record is the relative ease of sharing the typically extensive record with other providers. CYSHCN often have thick paper charts with volumes of information that are difficult to access and transfer to other providers. Electronic charts can provide appropriate retrieval of clinical information by providers through networks that are accessible via internet protocol (IP) based systems. Known as Regional Health Information Organizations (RHIOs),[23] these systems are the latest iteration of attempts to share health data among providers via secure, encrypted, authenticated connections. This concept has been incubating for nearly 3 decades, starting with Community Health Information Networks (CHINs) in the 1980s. Although conceptually sound, the first CHINs suffered from lack of ubiquity, concerns about security, and a general reluctance of health care organization to share any information. However, the resurgence of this approach has accompanied increasing pressure on the health care industry to reduce errors and rework, as well as the cost of managing individual patients. RHIOs may offer a solution to some of these issues.

Simply stated, RHIOs are regional networks of systems that assemble data about an individual patient into a searchable, secure record. The information comes from disparate computer systems, and so a common format is necessary to ensure that the data can be shared and is readable regardless of computer platform. RHIOs depend on intersystem compatibility that has become achievable because of improvements in web-based programming languages and interface standards, but creation of a RHIO still presents funding challenges. Several states and locales have formed

RHIOs, however, and the movement to increase information availability through this venue appears to be gaining momentum.

15.6   Case Study: Automating Referrals and Reports

Using the same five provider practice from the business case, let's assume that the practice has automated its medical record system. Each practitioner has a personal login, password, and specific "work areas" in the electronic record, as do all of the staff members. Access to laboratory tests and reports has improved greatly, usually requiring only a few mouse clicks to retrieve a wealth of patient information. For their CYSHCN, special reports are available that trend data, such as anticonvulsant drug levels, with prompts activating when levels are outside normal ranges for the reference lab. The providers have come to realize, however, that many of the physicians who comanage these children have significant information regarding care pathways and interventions, but relaying information from the subspecialists to the practice's EHR is tedious and error-prone. They create a process map (Fig. 15.1) that outlines the current process of referral and management of incoming reports. From the process diagram, the practice manager determined that a number of steps that required manual intervention in the system could be eliminated. For example, at node 1, two steps were needed to create a referral request and select a subspecialist based on the patient's need and payment profile. The EHR has the ability to match specialists with specific insurance plans, making these steps redundant. At nodes 2 and 3 in Fig. 15.1, the traditional method of making referrals and sending records to the subspecialist added additional costly manual steps, often requiring a nurse to effect the referral and ensure proper portions of the record are transferred. With the shortage and expense of nurses, these process steps are particularly problematic. Finally, at node 4, the paper document returned from the subspecialist is scanned and associated with the patient's record so that it is available to the practice's providers.

Using a lean process review, the staff identified several steps that could be eliminated or modified. First, the group determined which subspecialists received most of the practice's referrals. These physicians were invited to be "Practice Partners," which allowed secure connections to the EHR system and access to specific patient records. Practice Partners had to agree to a few process changes, however:

- Willingness to accept appointment requests by email or instant messaging, with a priority response within 5 min
- Willingness to submit reports electronically by uploading the report into the patient record on the practice's EHR
- Ability to function as a HIPAA compliant business associate
- Maintenance of at least one workstation compatible with current VPN and telecommunication standards

Practice Partners then receive "preferred" referrals from the practice, which should be financially beneficial.

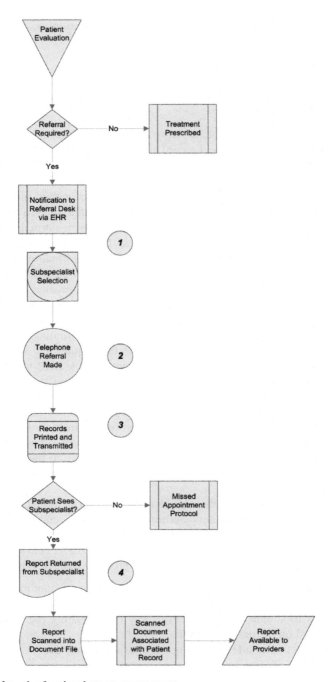

Fig. 15.1 Manual referral and report management

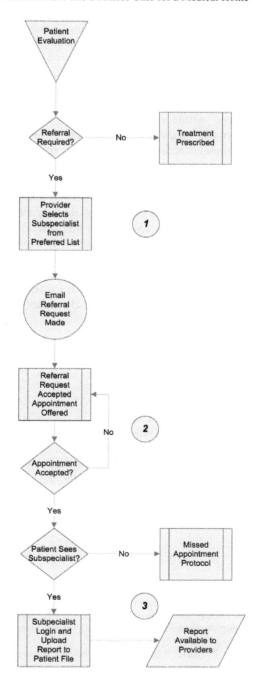

Fig. 15.2 Automated referral and report management

The automated system process is presented in Fig. 15.2. Several steps have been eliminated by the automated approach, with consequent savings in personnel time making telephone referrals and managing paper reports. Elimination of the three step process of referral is evident at node 1 in Fig. 15.2. The provider picks a sub-specialist from a dropdown list during the patient visit and immediately dispatches an email request for an appointment. In most cases, a reply with a time and date for an appointment returns within a couple of minutes, but if the process requires more time, the provider can "hand off" the process to one of the support staff (node 2). As the appointment is accepted, the provider can also click on a dropdown box to select the sections of the chart that are to be made available to the subspe-cialist for the consultation, and the consultant can connect at a convenient time to review those chart sections. After the patient has been evaluated by the consultant, (s)he can either enter the results of the consultation directly into the patient's EHR, or create a document file that can be uploaded to the patient's record as indicated at node 3. These improvements to the process not only expedite delivery of the information to practitioners, but they also reduce costs by eliminating much of the paper handling that requires expensive human resources. Cost avoidance benefits provide additional support for the business case made earlier to justify automation, as well as increase the quality of care by more timely access to information by all of the child's health care providers.

15.7 Summary

The information required to care for CYSHCN has increased exponentially in the last few years, and manual systems of recordkeeping are inadequate to the task. As EHR systems become ubiquitous, the needs of these children must be addressed if auto-mation is to be considered successful. By eliminating the costly and time-consuming human interventions in managing information transfer, the quality and cost of care can be enhanced, resulting in favorable financial and clinical outcomes.

References

1. American Academy of Pediatrics Medical Home Initiatives for Children With Special Needs Project Advisory Committee. The medical home. *Pediatrics*. 2002;110(1):184–186.
2. Lighter D, Fair D, eds. *Quality Management in Health Care: Principles and Methods*, Chapter 10: Making Quality Improvement in Health Care Work – Care Management. Sudbury, MA: Jones & Bartlett; 2004.
3. American Academy of Pediatrics Committee on Pediatric Emergency Medicine. Policy statement: overcrowding crisis in our nation's emergency departments: is our safety net unraveling? *Pediatrics*. 2004;114(3):878–888.
4. Brennan P. Winning the paper chase: bedside terminals help clear the record. *Health Prog*. 1980;70(8):66–68.

5. Luxenberg SN, DuBois DD, Fraley CG, Hamburgh RR, Huang XL, Clayton PD. Electronic forms: benefits drawbacks of a World Wide Web-based approach to data entry. *Proc AMIA Annual Fall Symposium.* 1997;804–808.
6. Nielsen PE, Thomson BA, Jackson RB, Kosman K, Kiley KC. Standard obstetric record charting system: evaluation of a new electronic medical record. *Obstet Gynecol.* 2000;96(6):1003–1008.
7. Bakker A. Digest of the discussion group sessions. Realising security of the electronic record. *Int J Med Inform.* 2004;73(3):325–331.
8. Hagland M. Electronic record, electronic security. *J AHIMA.* 2004;75(2):18–22.
9. France FH, Gaunt PN. The need for security–a clinical view. *Int J Biomed Comput.* 1994;35(suppl):189–194.
10. Walker K, Flanagan JR, Lane T. Lightening the burden of the heavy regulatory hand an incentive for outpatient computer patient record. *Proc AMIA Symp.* 2001;736–740.
11. Boaden R, Joyce P. Developing the electronic health record: what about patient safety? *Health Serv Manage Res.* 2006;19(2):94–104.
12. Microsoft Corp. Electronic medical record sets group apart as e-pioneers and delivers powerful advantages. Microsoft.net Enterprise Servers, Microsoft Customer Solution Healthcare Industry. Available at: http://download.microsoft.com/documents/customerevidence/6043_Holston_BDM_Healthcare_CS_Final.doc. Accessed December 21, 2008.
13. Grams RR, Moyer EH. The search for the elusive electronic medical record system–medical liability, the missing factor. *J Med Syst.* 1997;21(1):1–10.
14. Omura G. Electronic records in a private practice. Presentation given at Colorado Medical Society Tech Fair. Available at: http://www.cms.org/TechFair/Omura.ppt. Accessed December 21, 2008.
15. Guzick D. Electronic Records at URMC. University of Rochester Dean's Newsletter; 2006. Available at: http://www.urmc.rochester.edu/SMD/newsletter/article.cfm?id=57. Accessed December 21, 2008.
16. National Quality Forum Executive Institute's Task Force on Electronic Health Record Systems. CEO Survival Guide to Electronic Health Record Systems. National Quality Forum; 2006.
17. The Leapfrog Group. Leapfrog Group Website; 2008. Available at: http://www.leapfroggroup.org. Accessed December 21, 2008.
18. The Institute for Healthcare Improvement. IHI Website; 2008. Available at: http://www.ihi.org. Accessed December 21, 2008.
19. Office of the National Coordinator for Health Information Technology. ONC Website; 2008. Available at: http://www.hhs.gov/healthit/onc/mission/. Accessed December 21, 2008.
20. Gioia PC. Quality improvement in pediatric well care with an electronic record. *Proc AMIA Symp.* 2001;209–213.
21. Honigman B, et al. Using computerized data to identify adverse drug events in outpatients. *J Am Med Inform Assoc.* 2001;8(3):254–266.
22. Andreae MC, Fawley M, Freed GL. Hitting the mark… sometimes. Improve the accuracy of CPT code distribution. *MGMA Connex.* 2005;5(1):39–43, 1.
23. Office of the National Coordinator of Health Information Technology. Goals of Strategic Framework; 2004. Available at: http://www.hhs.gov/healthit/goals.html. Accessed December 21, 2008.

Additional Suggested Resources

Amatayakul M. *Electronic Health Records: A Practical Guide for Professionals and Organizations.* Chicago, IL: American Health Information Management Association; 2004.

Gartee R. *Electronic Health Records: Understanding and Using Computerized Medical Records*. Upper Saddle River, NJ: Prentice-Hall.

Johns M. *Health Information Management Technology: An Applied Approach*. Chicago, IL: American Health Information Management Association; 2002.

Lighter D, Fair D. *Quality Management in Health Care: Principles and Methods*. Boston, MA: Jones & Bartlett.

Chapter 16
Prioritizing Pediatric Investment for IT in Smaller Practices

Mark M. Simonian

Objectives

- To discuss IT investment for small practices from a pragmatic viewpoint
- To list the steps and issues of adoption
- To provide a description of a solo practice adopter

16.1 Introduction

Small practices are the least likely to adopt electronic health records.[1-4] Practical business decisions determine the choices that office-based physicians make in prioritizing information technologies purchases. Beyond basic clinical and clerical tools (stethoscope, typewriter, telephone, or fax), practices need to consider customer and market expectations, business efficiency, and regulatory issues to choose IT applications that impact on the quality of practice services and the bottom line.

16.2 Pressures in Small Pediatric Practices

16.2.1 Financial

Regardless of size and mission, pediatric practices are businesses, and as such, must build a loyal clientele with a steady stream of sustainable business. Practices have investments in licensing (for clinicians, offices, and point-of-care laboratories), labor (salaries and benefits for nursing and support staff) and equipment (overhead costs for rental, utilities, and supplies). They earn revenue by providing clinical services to patient groups and individuals (contracts and fee-for-service) and may provide pro-bono services. Practices also compete with other practices for patients in an era when reimbursement levels have decreased and documentation requirements have increased.

Some of these financial pressures may be mitigated by the size of an organization. Larger practices may have more resources to invest, but also have greater

C.U. Lehmann et al. (eds.), *Pediatric Informatics: Computer Applications in Child Health,* Health Informatics,
© Springer Science+Business Media, LLC 2011

organizational barriers to overcome, with added complexities including corporate taxation and labor issues. In contrast, small practices, with fewer resources, have greater flexibility and agility in making the necessary decisions for IT adoption.

Small practices must, out of survival, adhere to the maxim of "No margin, no mission." In addition to debts from medical education (many physicians are repaying educational debts of over \$200,000,[5] small practices must remain competitive (continuing education, new equipment), which increases burdens on practice owners. In smaller practices, practitioners must also stay current on effective coding and billing for rendered services to be productive and to maintain sufficient operational income.

In this context, IT can be an investment, but small practices must be much more cautious than larger ones due to smaller financial resources. To facilitate acquisitions, small practices may form purchasing groups with other practices or local medical associations. Even so, the benefits of IT purchases in reducing labor costs through increased efficiency are difficult to measure directly.

16.2.2   Quality Data Reporting

Increasing requirements for clinical data collection and reporting for quality assurance, continuous professional development and regulatory auditing place additional burdens on practices. Newer reporting requirements go beyond what is traditionally contained in claims data and into data that is available only in clinical records. Thus, IT systems provide an attractive possibility to reduce the burdens and costs (lost practice time and additional staff to collecting data).

16.2.3   Time Management

The combination of these pressures leads to higher demands for productivity: more patients seen per day, more time spent at the office, less time for family and other activities. IT tools can support efficient management of financial, documentation, and reporting functions to make time for other activities, including continuous professional development, advocacy, networking, and family.

16.3   Weighing Benefits and Costs

16.3.1   Benefits

In selecting IT for a practice, primary drivers (beyond cost) to adopt are ease of use and perception of usefulness of a technology.[6] Tasks for which IT may provide benefits include:

- Optimizing charge capture, coding, and billing
- Assuring complete documentation of encounters, procedures, and time

- Increasing efficiency through reduced paperwork and physical storage
- Providing reminders, alerts, and other decision support
- Reusing practice data for research and to understand and plan practice

16.3.1.1   Optimizing Charge Capture

Electronic health record tools and other tools can help improve the accuracy of coding, resulting in higher levels of reimbursement.[7] Coding tools can analyze documentation levels to suggest appropriate billing levels for the provided care and what is needed to optimize appropriate charges. The educational and remuneration value of such tools to a practitioner can be significant[8] and are a principal selling point for EHRs.

16.3.1.2   Assuring Complete Documentation

Improved charge capture depends on improved documentation. Handheld and mobile technology can streamline necessary documentation of clinical procedures and informed consent. Such tools can also accurately record time for encounters, such as behavioral counseling or complex disorder evaluations, which may be billed according to clinician time spent.

Documentation of encounters or consultations narratives is performed by transcription of dictation or use of template reports. Speech recognition technology, which has widespread use in radiology, is not used extensively in primary care, but the availability of low cost computer memory has made facilitated recording for transcription (leaving a copy of un-transcribed reports available). Templated reports, filled with data directly from an EHR database, may be created with standard word processor and spreadsheet merging tools to facilitate form completion. However, the majority of reports are still prepared by handwriting, typing, or word-processor.

16.3.1.3   Increasing Efficiency

Practice management systems can be used to retrieve and validate demographic and insurance information and update patient information as needed when telephone or patient portal requests are received. Other functions, such as medication reconciliation may also be performed easily.

Electronic prescribing (eRx, Chapter 19) and computerized prescription writers can improve the quality and safety of delivering drugs to patients. In both of these, electronic prescription template forms connect EHR problem, allergy, and medication lists and formularies to prevent illegibility, dosing errors, allergy identification, and drug interactions. More efficiency and checking can be added when eRx applications connect office to pharmacy, linking knowledge from both sides.

Other advantages of digital information include reduction or elimination of paper, resulting in more efficient use of office space. This benefit must be weighed against the costs of converting legacy documents and creating redundant access.

16.3.1.4 Providing Decision Support

Clinical decision support (CDS) tools, covered in greater detail elsewhere in the book (Chapters 10, 12, and 13) can provide clinicians with access to information (through online libraries), they can guide entry and choices (through template forms and clinical practice guidelines) for diagnosis and therapy, they can provide knowledge-based prompts (via alerts and reminders) and they can help clinicians understand practice.[9]

16.3.1.5 Reusing Practice Data

Most EHR systems allow filtering of data elements that can be configured by providers or practice managers. In addition to required reports, ad hoc queries may be generated to help identify patterns according to patient demographics, diagnosis (ICD) or therapy (CPT) codes. More complex queries can be used for quality improvement, practice planning, continuous professional development[10] and research.

16.3.2 Costs

The most critical issue and the principal barrier to small practice adoption of EHRs are the costs of a system. These costs include:

- Base costs of hardware, software, and training
- Costs to customize products
- Costs to interface/integrate systems
- Upgrade costs

16.3.2.1 Base Costs of Hardware, Software and Training

An example of cost ranges per provider of an EHR system is in Table 16.1.

Table 16.1 Cost range per provider of an electronic health record system[15]

	Base	Range
System costs		
Software (annual license)	$1,600	$800–3,200
Implementation	$3,400	
Support and maintenance	$1,500	$750–3,000
Hardware (three computers and network)	$6,600	$3,300–9,000
Induced costs		
Temporary productivity loss	$11,200	$5,500–16,500

16.3.2.2   Costs to Customize Products

Small practice decision makers must decide if "commercial off-the-shelf (COTS)" technology will meet practice needs or if customization is required. Customization may range from "built-in" specification of forms (low cost) to changes in the underlying data structures that require technologist intervention (high cost). In addition, practices need to determine the frequency of customization updates and how these will incur further costs.

16.3.2.3   Costs to Interface/Integrate Systems

In the same manner, practices must decide if "standalone" products will meet needs of if they must connect to other systems (and on what basis). Interface/integration considerations include the costs of interfaces (and functionalities) of an EHR to:

- Practice cost centers or management system
- Different office locations (and home/mobile)
- Commercial laboratory and imaging services
- New entities (How much will it cost to modify current interfaces)

The most useful interface is between clinical information tools (such as EHRs and eRx) to practice management systems to integrate clinical information with billing and scheduling functions. Interfaces that connect products from different vendors to form value-added integrated suites are available. Challenges to practices include decisions on how to transition from current management systems while minimizing costs of productivity loss and retraining of staff. Transitions may require operation of more than one system.

16.3.2.4   Upgrade Costs

Proprietary and customized systems are vulnerable to discontinuation by their vendors. Contractual negotiations with vendors should include contingency plans for continued service, including if needed, availability of code or interfaces for modification. All hardware and software have a life span and upgrades may include major changes, with accompanying costs. Tools are available that can help a provider look at individual pieces or the cost breakdown.[11]

16.4   Planning IT Adoption

16.4.1   The Steps

The steps in planning adoption for small practices may be less formal than for larger ones. These include:

- Outline practice information needs for now and the future
- Participate in different vendor displays or demonstrations
- Select vendor and product candidates
- Check the vendor performance and experience, especially in service and support
- Test drive products and ask around
- Narrow choice and make selection
- Negotiate the contract

16.4.2   Information Resources

Information sources on products may include other physicians and practices, vendors, and professional medical societies who have experience with specific products. Consultation with colleagues in close proximity to the office allows office staff access to what other groups or individuals are doing. First hand experience is also very helpful in providing lessons learned. If a paid consultant is used, the experience and recognized expertise of the consultant should be researched.

16.4.3   Deployment and Operation

Most practices will require help with installation. Tasks include: hardware configuration and networking, software installation and testing, data conversion, staff training, and rollout. Some vendors provide help themselves or contract with local technicians for setup and support of their system. Purchasers and staff should feel comfortable about operating the system (including remote access) and about finding support. This aspect of products should be explored with other practices that have experience with the system.

16.4.4   Expenses – Initial Setup

The most complex part of adoption is choosing how to finance the process for a given practice. Each practice must decide how to approach the decision and which approach is the best. Four general approaches (not including private development or open-source tools) include direct purchase, traditional loans, leasing, subscription (application service providers) and (if available) gift, grants or network membership benefit.

16.4.4.1   Direct Purchase

Some technology will not require much deliberation and can be purchased as a practice expense. These include office workstations, printers, wireless networking, and other inexpensive hardware. In this case, the practice owns the technology outright, eliminating monthly installments and interest.

16.4.4.2   Traditional Financing

Larger purchases, such as servers, electronic health record applications, interfaces to other systems and higher speed connectivity are often financed over time. Advantages include reduction of large upfront expenses to affordable monthly payments, minimization of the risk (due to obsolescence), preservation of capital and other assets for other investments. The time of the loan period is critical. Although most technology is relatively consistent for 2–5 year periods, the technology could become obsolete before the end of the financing period. In the first decade of the twenty-first century, financing costs are relatively low compared to the 1980s, with no expected changes in the foreseeable future.

16.4.4.3   Leasing and Subscribing (Application Service Providers)

In some tax situations, leasing might more advantageous (Tax advisors should be consulted to determine what is appropriate in each practice's financial situation). For some technologies (such as EHR systems), subscribing to an application service provider (ASP) may be preferable. These options reduce the burden of system ownership and allow earlier adoption than purchase or financing, however at a higher long term costs.

   Application Service Providers (ASPs)[12] provide on-demand computer services (such as EHRs, electronic prescribing or journal resources) to customers over a network (such as the Internet or other server-client model) as a subscription. ASPs own, operate and maintain the hardware and software for an application and provide access for a subscription fee. Practice advantages include no separate expense for hardware, third party software, system management, or maintenance. Practice disadvantages include the facts that over time total costs of operation are higher, that ownership is never achieved, that remote availability requires secure broadband connections.

16.4.4.4   Gifts or Grants

Some technologies may be "gifts" or trade-offs for participation in or adoption of another program-wide change. An example of this is provision of hardware and software by insurers for practices to support e-prescribing. Some state governments have subsidized EHR system and offered lower costs or repayment options as incentives (including tax savings) to increase adoption.

   Grant options may be available from regional health information organizations (RHIOs) or other programs (such as local registries) that might offer technology at low or no cost to providers for participation. The Agency for Healthcare Research and Quality (AHRQ) Web site has many grants for individuals interested in applying technology to their practice. Most involve studies using technology for certain clinical conditions. Others involve large organizations evaluating the effectiveness of technology to solve particular problems.[13]

16.4.4.5 Network Membership Benefit

Practices associated with multiple hospital systems often see value in using practice management and electronic health record systems that are compatible or interoperable with the systems used by those institutions. Mutual benefits between hospitals and office-based practices include sharing of demographic, billing and payment data and easier tracking of referrals and more accurate billing. After the initial costs of development by hospitals, technology becomes a marketing tool that can be used to build loyalty at low cost to private practices.

An issue that should be considered is the effect of Stark (or "anti-kickback") legislation[14] on adoption. Stark legislation had hindered growth of technology in practices that do not have the financial resources to invest. This is of significance in IT obtained as a network membership benefit. Again, legal counsel may be helpful in navigating these issues.

16.4.5 Expenses – Ongoing and Operational

16.4.5.1 Software Licenses

Software licenses are certificates, sometimes linked to access and services that allow practices to use purchased software (such as practice management and electronic health record systems, clinical decision support, periodicals, clinical journals, or diagnostic services). Group licenses (such as through professional associations or community practice consortia (IPAs) for a shared or commonly used application may reduce individual costs at a bulk rate.

16.4.5.2 Training and Technical Support

Training staff to use applications properly can be an additional expense if it is not included as part of the purchase price. Training costs may exceed the software costs when travel, housing, and consultation are included, but may be mitigated if online training is available.

Technical support should be considered in terms of how and when service is scheduled (Telephone? Online? 24/7/365? Workdays only? Immediate response? Can maintenance or repairs be handled online (onsite repair costs may be higher)?).

Other contingencies that must be planned include prolonged downtime (How does the practice operate when the system is nonoperational?) and recovery (How is data from downtime restored to the system? How is data loss or theft handled?). Practices must have a clear idea about how support will respond either to routine or urgent requests. Are they fast and dependable? Communication with previous users is essential because vendor promises might not be reliable.

16.4.5.3   Maintenance

In a paperless pediatric office the electronic data repository will be the life blood of the practice and it must be maintained. Information must be backed up on a regular basis. Technologies to automate this process include tapes, redundant hard drives, optical disks, etc. have been in use for practice management systems and can be applied to EHRs. This task can also be entrusted to an Application Service Provider to store data securely off site.

Most systems incorporate regular backup processing to multiple locations to provide redundancy. Assurance of the restoration (and retrieval) process, while the responsibility of the practice, requires guidance from vendors and purchasers should look for guarantees of rapid response in case of an emergencies. No office should be placed into the position of having to manage a restoration without help available.

Downtime policies for staff should be in place in case of a failure (system failure, power outage, misplaced record). This includes a mechanism to create a temporary record until updating the electronic systems can be restored and reincorporating interim records into the main system. These policies and procedures should be reviewed periodically by the practice.

System updates and repairs should be considered as part of service contracts for workstations, servers and other hardware. Upgrades should be considered in terms of compatibilities with other components of the system (operating system, network connection, control devices, and any system that cannot be updated easily should be questioned (as it may incur additional costs and upgrades).

16.4.6   Expenses – Nonmonetary

Important questions to ask about contingency procedures involve how data (or lack of data) is handled when the system does not function optimally.

16.4.6.1   Confidentiality and Security

What happens if information security is compromised (stolen or lost) due to any cause (malicious or otherwise)? What are ways of mitigating this compromise and its effects on care? What are the disclosure requirements and procedures as to patients affected by breaches? What are liability issues? Depending on the type of information compromised the technology vendor may help identify individuals affected (audit trails), and policy will be necessary to establish whether telephone, e-mail, paper or fax will be used to communicate to any potential harmed patients.

16.4.6.2 System and Data Integrity and Availability

What happens when the system (hardware or software) becomes nonfunctional and what is the ability of the user to replace or repair it in a timely way? Some repairs may be quick and simple (rebooting a server), some may be facilitated by online help (telephone, online, or network control) and others may require live service and time. Practices may require onsite backup replacements for hardware (extra printers, workstations) and ready access to expertise when needed. Some downtime is necessary for upgrades and backups and should be planned to minimize its impact (nighttime backups).

How will downtime data be handled? How will data captured on paper and pencil be recovered for electronic use? When data integrity is compromised, how will final authority be assured (human review, electronic backup, or a combination)?

16.5   Conclusion

Adoption of health IT for small practices is a big investment that is easier to navigate than previously. New opportunities exist for practices to incorporate electronic health records into their practices without large initial costs, but with some tradeoffs.

16.6   Case Study: A Solo Practitioner's Experience in EMR Adoption

In my one doctor practice with two support staff, workflow efficiency was the number one criteria when adopting an electronic medical record (EMR) and integrated practice management software (PMS). After moving to a new location with anticipation of greater patient numbers, I needed to be able to retrieve patient information and generate documentation with minimal additional operational costs and staff time.

As the primary financial decision maker, I chose to bring in about $25,000 through a home equity line (which was tax deductible) at relative low interest rates (4–5%). About $17,000 went into software and the remainder into hardware. The capital access allowed me to buy software licenses, associated additional application software like antivirus and antispam software, some decision support software, and hardware. The hardware costs covered two servers (one was a redundant system for emergency recovery), one workstation and a scanner for the front office, one laptop per exam room and one laser printer for each laptop.

DSL (broadband) connectivity was already covered in the practice overhead (no additional) costs. Training through Internet-based sessions (1 h every 3–7 days) was covered as part of the cost of the initial software license. Training covered the clinical EMR (which I use primarily) and the integrated practice management (which my biller uses). Training for simple "crossover" tasks (appointment scheduling, patient registration, vaccine entry, and encounter charges) was provided to all staff. Annual maintenance fees would start after the first year and were about 10% of the purchase price.

Transitioning our office charges and collections while we moved from the old PMS into the new integrated EMR/PMS required concurrent use of both systems. As new patients were added, we billed and charged them in the new system, with manual review and clearance of older charges (from the old system) as payments arrived. This dual system was maintained through two monitors, one to the old PMS and one to the new integrated system, and we maintained the dual system for about a year (although most of the payments were cleared within 6 months).

Since starting in the newer practice location patient numbers and income have almost doubled without requiring more staff. Setup of the EMR, hardware, and maintenance costs were recovered in less than 2 years.

16.7   Additional Resources: EMR Buyer Support Tools

- *EMR cost calculator*

URL: http://www.aafp.org/fpm/20020400/57howm.html
A spreadsheet tool from Family Practice to help compare long-term costs of an electronic health record for a small practice.

- *EHR Review*

URL: http://www.aapcocit.org/emr
A Website created and hosted by the American Academy of Pediatrics Council on Clinical Information Technology (COCIT) to help users discover and share experiences of peers with commercial EHR products.

- *Implementing an Electronic Health Record Toolkit*

URL: https://www.nfaap.org/netforum/eweb/DynamicPage.aspx?webcode = aapbks_productdetail&key = afd90736–5fad-4674-b909–5489e5553bee.
A CD-ROM toolkit consisting of the AAP Policy Statement on the "Special Requirements for Electronic Medical Records Systems in Pediatrics" and other information for adopting an EHR.

References

1. Simonian M. The electronic medical record. *Pediatr Rev.* 2007;28(10):e69–76.
2. Simon SR, Kaushal R, Cleary PD, et al. Correlates of electronic health record adoption in office practices: a statewide survey. *J Am Med Inform Assoc.* 2007;14(1):110–117.
3. Simon SR, McCarthy ML, Kaushal R, et al. Electronic health records: which practices have them, and how are clinicians using them? *J Eval Clin Pract.* 2008;14(1):43–47.
4. Gans D, Kralewski J, Hammons T, Dowd B. Medical groups' adoption of electronic health records and information systems. *Health Aff (Millwood).* 2005;24(5):1323–1333.
5. Morrison G. Mortgaging our future–the cost of medical education. *N Engl J Med.* 2005;352(2):117–119.
6. Chismar WG, Wiley-Patton S. Does the Extended Technology Acceptance Model Apply to Physicians. Proceedings of the 36th Hawaii International Conference on System Sciences (HICSS'03); 2003. Available at: http://www.hicss.hawaii.edu/HICSS36/HICSSpapers/HCDMG04.pdf. Accessed December 21, 2008.
7. Adler KG. Why it's time to purchase an electronic health record system. *Fam Pract Manage.* 2004;11(10):43–46.
8. Stausberg J, Koch D, Ingenerf J, Betzler M. Comparing paper-based with electronic patient records: lessons learned during a study on diagnosis and procedure codes. *J Am Med Inform Assoc.* 2003;10(5):470–477.
9. Perreault L, Metzger J. A pragmatic framework for understanding clinical decision support. *J Healthcare Inf Manage.* 1999;13(2):5–21.
10. Sectish TC, Floriani V, Badat MC, Perelman R, Bernstein HH. Continuous professional development: raising the bar for pediatricians. *Pediatrics.* 2002;110(1 Pt 1):152–156.
11. Valancy J. How much will that EMR system really cost? *Fam Pract Manage.* 2002;9(4):57–58. Available at: http://www.aafp.org/fpm/20020400/57howm.html. Accessed December 21, 2008.
12. Bush J. The Internet as cure for inefficient office business processes. *Med Group Manage J.* 2000;suppl:10–13.
13. Agency for Healthcare Research and Quality. Technology Assessments; 2008. Available at: http://www.ahrq.gov/clinic/techix.htm. Accessed December 21, 2008.
14. Strahan M. Seven years until electronic health records: the negative effects of the new Stark exceptions and anti-kickback safe harbors. *J Health Law.* 2007;40(2):291–303.
15. Wang SJ, Middleton B, Prosser LA, et al. A cost-benefit analysis of electronic medical records in primary care. *Am J Med.* 2003;114(5):397–403.

Chapter 17
Aligning Pediatric Ambulatory Needs with Health IT

Michael G. Leu, George R. Kim, Ari H. Pollack and William G. Adams

Objectives

- To outline the motivations for and clinical uses of health IT in the ambulatory care setting
- To describe the current state of ambulatory health IT adoption, and describe the effect of practice size on adoption decisions
- To illustrate organizational, financial, and technical considerations when adopting health IT

17.1 Introduction

Primary motivations for health IT adoption, from a federal policy level, are to improve quality and reduce costs in health care. In ambulatory care, incentive alignment among stakeholders is a major obstacle. While patients and payors benefit from adoption, it is the practices and provider groups that must bear the burdens of financial investment, workflow redesign, and organizational change. Even for institutions and practices skilled in managing the necessary changes, the task of health IT adoption is risky (Table 17.1).

17.2 Motivations for Health IT Use

Pediatric care is rendered primarily in ambulatory settings (private offices, urgent care centers, specialty clinics, emergency departments) by a variety of clinicians (including general and specialist pediatricians, general practitioners, nurse practitioners, physician assistants, and emergency physicians). There has been increased interest in using health IT to support efforts to implement evidence-based guidelines and indicators in pediatric ambulatory care to improve quality.[1] Health IT has also been viewed as a means to reduce costs.

C.U. Lehmann et al. (eds.), *Pediatric Informatics: Computer Applications in Child Health,* Health Informatics,
© Springer Science+Business Media, LLC 2011

Table 17.1 Motivations for and challenges to adoption of health IT

Motivations
Improved quality of care
Reduced cost of care
Administrative efficiencies
Savings from clinical redesign
Increased revenue and productivity

Challenges
Organizational factors
Requires executive leadership, support, and sponsorship
Practice must be receptive to change
Clinical processes must work before they can be automated with health IT
Education, training, and retraining of staff; support infrastructure

Cost
Large capital outlay with significant up front and ongoing costs
Uncertain or slow recovery of initial investment
Practices face risk, but cost savings realized by payors

Expertise
Requires significant technical infrastructure and IT expertise
Vendor evaluation and partnerships

17.2.1 *Improving Quality*

In the landmark report *To Err is Human*,[2] the Institute of Medicine (IOM) noted that "tens of thousands of Americans die each year from errors in their care, and hundreds of thousands suffer or barely escape from nonfatal injuries." Subsequent reports revealed that adults receive only 54.9% of recommended preventive services, and that children receive only 46.5% of indicated care.[3,4] Other reports demonstrate regional variability in care, and suggest that there is also variability in ambulatory care settings.[5]

Quality care is defined as care that is safe, effective, patient-centered, timely, efficient, and equitable (Table 17.2).[6,7] Systemic change has been recommended to improve quality.[7] According to the IOM, this change requires transformation of microsystems (patient populations, care provider teams, health information systems, and work processes) using the principles of quality as targets, guided by three high level philosophies and ten strategies (Table 17.3).[6,7]

To implement these strategies, the health care industry has incorporated ideas and lessons learned from other industries (such as aviation and manufacturing) to create resilient approaches to planning and process redesign. Included in these approaches are: focus on proactive and anticipatory problem-solving, creation of learning organizations, engagement of all levels in process improvement, creating a culture which values safety, and mitigation of system-based vulnerabilities that induce human error.[8]

Health IT can be used to standardize communication and to coordinate information flow throughout an organization, while simultaneously capturing transaction records. Information captured and stored in these systems is in itself a valuable resource for analyzing organizational and individual performance, tracking errors and providing

Table 17.2 Institute of Medicine principles of quality care[6,7]

Safety: Patients should be as safe in health care facilities as they are at home.

Effectiveness: The health care system should match care to science, avoiding both overuse of ineffective care and underuse of effective care.

Patient-centeredness: Health care should honor the individual patient, respecting the patient's choices, culture, social context, and specific needs.

Timeliness: Care should continually reduce waiting times and delays for both patients and providers of care.

Efficiency: The reduction of waste (and total cost of care) should be never-ending (e.g., waste of supplies, equipment, space, capital, ideas, and human spirit).

Equity: The system should seek to close racial and ethnic gaps in health status.

Table 17.3 Philosophies and strategies to transform health care

Philosophies[7]

Provide knowledge-based care. Use the best scientific and clinical information available in the service of the patient.

Provide patient-centered care. Respect the individuality, values, ethnicity, social endowments, and information needs of each patient; putting each patient in control of his or her own care and customizing care to respect individual needs, desires, and circumstances.

Provide systems-minded care. Coordinate, integrate, and foster efficiency across traditional boundaries of organizations, disciplines, and roles.

Strategies[6,7]

Base care on continuous healing relationships. Patients should receive care whenever they need it and in many forms, not just face-to-face visits. This rule implies that the health care system should be responsive at all times and that access to care should be provided over the Internet, by telephone, and by other means in addition to face-to-face visits.

Customize care according to patients' needs and values.

Have patients control care.

Share knowledge freely, with patients having unfettered access to their own medical information and to clinical knowledge.

Base decision-making on scientific evidence, to allow consistent care between clinicians and practice settings.

Treat safety as a system property, paying greater attention to systems that help to prevent and mitigate errors.

Support transparency, allowing patients and their families to make informed decisions (for areas such as health plans, hospitals, or clinical practice alternatives).

Anticipate patient needs instead of acutely reacting to events.

Continuously decrease the amount of wasted resources (be they tests, supplies, or patients' time).

Support collaboration and cooperation among care providers.

explicit quantitative data on the impact of organizational changes (such as the outcomes related to changes in clinical practice by adopting different care guidelines).

17.2.2 Reducing Cost

Cost reductions in health care can be derived from redesign of administrative and clinical workflows, augmented by technology.

17.2.2.1 Reductions Through Administrative Redesign

Computerized practice management systems (CPMS) perform essential business functions such as scheduling, registration and billing. CPMS are used nearly universally, with 84% of practices submitting claims electronically in 2005.[9] In addition to managing these functions, the administrative data stored in CPMS can measure practice efficiency (e.g., no-show rates) and effectiveness of resource allocation, allowing practices to optimize staffing and productivity. An example of technology-enhanced administrative redesign is the use of automated telephone appointment reminders in conjunction with letters to encourage childhood immunizations.[10]

CPMS can reduce paper use, decreasing on-site storage requirements and making information more readily accessible. Inventory management systems can help track vaccine and medication inventory to reduce waste. Online "dashboards" can keep managers informed by presenting real-time measures of operational efficiency, allowing timely focus on practice areas needing improvement.

17.2.2.2 Reductions Through Clinical Workflow Redesign

The "Medical Home" concept, first articulated in 1967 in *Standards of Child Health Care* published by the American Academy of Pediatrics (AAP),[11] is a partnership between the patient (a child with special health care needs), his/her family, and the primary care provider (PCP). This partnership originates in the clinical care provider's office. Within this model, the role of the PCP is to plan and ensure access to, and create linkage and coordination between the patient and a community of resources tailored to the patient's needs. The original model has been expanded[12,13] as the Advanced Medical Home in which primary care is transformed to emphasize preventive and chronic care management in the ambulatory care setting. Cost reductions are realized through prevention of hospitalizations and severe complications of chronic medical conditions.

One study suggests that adoption of electronic health records (EHRs) in conjunction with other health IT to facilitate prevention and chronic care management can result in a savings of more than $81 billion annually.[14] The central hypothesis of this study is that authenticated, ubiquitous access to medical records in electronic form will provide a better historical context for the patient's medical care, leading to reductions in unnecessary duplication of testing and services. In the ambulatory setting, it is postulated that reduced costs of transcription, chart pulls, laboratory testing, medication usage, and radiology may be as great as $159 billion over 15 years, with $20.4 billion saved annually when 90% of clinics have adopted health IT.

17.2.3 Increasing Revenue and Provider Efficiency

It is believed that health IT can increase provider efficiency, by allowing speedier access to information with less effort.[15] This increase in efficiency would lead to increased patient throughput and increased revenue. Theoretical modeling also suggests that benefits accrue from savings in drug expenditures, improved utilization, better charge capture, and decreased billing errors.[16] In current EHR systems, revenue has been derived primarily through improved documentation via electronic charting and coding optimization.[17] Under proposed Medical Home models, primary care clinicians may also be reimbursed at a higher rate for care continuity and coordination.

Although health IT has a great potential to improve quality and safety, actual improvements in efficiency are highly dependent on providers and existing practice workflows. For some, the increased efficiencies in performing some tasks are offset by additional tasks which they must now accomplish (for example, examining additional patient information that is available, or reviewing a more comprehensive set of lab results presented to them).[18]

17.3   Clinical and Workflow Impact of Health IT

Prior to health IT adoption, clinical and organizational leadership must have a clear and thorough understanding of the workflows and processes that will be affected. Inappropriate adoption, implementation and deployment of health IT will not "fix" dysfunctional workflows and processes, but may in fact reinforce and worsen them. A realistic accounting of organizational needs, coupled with organizational process and culture change is necessary. If these changes are overlooked or ignored, the technical deployment may take much longer than anticipated, and may ultimately fail.

The first step in adopting a health IT solution is formal exploration of existing workflows, problems, and potential technical solutions. With the exception of mandated (and proven) technical initiatives, practices tend to begin adoption initiatives with those that have minimal impact on clinician workflow and/or high probability of success ("low-hanging fruit"). With small successes, organizations gain internal structures and overcome organizational inertia, resulting in increased clinician participation and medical oversight (e.g., clinical committees, clinical champions), which allows for more ambitious projects to be undertaken with greater impact on clinician workflow (Table 17.4).[18]

17.3.1   Health IT with Minimal Impact on Clinician Workflow

Health IT that supports clerical functions has minimal impact on clinician workflow. This may include CPMS (as discussed previously); and practice Websites or portals that provide information and services for patients (e.g., contact information, provider lists, description of services the clinic can provide, office hours). Personal

Table 17.4 Clinical areas for health IT use, and available solutions (adapted from[18])

Area of Health IT use	Minimal/none	Impact on clinician workflow		
		Some	Moderate	Significant
Orders, results, and results management	Results for ordered tests printed or faxed (paper-based)	Online order sets, online results for clinicians of ordered tests	Online chart or results review between different care settings	Tools track and follow up preventive care needs, results, and outcomes
Intra-clinic communication	Providers and clinic staff communicate with e-mail, text messages; notes dictated	Clinical tasks assigned electronically, document imaging of paper notes (a.k.a., "Go paperless")	Electronic documentation by clinician (EHR, word processor)	Multidisciplinary coordinated care; specific fields in structured, analyzable format
Patient education and outreach	Practice website with educational materials, automated reminders for appointments	Automatically generated forms/care plans (e.g., asthma action plan)	E-mail with patients	Clinical care managed between visits (includes goal-setting and tracking)
Inter-clinic coordination	Paper immunization cards	Electronic referral paperwork	Information exchanges, provider-maintained personal health record systems	Referrals managed per electronically reinforced protocols; information exchanges
Medication management	Online drug reference	e-prescribing (with interaction checking), frequently used lists	e-prescribing with dose calculation, medication reconciliation	e-prescribing with diagnosis- and patient- based decision support
Provider education and feedback	Web site links, online clinic policy manuals	Integrated or handheld reference materials, online training	Clinical calculators	Integrated electronic clinical decision support; report cards, assessments

productivity tools which can be accessed independently of the patient visit (such as online medical reference materials) can support clinician work without forcing workflow to change.

Practices which use these technologies are likely to use paper-based medical records and personal health records (such as immunization cards). Electronic information exchange is likely to be limited to administrative data (billing and mandated reports).

17.3.2 Health IT with Some Impact on Clinician Workflow

When small gains, practices may advance to adopt health IT solutions that are considered to be "big wins" (high probabilities of success and/or that provide "instant gratification"), but which also have limited impact on clinician workflow. These solutions may require few simple changes in manual activities that save time for clinicians. These focused activities reduce the risk of failure, while increasing enthusiasm when gains are realized. Modules that fall under this category include: document imaging, electronic prescribing (e-Rx)/computerized provider order entry (CPOE), electronic results lookup, and intra-clinic communication.

17.3.2.1 Document Imaging

Purported advantages of "paperless" offices include: speedy access to up-to-date information, decreased staffing requirements, and decreases in filing errors.[19] One study suggests that document imaging may result in an ongoing net savings of over $9,000 per provider per year.[20] However, there are many hardware and operational requirements for in-house scanning solutions ([21] for a partial list), as well as limitations on full-text retrieval. Administrative costs of document imaging include the purchase of the scanning hardware and software, and the initial and ongoing costs of converting archived and new paper-only information, including faxes and paper communications from other practices or laboratories.

However, the impact of this technology may be limited. Although the technology itself has minimal effects on clinician workflow, scanned image data lacks the advantages of truly digital data. Scanned handwritten notes are searchable only by direct visualization. Scanned graphical data (x-rays, photos, electrocardiograms, etc.) are not amenable to electronic interpretation. In order for data to be analyzable, there must be a process to allow for discrete data elements to be created. Either these elements can be entered via structured data entry, or data conversion processes can be used. Some researchers use scanned mark-sense forms and optical character recognition (OCR) to perform these conversions.[22] However, these technologies are not yet in widespread use.

17.3.2.2 Electronic Prescribing and Computerized Provider Order Entry

Electronic prescribing (e-Prescribing, e-Rx), covered in greater detail in Chapter 19 and elsewhere[23], is currently being piloted in practices, supported by payors that plan to deploy this technology widely. e-Rx reduces prescription errors by increasing legibility, speed and accuracy. Specific applications also provide clinical decision support (checks for drug allergies, drug–drug interactions and formulary availability).[24] Considerations for pediatric e-Rx include[25]:

- Does the system support weight-based (or body-surface-area based) dosing?
- Does the system support remote (secure Internet) electronic prescribing (including access to the necessary patient data)?
- What education and user support is needed by the clinical and clerical staff to use the system?
- Does the system support paper prescriptions (fax and hand-carried prescriptions) with the recipient pharmacies as well as e-Rx?
- Does the system interface and integrate with the EHR and CPMS?

Ambulatory computerized provider order entry (ACPOE) provides a means for providers to choose groups of orders (order sets) for treatment. Order sets may include instructions for laboratory tests and procedures in addition to the medication orders (which are supported by e-Rx). An example of an order set is: a combination of an e-Rx for warfarin, laboratory studies for therapeutic drug monitoring, and scheduling of follow-up visits for a patient on anticoagulation therapy. A central consideration when considering an ACPOE product is detailed clinician knowledge (and/or review) of order sets, their source, and whether evidence based principles were used in their formulation. There is currently no standard for order sets, resulting in variation between implementations.

One pediatric study found approximately 15% of children may be dispensed medications with a potential dosing error.[26] It is generally believed that ACPOE can help to reduce these errors.[27] A study from the Center for IT Leadership (CITL) provides a cost–benefit analysis of ACPOE.[28] This study examined three tiers of ACPOE: basic (links to non-patient-specific clinical resources at point of care, printed orders), intermediate (order and patient-specific information brought to provider's attention, orders faxed or e-mailed), and advanced (intermediate + automated order transmission to labs and pharmacies). They found that advanced ACPOE may prevent nearly 2.1 million adverse drug events and more than 190,000 hospitalizations yearly (nine adverse drug events and six visits per year per provider), while eliminating an average of $10.55 in rejected claims per visit. This study also found that most of the financial benefits of ACPOE go to payors, with providers in smaller practices realizing a much higher relative financial cost (and correspondingly smaller net financial benefit) when compared with providers in large practices.

17.3.2.3   Electronic Results Lookup and Intra-clinic Communications

Clinicians believe that electronic medical records can help them to process ambulatory laboratory results more efficiently.[15] Many EHR products that support automated results lookup also support intra-practice communications (instructions for follow-up tasks to be performed by other staff). One example might be an electronic message from a pediatrician to a clinic nurse, to arrange home phototherapy for an infant with an elevated discharge bilirubin level. The EHR and the CPMS may facilitate this process by providing easy access to insurance and contact information. More sophisticated systems may allow future labs to be ordered, and communications about the patient's condition to be saved to their electronic record.

While many clinicians find these functions increase their efficiency, some may be overwhelmed by the new workflow. Receiving too many results may increase the potential for error or the likelihood that the physician will not process messages in a timely manner. In part, this may be addressed through effective clinician training and/or by a monitoring system that can identify providers who have problems (such as a large backlog of unchecked results) in using the system.

17.3.3   Health IT with Moderate Impact on Clinician Workflow

"Transitional" health IT is a class of applications that have a moderate impact the way clinicians work. These applications include clinical calculators, interfaces that allow users to access, create, and update electronic information and patient–provider e-mail. Currently there is little data on the clinical efficacy of these applications, but there is face validity to claims that increased information will lead to reduced duplication of services, increased accuracy, and improved care.[29] Because the impact on clinician workflow is more than minimal, individual variation in adoption and use of these technologies may result in significant variations in health care outcomes.

17.3.3.1   Clinical Calculators

Clinical calculators automate computations, but may require manual data entry. Most studies using them have been in academic or research settings, and these tools are not yet used in a widespread and standardized manner. Domains in which calculators have been developed include nephrology,[30] nutritional support (e.g., total parenteral nutrition[31]), and anthropometrics (weight, height, body mass index percentiles[32]). Calculation programs may reside on different platforms, including programmable calculators, mobile personal digital assistants (PDAs),[33] and Websites; they may also be integrated into electronic medical records. If calculators are to be effective in reducing error, human factors and clinical workflows must be considered when designing interfaces. Embedded calculators with minimal human interaction provide the fewest errors (e.g., automatic computation and display of weight, height, and body mass index percentiles when a child steps on a scale in the pediatrician's office).

17.3.3.2 Tools to Access, Create, and Update Information

EHRs make information available in a legible and accessible form, but this alone is not sufficient to improve the quality of care.[34] Users (patients, providers, and office staff) must also be able to interact with and control access to electronic health information. Important considerations include:

- *Data entry*. Some users find computer data entry to be difficult or cumbersome. Transitioning from handwritten to online notes may require adequate user interface design; or support for alternate forms of data entry such as audio-recording and transcription. Changes to user interfaces (such as larger, simpler forms) may be needed for users with visual impairment.[35]

  Another important consideration with regards to electronic data entry is *comprehensiveness*. Just as creating standardized forms for well child visits encourages uniform practice, easily updatable electronic templates or checklists can support the consistent practice of high quality, evidence-based care.
- *Data retrieval and review*. Currently, the way patient information is displayed may vary greatly between EHR systems. There are no standards for retrieval and visualization functions between EHR systems in the U.S. (although the U.K. National Health Service is deploying a Common User Interface for use across all EHRs[36]). Using a system with a well designed user interface which supports appropriate clinical workflows is particularly important in the fast-paced, high-volume ambulatory care setting. The user model for the system, including design considerations such as layout of information, intuitiveness, specific language used, and level of detail required for interaction may all dictate whether the system improves provider productivity, or the implementation fails.

  Properly designed electronic health record systems provide a longitudinal (over time) view of a patient, which allows providers to provide better care. Tests can be reviewed instead of being reordered, and providers can take historical information such as allergies or treatment failures into consideration. However, common trend views, such as growth charts, may not be readily available in all products. It is important to know which displays and reports that are available and which need to be constructed when considering the purchase of an EHR system.
- *Data security*. Tools and interfaces must guarantee information assurance (confidentiality, integrity and availability) and adhere to HIPAA privacy and security rules.[37] In addition to technical approaches (e.g., secure interfaces, time-limited user authentication), practices must have policies in place that define appropriate staff use of information, penalties for violations, and protocols for reporting

and recovering from information breaches. It is imperative for practices to have a global knowledge of these policies and protocols.

17.3.3.3   Patient-Provider Electronic Mail/Secure Messaging

It has been estimated that about 7% of all ambulatory visits in the US are to providers that use electronic mail to communicate with patients.[38] Some providers provide this service as an adjunct to telephone care, and often will place restrictions on what may be discussed with patients through this medium.[39-41] One study found that providing electronic consultation through secure messaging led to decreased overall messages to the practice, with increases in both patient and provider/staff satisfaction. It has been inferred that secure messaging may decrease provider/staff interruptions, and increase clinical efficiency.[42]

17.4   Health IT with Significant Impact on Provider Workflow

Progressive practices and organizations seek to improve by creating new relationships between care teams and patients, in contrast to the one provider-one patient model. In these newer models, clinical information systems support team communication and patient care coordination. They may also be used to report performance measures which underscore successes while simultaneously identifying areas for improvement.

17.4.1   Redefining the Patient–Clinician Relationship

Health IT can be used to improve health status and outcomes in complex patients by coordinating their interactions with care teams (as in the Chronic Care Model[43]), and by supporting patients' self-management activities.[44] Specific software applications can enhance care provided between visits through remote communication, monitoring, and feedback.[45,46]

One study simulated potential cost-benefits of different health IT-enabled approaches to diabetes management.[47] They examined (1) provider-focused (disease registries and clinical decision support systems), (2) patient-focused (self-management and remote monitoring systems), (3) payor-focused (claims-data monitoring systems) and (4) patient–provider focused systems (an integration of the patient and provider systems mentioned above). While all intervention types improved care and prevented complications, provider-focused forms of disease management were the most cost-beneficial. In all situations, disease-specific registries (providing performance measurement and feedback to clinicians) were cost-beneficial; and clinical decision support systems were only beneficial for large provider organizations. The other interventions were not cost-beneficial. Despite these findings, provider-focused disease management systems may prove to be the least likely to be adopted given existing incentive structures.

17.4.2 Providing Performance Measures and Feedback to Clinicians

In many health care organizations, the process of clinician performance management and feedback exists on a small scale (periodic random selection and manual review of charts). Some practices (such as federally-funded community health centers) are required to submit structured quality measures to external agencies for review (e.g., the Health Disparities Collaboratives, public health agencies), and in many cases, this data abstraction is performed manually.

The use of electronic reporting tools that extract data electronically from records is generally restricted to large practices and organizations (that can afford them). As the health industry moves to pay for performance measures for remuneration of services,[48] the automated collection of data from EHRs will become increasingly desirable if not mandatory. Research also suggests that health IT-supported performance monitoring may improve adherence to clinical practice guidelines.[49] Such performance monitoring requires basic functionalities:

- Identification of patients to whom clinical practice guidelines apply
- Linkage of identified patients to clinicians responsible for their care
- Assurance that data integrity is sufficient for analysis
- Control of identification/de-identification of data
- Assimilation of relevant patient historical data
- Incorporation of additional measures
- Creation and dissemination of reports

Once these functions are realized, practices can derive performance measures to examine the appropriateness and impact of practice guidelines on their own practices.[18]

17.4.2.1 Identification of Patients to Whom Clinical Practice Guidelines Apply

With the increasing desire to use evidence-based clinical practice guidelines, and to comprehensively manage patients with chronic medical conditions through health IT (e.g., with automated reminder and recall systems, or with remote communication, monitoring and feedback systems), it is important to be able to easily identify patients which may benefit from these interventions.

Performance monitoring systems must be able to link guideline or intervention parameters to specific patient records. For example, if patients with asthma are to be prioritized for influenza vaccinations, it must be easy to find the patients in the practice with asthma. Such applications should also be able to be used to prospectively identify patients at risk for medical conditions. For example, all patients with a high body mass index and laboratory abnormalities may be identified for prospective diabetes screening. In current systems, the absence of linkages between administrative data (from a CPMS) and clinical data (from EHR systems) may make these tasks difficult.

17.4.2.2   Linkage of Identified Patients to Clinicians Responsible for Their Care

Identified at-risk patients (those eligible for guideline-based care) must be able to be linked to their primary care providers (PCPs). This linkage provides accountability for patient care and gives providers an incentive to be active in managing these patients. Performance measures are generally associated with individual providers or teams, which for pediatrics is the provider who manages the patient's well child visits (the PCP). Integrated performance measurement systems should support and give feedback on PCPs' management of chronic conditions by tracking patient visits and reminding providers of scheduled or overdue preventive care tasks.

17.4.2.3   Assurance That Data Integrity Is Sufficient for Analysis

Data from Health IT applications such as CPMS and clinical systems (EHR, laboratory, pathology, or imaging) may be collected and transmitted to regulatory or reporting systems (regional registries, data warehouses). For performance measurement and other analytical activities, this data must be of high integrity (trustworthiness and consistency). Data collected by manual data entry processes is often not suitable for analysis. If data is to be reused, it should be validated and/or normalized. For pediatric performance measures, this task may be more difficult than for adults because of the need to consider additional attributes – norms may be dependent on patient age, size, and/or maturity.

17.4.2.4   Control of Identification/De-Identification of Data

Performance measurement tools and systems must be able to maintain the one-to-one linkage between clinical data and its source, while de-identifying data for specific projects and reports.[50] Data de-identification should be accompanied by protocols and procedures for data access rights, for human subjects/institutional review (for research projects), for improving safety,[51] and for digital discovery and disclosure.[52]

17.4.2.5 Assimilation of Relevant Patient Historical Data

When a new EHR system is implemented, migration of historical clinical data (from paper or electronic formats) into the EHR system should be considered. This will allow patients to be correctly targeted for practice guidelines, and to be included when adherence to these guidelines is being evaluated. Some performance measures may require an accurate historical record (such as immunization histories or history of exposures to radiation, environmental, or chemotherapeutic agents). The assimilation of historical data may require time-intensive manual entry, so practices may need to prioritize which records are of greatest importance.

17.4.2.6 Incorporation of Additional Measures

As performance indicators evolve, including those for pay-for-performance, practices and measurement systems must be able to adapt to changes quickly and gracefully. EHRs and performance measurement systems need to be easily configurable, so that new data items can be created for collection. These items should be stored in formats which allow for ready retrieval and subsequent analysis.[53]

17.4.2.7 Creation and Dissemination of Reports

Clinical analytics,[54] the linkage of clinical and financial outcomes, involves using tools developed for business intelligence[55] to measure, then to optimize performance. *Dashboards*, visualizations which provide real-time data "at-a-glance," can be configured to track key clinical and performance indicators for the organization. The automated generation of these graphically summarized performance measures has been exploited in business, and prototypes have been developed for the clinical setting.[56,57]

17.5 Current Statistics and Observations on Ambulatory Health IT Adoption

In the United States, it is estimated that 29.2% of practices had electronic health record systems in 2006.[58] From a study in Florida, the overall pediatric ambulatory EHR adoption rate is estimated to be about 16%.[59] These adoption rates are far lower than those in the Netherlands (98%), New Zealand (92%), the U.K. (89%), and Australia (79%).[60,61]

Studies suggest that only 12.4% of U.S. practices (slightly more than a third of the self-reported EHR adoption rate) have adopted comprehensive EHR systems (defined by the IOM as systems which support e-Rx, computerized test ordering, online test results, and clinical notes[29]). Other countries also report lower rates of adoption for comprehensive systems. Reported rates include: New Zealand (33%), Australia (10%), the U.K. (5%), Germany (4%), Canada (2%), and the Netherlands (1%).[61,62]

During the first 6 months after deployment of an ambulatory EHR, most practices report decreases in the number of patients seen while providers ramp up on the system. In one study,[17] one practice reported almost 18 months before productivity with the new system returned to normal. Larger practices may choose to migrate to the EHR in small subgroups of physicians, to minimize productivity loss.[18]

Smaller practices represent a significant portion of community (and pediatric) practices.[63] The self-reported EHR adoption rate across solo practices was about 14% in 2003,[64] which is a much lower rate than for their larger counterparts.[58,63] Small practices face much greater individual risks when they do adopt EHRs, including a higher cost per full-time physician,[65] and a higher impact of income loss per clinician during initial deployment – which magnifies risks of failure, frustration and stress.

Perceived barriers to adopting EHRs are many, including financial costs, expertise (hardware, software, IT), training and maintenance needs, and loss of income during deployment. These barriers are compounded by uncertainty about data becoming unavailable if a vendor goes out of business.[65] In response to this, collective efforts to reduce these uncertainties have been launched.

- To reduce the risk in purchasing a system, a recognized certification body (CCHIT, the Certification Commission for Healthcare Information Technology[66]) provides certification of EHR products, but does not reduce the cost, which may be several thousand dollars per provider.[67] More certified products are providing pediatric-related features (such as weight based dosing, preventive care reminders, and growth charts), and CCHIT is in the process of developing a pediatric-specific certification for EHR products to accelerate this process.
- To allow pediatricians to "compare notes" on specific pediatric EHR products, the American Academy of Pediatrics Council on Clinical Information Technology (COCIT) has established an Electronic Medical Record Review Website,[68] a free online resource for pediatricians to share their experiences concerning EHR products and vendors.

17.6 Conclusion

In the ambulatory setting, health IT adoption is increasingly being driven by the desire for decreased cost, increased quality with respect to performance measures, and increased clinical productivity. These aims are in their early stages of realization, as EHR adoption rates are low in pediatric ambulatory settings, especially in the setting of small practices. Adoption is a complex process, with initial and ongoing financial, organizational, and technical investments required; and the potential for revenue loss during deployment. The strategy of adopting health IT solutions with low impact on clinicians' workflow but high returns first may prove to be a useful strategy towards the eventual widespread implementation of comprehensive EHR systems.

17.7 Case Study: Implementing ACPOE at Seattle Children's Hospital

17.7.1 Background

Seattle Children's Hospital is a 250-bed pediatric hospital located in the idyllic setting of the Pacific Northwest in Seattle, Washington. The hospital is the primary pediatric teaching site for the University of Washington School of Medicine, and serves as both the tertiary care referral hospital to a four-state region as well as the primary pediatric hospital for the Puget Sound area. Children's subspecialists also see patients in the ambulatory setting (170,000 visits annually).

The organization decided in the early 1990s not to pursue a multi-vendor best-of-breed approach, and sought instead to use a single vendor solution to meet all clinical information needs. Over a single weekend in November, 2003, inpatient CPOE had been implemented with support for laboratory, radiology, nursing and ancillary department (e.g., speech, physical therapy) orders. By the time of the planning stages for ambulatory CPOE, the laboratory results review system, pharmacy, radiology, and pathology systems had all been replaced by this vendor's solutions. In the ambulatory clinics, e-Rx was in place, with all non-chemotherapeutic medications being written in the clinical information system and charted electronically when given, with dose-range checking.

A summary of electronic capabilities of these clinics, in 2003, can be found in Table 17.5.

17.7.2 Pre-implementation

In the ambulatory clinics prior to ACPOE, there was a strong culture of informality. Providers would stop staff in the hallway, with a simple "Hey, can you get this for me?" and verbally communicate orders, which would be checked off or written on

Table 17.5 Seattle Children's Hospital ambulatory information infrastructure in 2003

Information function	2003 capability
Orders, results, and results management	Clinicians could receive online results for ordered tests
Intra-clinic communication	Providers and clinic staff communicate with e-mail, notes dictated
Patient education and outreach	Patients handed paper-based instructions
Inter-clinic coordination	Paper records
Medication management	Online drug reference
	e-Rx with some dose-range checking
Provider education and feedback	Web site links, online clinic policy manuals
	Handheld reference materials, some online training

a lab requisition form. These lab requisitions would sometimes exhibit the usual problems with handwritten documents: abbreviations, illegible entries, and missing or illegible signatures. There was no guarantee of clinical consistency (e.g., if a patient presented with a diagnosis, different providers could easily take many different approaches). Also, different subspecialty clinics approached ordering with differing work patterns.

Given the state of affairs, it became clear that ACPOE would force the entire process of ordering in the ambulatory clinics to be significantly redesigned. To help focus this redesign, the organization explored project justifications (e.g., "Why ACPOE?"). There were four specific reasons: compliance, patient safety, workflow, and revenue. The first two deal with the Institute of Medicine's philosophies and strategies to transform health care and reduce medical errors while the latter two address institution specific needs and goals (Table 17.6).

Given the significant CPOE infrastructure present available from the previous inpatient CPOE implementation, the decision was made for ambulatory CPOE to be far reaching and all inclusive from the very start. All staff members were required to use the new system, except two practitioners in their eighties.

17.7.3 Organizational Features

The ACPOE project was sponsored by the hospital leadership, and fully funded. This executive support was so prominent that during the critical periods in the project, all ACPOE-related meetings had priority, ensuring that staff would be available as needed.

Communication of ACPOE decision making started almost 1 year prior to the targeted implementation date, and increased throughout the year internally and even externally. As the implementation date neared, regular project meetings occurred with more frequency and included the Chief Operating Officer, Vice President of Ambulatory Services, Chief Information Officer, Chief Medical Information Officer, Medical Director, Nursing Director, Director of Clinical Information Services, the project sponsors and other key project team members. These meetings ensured that the appropriate people were available to make time-critical decisions, keeping the project both on time and on track. These decisions, as well as other important project related details, were presented at regularly scheduled

Table 17.6 Justifications for ambulatory CPOE implementation

Compliance	Joint Commission requirements for legibility, and for staff not to use unapproved abbreviations
Patient safety	Automation improves accuracy of which labs are drawn on which patient
Workflow	Providing point-of-care reference to consensus best practice makes it efficient to provide this care
Revenue	Automated system can reinforce correct billing practice leading to improved collection of payment

director-level meetings throughout the organization. This massive coordinated effort would not have been possible without the support provided by the hospital leaders.

In addition to hospital leadership, there was significant investment by the clinical divisions and staff. Prior to go-live, 100 ambulatory CPOE super-users were identified, with a broad representation of at least one physician, nurse, medical assistant, and ancillary staff member for every clinic. These individuals were involved with writing testing and training scenarios, conducting local site training as needed, and with providing support during and after go-live.

17.7.4 Design of Clinical Content

Concurrent with important process- and system-related decisions being made, two informatics physicians led an effort to design the order sets. A multistep development process was employed to design, build, test, and implement order sets (Table 17.7).

The first step of the process involved determining the current state and identifying key departmental clinician champions. As ACPOE was a hospital priority, these clinicians enjoyed the strong support of their departments. In the next step, institutional order set standards were defined, with a basic order template being created. This template was then sent to the clinician champions, in conjunction with a list of the "top ten" diagnoses seen in their specialty area and instructions for how to create the desired specialty-specific order sets. Clinicians were asked to use evidence-based standards where available, and otherwise to send consensus-based recommendations from their department.

Once received, the informatics physicians converted the content into a standard format. The clinical content of the order sets then underwent a multidisciplinary review with representatives from pharmacy, laboratory, radiology, nurses, and medicine. The revised order sets were sent back to the originating departments for a final signoff, and the order sets were then incorporated into the test system. After testing and additional user feedback, the order sets were fine-tuned prior to go-live.

Table 17.7 Order set development and deployment process

1. Define organizational order set standards, create basic template
2. Review current state of clinic orders, top ten diagnoses
3. Identify clinical champions (physicians) in each division
4. Send information collected in #2 to departments via clinical champions and collect proposed order sets
5. Multidisciplinary review of order sets
6. Finalize order sets and obtain divisional sign-off
7. Incorporate order sets into testing environment, test order sets
8. Refine order sets based on testing and feedback
9. Train users
10. Go-live with order sets and continually refine based on user feedback

17.7.5   Support and Training Infrastructure

A computer-based training program was created, as well as a required formal classroom training curriculum. Training took place in multiple 4-h instructor-led training sessions over a 6 week period. Physicians, nurses, medical assistants, and front desk staff were scheduled to be in classes by clinic, promoting multidisciplinary team building. Instruction covered both the system and the new processes needed to support it.

During go-live the project team was available around the clock. This high level of support ensured that end users would be able to care for their patients with minimal inconvenience. Go-live team members included clinicians, system analysts (both internal and vendor-provided), and project and hospital leadership. Divisional super-users assisted with the initial training, and continued to provide ongoing support after go-live.

17.7.6   Results

- Successful construction and deployment of several hundred disease- and specialty-specific order sets to help facilitate efficient, consistent, and consensus/ evidence based practice
- Clinical decision support provided, including pediatric-appropriate alerts and dose range checking
- Over 1,000 users successfully trained and using the system
- All orders including future visit orders and order management between clinic visits were online and available for any user to see

17.7.7   Lessons Learned

- Training, communication, and organizational support to shepherd the culture change were critical to the success of this project.
- The most difficult aspect of the project was developing standards and consistencies within the organization from nonstandardized ambulatory processes, which differed between clinics. Health IT systems do not handle ambiguity well and cannot be relied upon to correct broken or inconsistent processes. ACPOE helped to stimulate discussion and planning towards standardizing best practices at Children's.
- Ambulatory care by definition occurs in fragmented intervals over time, and this episodic care formed the basis of the system's data models. However, patients live and take actions in-between these episodes. Providers need a system that supports patients whenever they need care (e.g., lab draws between visits).

- As one of the first institutions to use the vendor's order set creation scheme, the order set development tools required refinement; and resultant order sets produced by these tools required extensive testing.
- Making information electronic increases its transparency. Being able to view care plans made by other subspecialists helped to streamline labs and make potential incompatibilities more apparent. The automatic generation of a clinic visit summary with patient instructions for families has also helped this process.
- It is possible to successfully implement CPOE in the ambulatory setting. Having a well structured project team, with a clearly defined escalation path to the hospital leadership, is essential. Despite challenges, frustrations, and at times, setbacks, keeping focused on priorities and guiding principles can lead to success.

Acknowledgements The authors would like to thank the Robert Wood Johnson Clinical Scholars Program at Yale University and our employers for supporting our time. We would like to acknowledge Dr. Richard Shiffman for his review and constructive feedback on early drafts, and Dr. Mark Del Beccaro for his careful review and comments on the case study. We would like to thank our families for their ongoing support.

References

1. Grimshaw JM, Russell IT. Effect of clinical guidelines on medical practice: a systematic review of rigorous evaluations. *Lancet*. 1993;342:1317–1322.
2. Institute of Medicine. *To Err is Human: Building a Safer Health System*. Washington, DC: National Academies Press; 2000.
3. McGlynn EA, Asch SM, Adams J, et al. The quality of health care delivered to adults in the United States. *N Engl J Med*. 2003;348:2635–2645.
4. Mangione-Smith R, DeCristofaro AH, Setodji CM, et al. The quality of ambulatory care delivered to children in the United States. *N Engl J Med*. 357:1515–1523.
5. Wennberg JE, Fisher ES, eds. The Care of Patients with Severe Chronic Illness: A Report on the Medicare Program by the Dartmouth Atlas Project. The Center for the Evaluative Clinical Sciences, Dartmouth Atlas Project, Hanover, New Hampshire; 2006. Available at: http://www.dartmouthatlas.org. Accessed December 20, 2008.
6. Institute of Medicine. *Crossing the Quality Chasm: A New Health System for the 21st Century*. Washington, DC: National Academies Press; 2001.
7. Berwick DM. A user's manual for the IOM's 'Quality Chasm' report. *Health Aff*. 2002;21:80–90.
8. Provnost PJ, Berenholtz SM, Goeschel CA, et al. Creating high reliability in health care organizations. *Health Serv Res*. 2006;41:1599–1617.
9. Cherry DK, Woodwell DA, Rechtsteiner EA. *National Ambulatory Medical Care Survey: 2005 Summary*. Advance Data from Vital and Health Statistics; No. 387. Hyattsville, MD: National Center for Health Statistics; 2007.
10. Lieu TA, Capra AM, Makol J, et al. Effectiveness and cost-effectiveness of letters, automated telephone messages, or both for underimmunized children in a health maintenance organization. *Pediatrics*. 1998;101:e3.
11. Sia C, Tonniges TF, Osterhus E, Taba S. History of the medical home concept. *Pediatrics*. 2004;113:1473–1478.
12. Wagner EH. Chronic disease management: what will it take to improve care for chronic illness? *Eff Clin Pract*. 1998;1:2–4.

13. Barr M, Ginsburg J. The advanced medical home: a patient-centered, physician-guided model of health care. *A Policy Monograph*. Philadelphia, PA: American College of Physicians; 2006.
14. Hillestad R, Biegelow J, Bower A, et al. Can electronic medical record systems transform health care? Potential health benefits, savings, and costs. *Health Aff*. 2005;24:1103–1117.
15. Joos D, Chen Q, Jirjis J, Johnson KB. An electronic medical record in primary care: impact on satisfaction, work efficiency and clinic processes. *AMIA Annu Symp Proc*. 2006;394–398.
16. Wang SJ, Middleton B, Prosser LA, et al. A cost-benefit analysis of electronic medical records in primary care. *Am J Med*. 2003;114:397–403.
17. Miller RH, West C, Brown TM, et al. The value of electronic health records in solo or small group practices. *Health Aff*. 2005;24:1127–1137.
18. Leu MG, Cheung M, Webster TR, et al. Centers speak up: the clinical context for health information technology in the ambulatory care setting. *J Gen Intern Med*. 2008;23:372–378.
19. Cisco SL, Wertzberger J. Indexing Digital Documents – It's NOT an Option. Pay Now or Pay (More) Later. *Inform*. 1997;11(2):12–20.
20. Grieger DL, Cohen SH, Krusch DA. A pilot study to document the return on investment for implementing an ambulatory electronic health record at an academic medical center. *J Am Coll Surg*. 2007;205:89–96.
21. Healthcare Reports. Traditional In-House Document Imaging Implementation Costs; 2006. Available at: http://www.healthcarereports.com/di-costsdetail.htm. Accessed December 21, 2008.
22. Biondich PG, Downs SM, Anand V, Carroll AE. Automating the recognition and prioritization of needed preventive services: early results from the CHICA system. *AMIA Annu Symp Proc*. 2005;51–55.
23. Gerstle RS, Lehmann CU. AAP Council on Clinical Information Technology. Electronic prescribing systems in pediatrics: the rationale and functionality requirements. *Pediatrics*. 2007;119: e1413–1422.
24. Marcus E. E-prescribing can add quality, safety to patient care. *AAP News*. 2005;26:15.
25. Gerstle RS. Practices should seriously consider e-prescribing systems. *AAP News*. 2007;28:33.
26. McPhillips HA, Stille CJ, Smith D, et al. Potential medication dosing errors in outpatient pediatrics. *J Pediatr*. 2005;147:761–767.
27. Sittig DF, Stead WW. Computer-based physician order entry: the state of the art. *J Am Med Inform Assoc*. 1994;1:108–123.
28. Johnston D, Pan E, Walker J. The value of CPOE in ambulatory settings. *J Healthcare Inf Manage*. 2003;18(1):5–8. Available at: http://www.himss.org/content/files/ambulatorydocs/ValueOfCPOEInAmbulatorySettings.pdf. Accessed 21 December 2008.
29. Institute of Medicine. Key Capabilities of an Electronic Health Record System: Letter Report. Washington, DC: National Academies Press; 2003. Available at: http://www.nap.edu/catalog.php?record_id=10781. Accessed December 21, 2008.
30. Sanfelippo ML, Walker WE, Hall DA, Swenson RS. Clinical application of a single compartment model to urea and creatinine kinetics in dialysis therapy. *Comput Programs Biomed*. 1978;8:44–50.
31. Lehmann CU, Conner KG, Cox JM. Preventing provider errors: online total parenteral nutrition calculator. *Pediatrics*. 2004;113:748–753.
32. Centers for Disease Control. Other Growth Chart Resources. Available at: http://www.cdc.gov/nccdphp/dnpa/growthcharts/resources/index.htm#BMI. Accessed December 21, 2008.
33. Stockwell DC. Pediatrics on hand; 2008. Available at: http://www.childrensnational.org/pdas. Accessed December 21, 2008.
34. Linder JA, Ma J, Bates DW, Middleton B, Stafford RS. Electronic health record use and the quality of ambulatory care in the United States. *Arch Intern Med*. 2007;167:1400–1405.
35. Scott IU, Feuer WJ, Jacko JA. Impact of graphical user interface screen features on computer task accuracy and speed in a cohort of patients with age-related macular degeneration. *Am J Ophthalmol*. 2002;134:857–862.

36. Microsoft Corporation. Microsoft Health Common User Interface; 2007. Available at: http://www.mscui.org/. Accessed December 21, 2008.
37. Department of Health and Human Services. Office for Civil Rights – HIPAA; 2008. Available at: http://www.hhs.gov/ocr/hipaa/. Accessed December 21, 2008.
38. Sciamanna CN, Rogers ML, Shenassa ED, et al. Patient access to U.S. physicians who conduct internet or E-mail consults. *J Gen Intern Med.* 2007;22:378–381.
39. Stone JH. Communication between physicians and patients in the era of e-medicine. *N Engl J Med.* 2007;356:2451–2454.
40. Anand SG, Feldman MJ, Geller DS, et al. A content analysis of e-mail communications between primary care providers and parents. *Pediatrics.* 2005;115:1283–1288.
41. Kane B, Sands DZ. AMIA Internet Working Group. Guidelines for the clinical use of electronic mail with patients. *J Am Med Inf Assoc.* 1998;5:104–111.
42. Liederman EM, Lee JC, Baquery VH, et al. Patient-physician web messaging: the impact on message volume and satisfaction. *J Gen Intern Med.* 2005;20:52–57.
43. Wagner EH, Austin BT, Davis C, Hindmarsh M, Schaefer J, Bonomi A. Improving chronic illness care: translating evidence into action. *Health Aff.* 2001;20:64–78.
44. Lorig KR, Ritter PL, Laurent DD, Plant K. Internet-based chronic disease self-management: a randomized trial. *Med Care.* 2006;44:964–971.
45. Leu MG, Norris TE, Hummel J, Isaac M, Brogan MW. A randomized, controlled trial of an automated wireless messaging system for diabetes. *Diabetes Technol Ther.* 2005;7:710–718.
46. Logan AG, McIsaac WJ, Tisler A, et al. Mobile phone-based remote patient monitoring system for management of hypertension in diabetic patients. *Am J Hypertens.* 2007;20:942–948.
47. Bu D, Pan E, Johnston D, et al. The Value of Information Technology-Enabled Diabetes Management. Center for Information Technology Leadership. Charlestown, MA; 2007.
48. Rosenthal MB, Dudley RA. Pay-for-performance: will the latest payment trend improve care? *JAMA.* 2007;297:740–744.
49. Landon BE, Hicks LS, O'Malley AJ, et al. Improving the management of chronic disease at community health centers. *N Engl J Med.* 2007;356:921–934.
50. Agrawal R, Johnson C. Securing electronic health records without impeding the flow of information. *Int J Med Inform.* 2007;76:471–479.
51. Grzybicki DM, Turcsanyi B, Becich MJ, Gupta D, Gilbertson JR, Raab SS. Database construction for improving patient safety by examining pathology errors. *Am J Clin Pathol.* 2005;124:500–509.
52. Dimick C. E-discovery: preparing for the coming rise in electronic discovery requests. *J AHIMA.* 2007;78:24–29.
53. Chen R, Enberg G, Klein GO. Julius–a template based supplementary electronic health record system. *BMC Med Inf Decis Mak.* 2007;7:10.
54. Hammarstedt R, Bulger D. Performance improvement: a "left brain meets right brain" approach. *Healthcare Financ Manage.* 2006;60:100–4, 106.
55. Luhn HP. A business intelligence system. *IBM J.* 1958;2:314–319.
56. Olsha-Yehiav M, Einbinder JS, Jung E, et al. Quality dashboards: technical and architectural considerations of an actionable reporting tool for population management. *AMIA Annu Symp Proc.* 2006;1052.
57. Jung E, Li Q, Mangalampalli A, et al. Report central: quality reporting tool in an electronic health record. *AMIA Annu Symp Proc.* 2006;971.
58. Hing ES, Burt CW, Woodwell DA. Electronic medical record use by office-based physicians and their practices: United States, 2006. Advance Data from Vital and Health Statistics; No. 393. Hyattsville, Maryland, MD: National Center for Health Statistics; 2007.
59. Menachemi N, Ettel DL, Brooks RG, Simpson L. Charting the use of electronic health records and other information technologies among child health providers. *BMC Pediatr.* 2006;6:21.
60. McInnes DK, Saltman DC, Kidd MR. General practitioners' use of computers for prescribing and electronic health records. *Med J Aust.* 2006;185:88–91.
61. Schoen C, Osborn R, Huynh PT, Doty M, Peugh J, Zapert K. On the front lines of care: primary care doctors' office systems, experiences, and views in seven countries. *Health Aff.* 2006;25:w555–w571.

62. Jha AK, Ferris TG, Donelan K, et al. How common are electronic health records in the United States? A summary of the evidence. *Health Aff.* 2006;25:w496–w507.
63. Simon SR, Kaushal R, Cleary PD, et al. Correlates of electronic health record adoption in office practices: a statewide survey. *J Am Med Inf Assoc.* 2007;14:110–117.
64. Audet AM, Doty MM, Peugh J, Shamasdin J, Zapert K, Schoenbaum S. Information technologies: when will they make it into physicians' black bags? *MedGenMed.* 2004;6:2.
65. Bates DW. Physicians and ambulatory electronic health records. *Health Aff.* 2005; 24:1180–1189.
66. Certification Committee on Healthcare Information Technology. CCHIT Website; 2008. Available at: http://www.cchit.org/. Accessed December 21, 2008.
67. American Academy of Family Physicians Center for Health Information Technology. Partners for patients electronic health record market survey; 2005. Available at: http://www.center forhit.org/PreBuilt/chit_2005p4pvendsurv.pdf. Accessed December 21, 2008.
68. American Academy of Pediatrics Council on Clinical Information Technology. EMR Review Project Website; 2006. Available at: http://www.aapcocit.org/emr/. Accessed December 21, 2008.

Chapter 18
Electronic Health Records and Interoperability for Pediatric Care

George R. Kim and Christoph U. Lehmann

Objectives

- To state working definitions for electronic health records (EHRs), electronic health record systems (EHR-S) and interoperability
- To provide a brief overview of current efforts to define pediatric health data needs to guide EHR and EHR-S development
- To provide linkages to current information resources on pediatric EHRs

18.1 Introduction

Electronic health records (EHRs) are a central structure in the improvement of the quality and safety of medical care. Set as a national goal for 2014,[1] universal adoption of EHRs has been cited as a chief pathway by which medical errors can be reduced and costs saved.

18.2 Definitions

18.2.1 Electronic Health Records (EHR)

An EHR, in its "basic generic" form, is defined as "a repository of information regarding the health status of a subject of care [a patient], in computer processable form." Historical, regional and contextual variants which refer to the same or related concepts include:

- Electronic medical record (EMR), used in North America and Japan, to include patient-focused clinical information (from ONE functional medical unit, such as a hospital, clinical department)[2] EMR is described as interchangeable with EHR (but is regarded as an outdated term by many)

C.U. Lehmann et al. (eds.), *Pediatric Informatics: Computer Applications in Child Health,* Health Informatics,
© Springer Science+Business Media, LLC 2011

- Electronic patient record (EPR), used by the English National Health Service (NHS) as "an electronic record of periodic health care of a single individual, provided mainly by one institution,"[3] typically by acute care hospitals or specialist units
- Computerized Patient Record (CPR) used in the US to denote either EMR or EPR[4]
- Personal Health Record (PHR) used to describe a longitudinal record of health and wellness information for an individual patient that is under the control of the patient (Chapter 21)

EHRs may be classified according to their ability to share information: to exchange information with other systems (functional interoperability) that is understandable (semantic interoperability) within a formally defined domain. Shareable (as opposed to standalone or non-shareable) EHRs facilitate longitudinal and integrated coordination of multidisciplinary team care of patients over time and assure ubiquitous availability of information.

A modification of the "basic generic" definition of an EHR for use in integrated care (ICEHR) is "a repository of information regarding the health of a subject of care in computer processable form, stored and transmitted securely, and accessible by multiple authorized users. The ICEHR has a standardized information model which is independent of EHR systems. Its primary purpose is the support of continuing, efficient and quality integrated healthcare and it contains information which is retrospective, concurrent and prospective."[4]

An EHR may also be described in term of its scope. A Core EHR "concerns a single subject of care [patient], has as its primary purpose the support of present and future health care of the subject, and is principally concerned with clinical information," while an Extended EHR concerns all health information: including administration (scheduling, billing, demographics, insurance, and payer information), practice management (health professional service/business operations recording, querying, and analysis and resource allocations), clinical knowledge infrastructure (decision support, guidelines, terminology, order management, population health recording) and information assurance (access control and policy management). The Core EHR is a subset of the Extended EHR and both may form the basis of a comprehensive health information system.[4]

18.2.2   Electronic Health Record Systems (EHR-S)

EHR systems (EHR-S) are defined as "the set of components that form the mechanism by which EHRs are created, used (accessed, edited, and amended), stored and retrieved... including people, data, rules and procedures, processing and storage devices, and communication and support facilities"[5] or as "a system for recording, retrieving, and manipulating information in EHRs."[6] "Critical building blocks of an EHR-S are the electronic health records (EHR) maintained by providers (e.g., hospitals, nursing homes, ambulatory health care settings such as physician offices) and by individual patients (the last also called personal health records (PHRs))."[7]

EHR-S functionalities include:

1. Longitudinal collection of electronic health information for and about persons, where health information is defined as information pertaining to the medical and psychiatric health and wellness status of an individual or to care provided to an individual
2. Immediate electronic access to person- and population-level information by authorized, and only authorized, users
3. Ability to provide access to the same information in multiple physical locations
4. Provision of knowledge and decision-support that enhance the quality, safety, and efficiency of patient care and
5. Support of efficient processes for health care delivery and administrative tasks[7]

The EHR-S Functional Model (EHR-S FM) developed by Health Level Seven divides EHR-S functions (from a user's perspective) into three groups: direct care, supportive, and information infrastructures (Fig. 18.1).[8] "Functional profiles" are functions selected from the reference list that are applicable for a particular purpose (user, care setting, domain, or other criteria) and may apply to a given EHR-S.

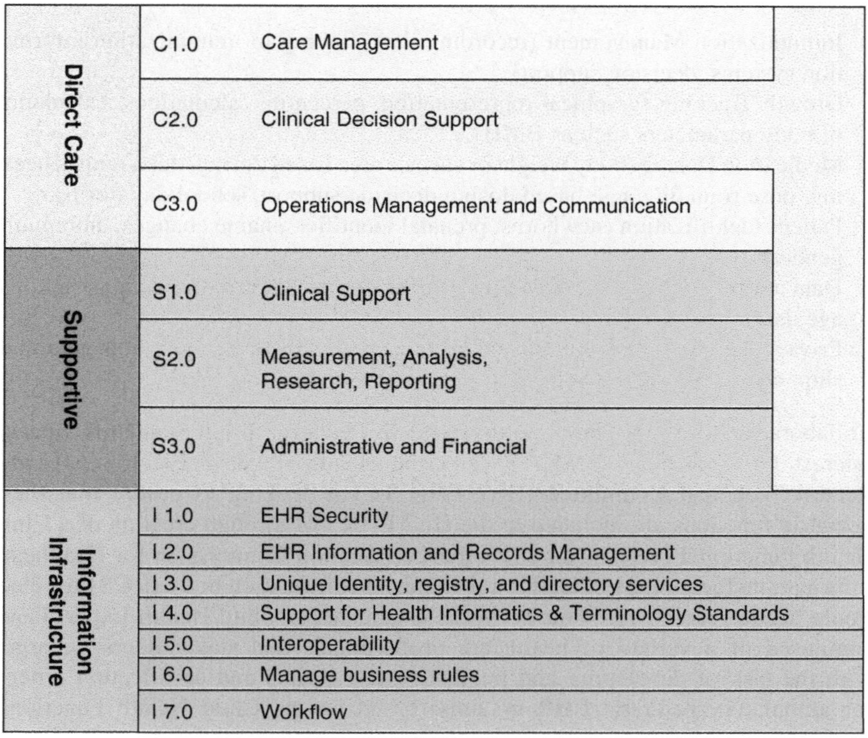

Direct Care	C1.0	Care Management
	C2.0	Clinical Decision Support
	C3.0	Operations Management and Communication
Supportive	S1.0	Clinical Support
	S2.0	Measurement, Analysis, Research, Reporting
	S3.0	Administrative and Financial
Information Infrastructure	I 1.0	EHR Security
	I 2.0	EHR Information and Records Management
	I 3.0	Unique Identity, registry, and directory services
	I 4.0	Support for Health Informatics & Terminology Standards
	I 5.0	Interoperability
	I 6.0	Manage business rules
	I 7.0	Workflow

Fig. 18.1 The Electronic Health Record System Functional Model (EHR-S FM)

18.2.3 Interoperability

Beyond shareability, "interoperability of healthcare information (in the form of data and records [stored in an EHR])" has three primary aspects: technical (assurance of structure, syntax, and reliable communication), semantic (preservation of full meaning) and process (integration to health care delivery process and work flow).[9] An EHR interoperability model (EHR-IM) also in development by HL7 is complementary to the HL7 EHR-S FM in describing specific profiles.

18.3 Pediatric Aspects

18.3.1 Functionality Needs

Critical pediatric "direct care" functionality areas for EHR-S have been described in a policy statement by the American Academy of Pediatrics[10] and include special functionalities (among others) for:

- Immunization Management (recording data, linking to immunization information systems, decision support)
- Growth Tracking (graphical representation, percentile calculations, calculation of body parameters such as BMI)
- Medication Dosing (body weight or surface area based dosing, dose-range checking, dose rounding, age-based dosing decision support, school day dosing)
- Patient Identification (newborns, prenatal identifiers, name changes, ambiguous gender)
- Data norms (numeric and nonnumeric data, complex normative data, gestational age data)
- Privacy (adolescents, foster/custodial care, consent by proxy, adoption, guardianship, emergent care, Chapter 22)

Collaborative work by the Health Level 7 Pediatric Data Standards Special Interest Group (HL7 PeDSSIG)[11] and the Health Level 7 Electronic Health Record Technical Committee (HL7 EHR TC) is seeking to ensure that these pediatric functions are included in the HL7 EHR FM through creation of a Child Health Functional Profile.[12] In 2007, the Certification Commission for Healthcare Information Technology (CCHIT, a recognized certification body (RCB) for electronic health records and their networks established a Child Health Expert Panel composed of a variety of healthcare professionals and stakeholders[13] charged with the task of developing and publishing test scripts and certification criteria for ambulatory pediatric EHR systems (based on the Child Health Functional Profile).[12]

18.3.2   Interface Needs

Pediatric EHRs may require interfaces to other information systems to share information needs. These include:

- Ambulatory EHRs to:
  - Practice management and billing systems
  - Public health agencies (Immunization information systems, newborn screening registries, regional health information networks)[14]
  - Inpatient hospital discharge records, including newborn discharges
  - Pharmacy, laboratory and imaging information systems
  - Patient portals and personal health records
  - Foster care and guardianship programs
  - School health record systems
- Hospital and Emergency Department EHRs to:
  - Maternal records for prenatal data, including prenatal screening and diagnoses, genomic data, risk factors, and in-utero procedures
  - State newborn screening registries and programs
  - Ambulatory (Medical Home) EHRs for follow up care
  - Long-term care facility EHRs for convalescent care
  - Specialty care and research programs
  - Breast milk banking programs
  - Error reporting systems
- Pediatric specialty EHRs to:
  - Biological resource registries (cord blood and tissue registries, organ banks)
  - Clinical trial databanks
  - Emergency medical services for children
  - Injury, poisoning, and other reporting registries

A practical articulation of both functionality and interface needs for a primary care practitioner's office may include a mix of functions and interfaces including telephone systems.[15]

18.3.3   Other Interoperability Needs

Beyond functional and interface needs, there is a need to develop standards that adequately and accurately represent pediatric entities and events (when communicating in electronic environments) with the appropriate concepts, to the appropriate granularity or level of detail and in the correct context in a form that can be encoded for use in computerized environments. Many current content standards lack this pediatric focus.[10] Considerations for data and terminology standards for pediatrics are covered in Chapters 32 and 33.

There is also a need for standard structures in which to package information for clinical use. These standards specify the order and attributes of data as they are to be specified when sending messages that represent specific entities. Perhaps the most visible effort at common standards by physician organizations in this regard has been in the creation of a standard for the ASTM's Continuity of Care Record (CCR). See Case Study.

18.4 Conclusion

At present, only about 20% of pediatricians use an EHR.[16] Technical barriers to pediatric adoption of EHRs have included the lack of definition of pediatric functionalities required of EHR systems as well as a lack of standards for EHR interoperability.[26] However, work in these areas is progressing with increasing participation of child health professionals in organized and academic medicine to define these standards (in cooperation with standards development organizations) and their place in certifying products that meet the needs of the pediatric workplace. A major challenge to academic pediatrics is to prove that data standards can lead to improved health outcomes for children.

18.5 Case Study: The Evolution of an EHR Standard – CCR/CDA to CCD

The Continuity of Care Record (CCR, "Specification for Continuity of Care Record, E2369-05"[17]) is an American National Standards Institute (ANSI[18])-accredited health information technology standard developed and maintained by volunteers from both health care and technology professions, under the auspices of the American Society for Testing and Materials (ASTM International, the world's largest standards development organization (SDO)). Development began in August, 2003, and the standard was published in January, 2006.[19]

The purpose of the CCR standard was/is to make it possible for a digital summary of relevant administrative and clinical health information about an individual to be created, stored, and passed from one computer system in a standardized electronic format. The problem that the CCR standard was developed to address is the pervasive lack of interoperability standards among health care computer software (including electronic health record systems). The CCR gained the sponsorship and endorsements of a number of professional organizations, including the American Academy of Pediatrics.[20]

However, the development of a Clinical Document Architecture (CDA) by Health Level Seven (also an ANSI-certified standard first released in 2000[21] and updated in 2005[22]) posed a problem of two standards for the same purpose that were not interoperable. Although there were distinctions (The CCR was not a complete record as was the CDA and the intended uses ("use cases") for the two formats differed), what ensued was a critical analysis to determine the problems with interoperability of the two standards.[23] Collaboration between HL7 and ASTM led to a mapping between the two standards that preserved interoperability[24] to create a new harmonized standard: the Continuity of Care Document (CCD)[25] that was accepted by both organizations with the endorsement of the Healthcare Information Technology Standards Panel (HITSP), a volunteer group created in 2005 by the Office of the National Coordinator for Health Information Technology (part of the US Department of Health and Human Services) to promote interoperability in healthcare by harmonizing health information technology standards.

Acknowledgment Acknowledgement and thanks are given to S. Andrew Spooner, on whose efforts much of the content of this chapter is based, for providing comments and review.

References

1. Bush GW. *State of the Union Address.* Washington, DC: US Capitol; 20 Jan. 2004.
2. Japanese Association of Healthcare Information Systems. Classification of EMR systems. *JAHIS*; 1996;V1.1.
3. NHS Executive. Information for Health: An Information Strategy for the Modern NHS 1998–2005; 2005.
4. International Standards Organization. Health Informatics – Electronic Health Record – Definition, scope and context. ISO/TR 20514:2005(E).
5. Dick R, Steen E. The computer-based patient record: an essential technology for health care. US National Academy of Sciences, Institute of Medicine.
6. Committee European Normalisation Health Informatics Technical Committee. Health Informatics – Electronic healthcare record communication – Part 1: Extended architecture. ENV13606–1, CEN/TC 251; 2000.
7. Institute of Medicine. *Key Capabilities of an Electronic Health Record System: Letter Report.* Washington, DC: National Academies Press; 2003. Available at: http://www.nap.edu/catalog. php?record_id=10781. Accessed December 21, 2008.
8. Health Level 7 Electronic Health Record Technical Committee (HL7 EHR TC). Electronic Health Record-System Functional Model, Release 1, February 2007. Available at: http://www. hl7.org/ehr/downloads/index_2007.asp. Accessed December 21, 2008.
9. Health Level 7 Electronic Health Record Technical Committee (HL7 EHR TC). EHR Interoperability Model with EHR Data Exchange Criteria: Draft Standard for Trial Use, Release 1, February 2007. Available at: http://www.hl7.org/ehr/downloads/index_2007.asp. Accessed December 21, 2008.
10. Spooner SA, Council on Clinical Information Technology, American Academy of Pediatrics. Special requirements of electronic health record systems in pediatrics. *Pediatrics.* 2007;119(3):631–637.
11. Health Level Seven Pediatric Data Standards Special Interest Group (PeDSSIG). HL7 Child Health; 2008. Available at: http://www.hl7.org/Special/committees/pedsdata. Accessed December 21, 2008.
12. Health Level Seven Child Health Functional Profile Workgroup Pediatric Data Standards Special Interest Group (PeDSSIG). Health Level Seven. Child Health Functional Profile, Final Version 1.0. National Institute of Standards and Technology. Functional Profile Registry; 2007. Available at: http://xreg2.nist.gov:8080/ehrsRegistry/faces/view/detailFunctionalProfile. jsp?id=urn:uuid:6f4d2971-e61f-458d-8aa8-878d6c9dea06. Accessed December 21, 2008.

13. Child Health Expert Panel, Certification Commission for Healthcare Information Technology (CCHIT). Child Health Expert Panel Website; 2008. Available at: http://www.cchit.org/childhealth/. Accessed December 21, 2008.
14. Orlova AO, Dunnagan M, Finitzo T, et al. Electronic health record - public health (EHR-PH) system prototype for interoperability in 21st century healthcare systems. *AMIA Annu Symp Proc*. 2005;575–579.
15. Simonian M. The electronic medical record. *Pediatr Rev*. 2007;28(10):e69–76.
16. Kemper AR, Uren RL, Clark SJ. Adoption of electronic health records in primary care pediatric practices. *Pediatrics*. 2006;118(1):e20–24.
17. ASTM International. E2369-05 Standard Specification for Continuity of Care Record (CCR). ASTM International, West Conshohocken, PA; 2007. Available at: http://enterprise.astm.org/REDLINE_PAGES/E2369.htm. Accessed December 21, 2008.
18. American National Standards Institute. ANSI Website; 2008. Available at: http://www.ansi.org/. Accessed December 21, 2008.
19. Kibbe DC. The ASTM Continuity of Care Record, CCR, Standard: A Brief Description for a Non-Technical Audience. Continuity of Care Standard Resource Site; 2007. Available at: http://www.ccrstandard.com/TheASTMCCRdefinition2.pdf. Accessed December 21, 2008.
20. Schneider JH. Continuity of care record aims to ease transfer of patient information. *AAP News*. 2004;24:222.
21. Dolin RH, Alschuler L, Beebe C, et al. The HL7 Clinical Document Architecture. *J Am Med Inform Assoc*. 2001;8(6):552–569.
22. Dolin RH, Alschuler L, Boyer S, et al. HL7 Clinical Document Architecture, Release 2. *J Am Med Inform Assoc*. 2006;13(1):30–39.
23. Ferranti JM, Musser RC, Kawamoto K, Hammond WE. The clinical document architecture and the continuity of care record: a critical analysis. *J Am Med Inform Assoc*. 2006;13(3):245–252.
24. Altshuler L. Health Level Seven Content and Interoperability Standards Panel. HL7 Clinical Document Architecture (CDA::CCR::CCD). American Health Information Management Association Long Term Care Health Information Technology Summit, June 9, 2006, Baltimore, MD; 2006. Available at: http://www.ahima.org/meetings/ltc/documents/Alschuler_HITinLTCPanel.June06.rev.ppt. Accessed December 21, 2008.
25. Health Level Seven, ASTM International. HL7 Continuity of Care Document, a Healthcare IT Interoperability Standard, is Approved by Balloting Process and Endorsed by Healthcare IT Standards Panel, Press Release; February 12, 2007. Available at: http://www.hl7.org/documentcenter/public/pressreleases/20070212.pdf. Accessed December 21, 2008.
26. Kim GR, Lehmann CU and the Council on Clinical Information Technology. Pediatric Aspects of Inpatient Health Information Technology Systems. *Pediatrics* 2008;122(6):e1287–e1296.

Chapter 19
Ambulatory Computerized Provider Order Entry (ACPOE or E-Prescribing)

Kevin B. Johnson and Carl G.M. Weigle

Objectives

On completing this chapter, the reader should be able to formulate and discuss important questions about ambulatory computerized provider order entry (ACPOE), including:

- Quality, safety, and process issues in ordering medications, tests, and procedures in ambulatory settings
- Requirements for using ACPOE to assure quality and safety in pediatrics
- The roles of pediatricians in using and adopting ACPOE

19.1 Introduction

Medical errors arise in part from variations in clinical care. Two broad sources of variations in care are: (a) the progressive complexity of health care (providers caring for more patients with multiple and/or chronic medical needs, less time in which to see them, fragmentation and lack of coordination of care) and (b) barriers (internal and external) that practitioners face in adhering to evidence-based treatment guidelines.[1-3]

Since the 1970s, patient safety has embraced computerized order entry (among other technologies) as a way to reduce medication errors and improve guideline compliance. Order entry for medication delivery to patients has been studied extensively.[4-13]

Early studies from the Regenstrief Institute in Indiana demonstrated significant reductions in ordering errors and have contributed to the recommendation that order entry (also known as CPOE (Chapter 26)) be used in all hospitals[14] and ambulatory settings[15] as a path to improving quality and safety. Although adoption is still limited (under 30% of ambulatory settings use order entry,[16-18]) ambulatory computerized provider order entry (ACPOE) systems, the focus of this chapter, continue to evolve.

C.U. Lehmann et al. (eds.), *Pediatric Informatics: Computer Applications in Child Health,* Health Informatics,
© Springer Science+Business Media, LLC 2011

## 19.2	Definitions and Classification of ACPOE

### 19.2.1	Ambulatory Computerized Provider Order Entry (ACPOE)

Ambulatory computerized provider order entry (ACPOE) is defined as "clinicians' use of computers to order and transmit [testing, procedure and] medication regimens for individual patients"[17] in outpatient care. When used to prescribe medication regimens, ACPOE is also known as electronic prescribing, e-Prescribing and/or eRx). ACPOE systems can be classified in terms of functionality (electronic prescribing (eRx) and/or electronic test and procedure scheduling/ordering (eDx)) and integration with other clinical information systems (electronic health records, pharmacy benefit and management systems, and clinical decision support systems).[15]

### 19.2.2	Electronic Prescribing (ERX)

Electronic prescribing (eRx) systems can be classified according to their level of sophistication:

- *Basic eRx only*: guides users in creating structured prescriptions and provides passive references (lookup tools)
- *Intermediate eRx only*: provides Basic eRx plus basic decision support (alerts and reminders) for orders, using some patient data
- *Advanced eRx only*: Basic eRx plus sophisticated decision support, using most patient data plus electronic data interchange
- *eRx-eDx*: eRx may also be combined with diagnostic tests/procedure ordering (eDx) (This is covered in the following section)

eRx application interfaces (Fig. 19.1) guide prescribers in: (a) constructing new prescriptions and (b) refilling/renewing prescriptions. According to the level of sophistication, eRx may provide access to information on current medications and tests, active orders, medication administration records for a patient, automated reports, and/or decision support (checks, alerts, and reminders for dosing errors, potential drug allergies, and interactions).

### 19.2.3	Electronic Diagnostic Test/Procedure Ordering (EDX)

Diagnostic test/procedure ordering (eDx) is similar to eRx, with some distinctions. Similarities include: an authorized prescriber's construction and encoding of an order (a test/procedure/medication) for a specific patient, transmission of the order to an agent (laboratory staff/nurse/pharmacist) who decodes and carries out the order (or fills the prescription) for the specified patient and documentation. Distinctions include: the need to link an order to (and therefore the capability to

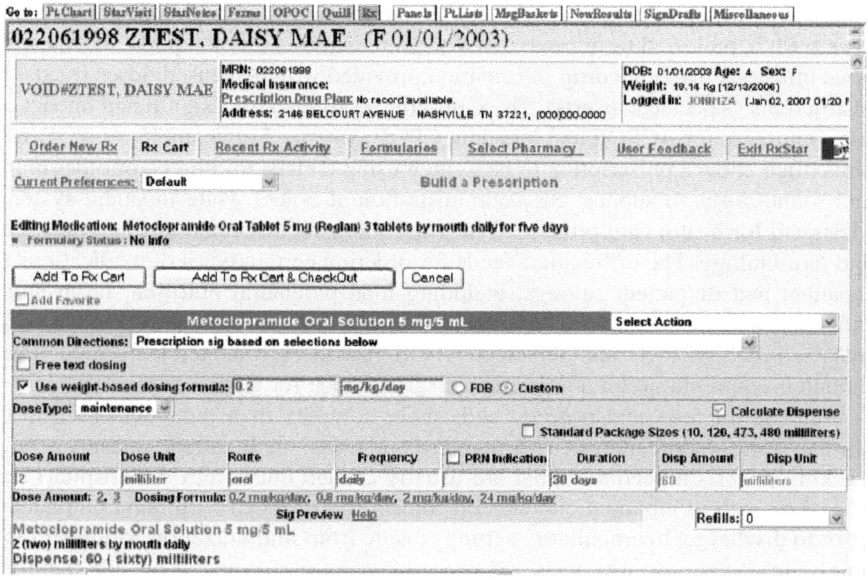

Fig. 19.1 Typical eRx interface: Vanderbilt RxStar System: This eRx application guides prescribers in: (a) constructing new prescriptions and (b) refilling/renewing prescriptions. eRx systems may feature: access to medications and tests, active orders, medication administration records, automated reports, and decision support (checks, alerts, and reminders for dosing errors, potential drug allergies, and interactions)

collect, preserve/store, and send) a biological or clinical sample for analysis, the need for a trained medical professional to perform an ordered test/procedure (blood drawing), documentation of clinical findings that justify the test/procedure (such as a referral), tracking and communication of the performance/cancellation of the procedure/test and the results of the procedure/test. Completion of all the necessary steps of this process is termed *fulfillment* (of the order).

It is important to note that fulfillment is a component of both eRx and eDx, but that because of the physical separation of most pharmacies from clinic sites, the fulfillment component (whether the prescription has been picked up) has traditionally been retained in the pharmacy information system. This distinction is also under scrutiny—many new systems exploit data feeds from retail pharmacies (e.g., SureScripts™) or insurers (e.g., RxHub™) to inform payors and clinicians about prescription fulfillment.

19.2.4 ACPOE Versus Inpatient CPOE

Ambulatory prescribing is largely similar to inpatient prescribing (Chapter 26) in most ways. Differences include: workflow role-based tasks (differential roles of nurses and pharmacists in dispensing and administration), the use of dosing guidelines (differential allowances for dosing intervals: "three times a day" vs "every 8 h"), preferred forms and routes of administration ("oral liquids" vs "intravenous infusions") and the drug information provided with dispensed doses (readable instructions vs package inserts). These differences often have a significant impact on user interfaces for ACPOE and inpatient CPOE systems. For example, ACPOE systems often allow a prescription to be written using tablets, milliliters, or other units, and round doses to support easy administration at home, while inpatient systems (designed for health care providers) may use more sophisticated dosing guidelines and terminology. The differential needs for ordering certain types of medications in inpatient and outpatient settings, including total parenteral nutrition, intravenous infusions, and specifically timed sequences of medications (such as chemotherapy) make current ACPOE and inpatient CPOE interfaces noninterchangeable (even though users might prefer a single universal interface for all prescriptions).

ACPOE for tests and procedures is more complex than inpatient ordering of similar tests or procedures. The "captive audience" of inpatient settings allows tracking of tests/procedures (that are usually carried out within the hospital) and review (as part of inpatient clinician responsibility) of order fulfillment on patients prior to discharge. In ambulatory settings (aside from immunization administration and point-of-care testing), tests and procedures are performed at outside facilities (that may provide services for many ambulatory practices). Ambulatory orders for testing will be fulfilled after the patient encounter is over and the patient has left the office. Routing of test/procedure information (date and location of test, completed, missed or rescheduled appointment, test result or interpretation) may be complex, and tracking a test/procedure or its result may be vulnerable to being missed.

In organizations where ACPOE is part of a larger EHR system that serves both inpatient and ambulatory settings, there are typically benefits of electronic linkage of patient information (to shared laboratory and radiology information systems) across clinical settings (that may facilitate clinical follow-up of test results), but there may also be challenges with regard to regulatory issues on referrals. Small group practices (including many pediatric practices) still using paper records will most likely adopt freestanding (standalone) EHR systems with or without an ACPOE system (unconnected to large organizations). Relaxation of Stark and "anti-kickback" regulations to create a safe harbor for larger organizations to provide information technology (such as interoperable EHRs) to referring physicians (to increase EHR adoption)[19] may help to realize the benefits.

19.3   General Considerations in ACPOE Adoption

Although numerous studies support the use of ACPOE system, less than one third of practices have integrated this technology into their workflow. There are many reasons for this low adoption rate, including:[20]

- Early adopter experience—may catalyze or impede adoption
- Legacy systems

- Inadequate standards (to support data exchange among systems)
- Lack of capital and implementation resources
- Operating costs
- Lack of incentives/reimbursement
- Risk-reward perception

Pediatric experience with ACPOE systems will likely be mixed or generally negative, given the state of these systems in the recent past. Therefore, early adopter experience may be a significant factor. Furthermore, legacy practice management systems may decrease willingness to adopt EHR and ACPOE systems.

19.3.1 Supporting Evidence

Knowledge about benefits of ACPOE may offset the risks for its adoption, especially in child health care settings. The evidence, as noted by the Institute of Medicine in their *Preventing Medication Errors* report,[21] is scant for pediatrics, but may be inferred from the evidence in family and adult medicine.

One study of outpatient laboratory test ordering errors revealed that 4.8% of paper-based test requisitions were mis-transcribed into laboratory information systems.[22] Of 643 institutions in the analysis, 0.5% employed ACPOE. The most frequent transcription error type was misidentification of the physicians to whom the reports were to be sent. Recent data (from an academic pediatric ambulatory center study by one of the authors (KBJ)) showed 39% of prescriptions were written with missing information. Another study[23] reported that information known to exist but not available to the provider at the time of care included laboratory test results (6.1% of visits) and radiology test results (3.8% of visits) and suggested that a full electronic record reduced episodes of care with missing information (Odds Ratio 0.4, 95% confidence interval 0.17–0.94). ACPOE reduction of transcription errors and assurance of information completeness in ordering are just two of its benefits.

19.3.2 Incentives and Return on Investment

In addition to the benefits of ACPOE functions, incentives to its adoption and use, particularly for eRx, include: the development of pharmacy benefits management (PBM) systems that facilitate prescription and formulary information management for both prescribers and patients, the promise of being able to use data from eRx and other EHR systems to help assess and improve quality of practice and the pressure of EHR adoption as a part of pay-for-performance.

Return on investment analyses have been performed by the Center for Information Technology Leadership[15] and are summarized in Fig. 19.2.

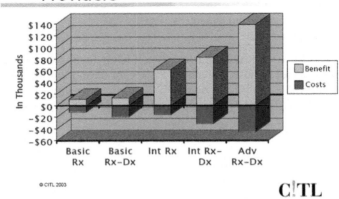

Fig. 19.2 Return on investment of ACPOE over 5 years[15]: Return on investment increases as system functionality increases. Systems capable of detecting potential adverse medication events and that are integrated into EHRs are the most costly, but are still able to realize a return on the investment within 5 years after purchase

19.3.3 Challenges

One study of an eRx pilot[24] involving three sites in Massachusetts identified ten key barriers to adopting ACPOE: (1) previous negative technology experiences, (2) initial and long-term cost, (3) lost productivity, (4) competing priorities, (5) change management issues, (6) interoperability limitations, (7) information technology (IT) requirements, (8) standards limitations, (9) waiting for an "all-in-one solution," and (10) confusion about competing product offerings. Many of these barriers and their perceptions are magnified in small pediatric practices that have had poor experiences in finding systems that conform to their needs.[25,26]

Other pediatric issues include:

- *Inadequate knowledge by physicians about benefits of order entry.* Many clinicians believe that order entry provides more of a clerical than a decision support function.[25,27]
- *Mismatches between cognitive workflow and current user interfaces.* Existing order entry interfaces add steps to a well-ensconced (though error-prone) process, shifting much of the cognitive burden that had previously been borne by clerks and nurses back to the prescriber (who may be preoccupied by a patient's immediate clinical condition).[28–30]
- *Cultural barriers.* Changes in long-term work habits may be difficult to introduce.
- *Decreased provider productivity.* Practitioner concerns of decreases in income and productivity over the short term (particularly with electronic records) are

related to adaptations in workflow, but evidence from one study shows that interim losses may be less and shorter than believed.[31] For eRx, it is high-volume prescribers (including pediatricians) who see earlier benefits in productivity.

19.3.4   Change Management

Adoption of eRx/eDx (or of any health technology) requires change management of the clinical work environment, which in turn requires understanding of the structures, processes, and culture of clinical work as well as the ways in which information is created, stored, and communicated among workers to accomplish clinical tasks. One such model, the Systems Engineering Initiative for Patient Safety (SEIPS),[32] identifies the interdependence of five major aspects of a clinical setting (Fig. 19.3):

- A *care provider* (such as a pediatrician) performing
- Various *tasks* (ordering ambulatory prescriptions, tests, and procedures) using
- *Tools and technology* (ACPOE) within
- A given *environment* (a pediatric office) within
- An established *organization* (a primary care practice)

Changes that must be considered include: cognitive needs of the workers using the new system (How does a physician/nurse/clerk use the interface to create/renew a

SEIPS Model Conceptual Framework is based on the Balance Theory of Job Design©
(Smith & Carayon, 1989, 1995; Carayon & Smith, 2000) and the concept of Healthy Organizations
(Sainfort, Karsh, Booske and Smith, 2001)

© The Board of Regents of the University of Wisconsin System

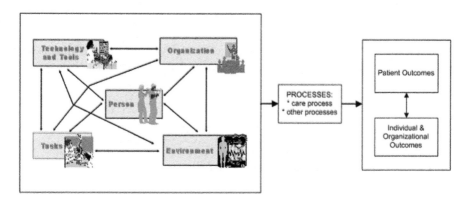

Fig. 19.3 Systems Engineering for Patient Safety Model[32]: Introducing a new component (such as ACPOE) into a system (such as a busy pediatric practice) significantly affects all other parts of the model (patients, staff, and outcomes) that must be considered with regard to patient safety (the Balance Theory of Job Design)

Financial

• Cost reductions from decreased administrative, clinical staffing, and resource requirements
  (i.e., elimination of paper chart pulls and transcription services).

• Revenue enhancements from improved charge capture and charge entry to billing times.

• Productivity gains from increased procedure volume, reductions in average length of stay, and increased transaction processing rates.

Clinical

• Care process advances from better adherence to clinical protocols and improvements in the stages of clinical decision-making
  (i.e., initiation, diagnostics, monitoring and tracking, and acting).

• Improved patient outcomes from reductions in medical errors, decreases in morbidity and mortality, and expedited recovery times.

Organizational

• Stakeholder satisfaction improvements from improved access to healthcare information, decreased wait times, and more positive
  perceptions of care quality and clinician efficacy.

• Risk mitigation from decreases in malpractice litigation and increased adherence to federal, state, and accreditation organization standards.

Fig. 19.4 ACPOE value dimensions[15]

prescription?), their task needs (How will ACPOE streamline/hinder specific steps in e-prescribing in a small/medium/large practice and how will it affect the error rate?) and their information needs (What specific medical and practical knowledge is needed to assure safe prescribing (pediatric-specific and appropriate drug forms (oral liquid availability) and test options (micro methods for infants)?). Consideration of provider culture is essential. As has been shown by Lorenzi and Ash, transformational impacts of ACPOE and other health information technology may be both recognized and mitigated using established approaches (Fig. 19.4).[27,33–35]

19.4 Recent Advances

Ambulatory order entry systems have become increasingly sophisticated to the point where the Institute of Medicine and the Leapfrog Group have advocated for eRx for use by all clinicians by 2010. A framework for measuring the impact (and value) of ACPOE in terms of financial, clinical, and organizational dimensions has been developed,[15] with the demonstration of significant benefits to patients as a result of eRx and medication management data inoperability.

19.5 Pediatric Issues in ACPOE Adoption

19.5.1 Pediatric Practitioners' Needs

Practitioners' needs for ACPOE are pragmatic: Does it make prescribing safer than without it? If it does not and if it is required for practice, how can it be adapted to meet practitioners' needs? How is return on investment in a product assured?

Availability of pediatric-specific functions: As shown in Fig. 19.1, basic pediatric-specific data and functions include patient weight, age, body-mass index, weight-based dosing information for drugs, and automated dose calculation. Additional information (to assure safety) may include: indications for therapy, dosing intention (formula used in prescribing), and contact information for the provider and patient in case of a need to discuss the prescription. Table 19.1 lists other "best practices" for prescription writing (with or without **eRx**).

Advocacy for pediatric needs in technology development: Not all products support pediatric-specific data fields or functions (such as weight-based dosing and checks), and advocacy for their inclusion in settings where children and adults receive care may be required. Support for some functions is more important in pediatrics than for adult medicine, such as immunization management[26] (which has become progressively complex as the number, variations, and frequency of updates on immunizations and the need to ration doses during shortages increase).

Certification of products and return on investment: Data about pediatric adoption of eRx are lacking. A recent study showed only 21% of the respondents had an electronic record in their practice.[37] While this study did not directly address eRx, only a subset of electronic health record (EHR) systems supports this functionality. Pediatric practices want assurances that they will have return on their investments in eRx and that the products they use will adhere to federal and local regulations. To this end, programs are in the process of developing consensus and evidence based criteria for certifying HIT products (including ACPOE) for use in different environments (such as pediatric ambulatory settings).

19.5.2 Pediatricians' Roles

The pediatrician's primary roles in ACPOE adoption are as child advocates and clinical technology user. Clinical and informatics expertise and/or experience, while essential, are not sufficient to fulfill these roles. Pediatric champions must

Table 19.1 Safe prescribing practices[36]

All orders must be legible
Avoid prescribing units such as teaspoons or dropperfuls
Include patient weight and age
Include dosing formula on prescription
Make sure patient's name and medical record number are on the order sheet
Include the date, time, physician signature, and physician pager number on all orders
When possible, include the purpose of the order (e.g., for cough)
All orders should be written in the metric system, except for therapies that use standard units (e.g., insulin, vitamins)
Spell out "units" rather than using "U"
Orders should be written in total dosage amount, rather than by volume or as a amount per weight (e.g., mg/kg)
All medications should always include drug name, exact metric dose and concentration, and dosage form
A leading zero should always precede a decimal expression of less than one (e.g., 0.1 mg)
Trailing zeros should never be used (e.g., 1.0 vs. 10 mg)

also possess team-building and leadership skills to achieve consensus among disparate stakeholders.

Pediatricians as liaison: Pediatricians are the link between children and pediatricians and the leadership of the clinical enterprise, institution, and between clinicians and the leadership of the health information technology infrastructure (usually a CMIO, industry group or regulatory agency). In this role, pediatricians, especially pediatric informatics experts can: articulate clearly the needs of children and pediatricians in terms of patient safety, influence decisions in executive HIT choices, guide application development, deployment, and educational programs to optimize safe ordering. Pediatricians must represent the needs of children on local, national, and industry levels.

Pediatricians as facilitators: The most vital roles for pediatricians and pediatric informatics experts are: to recognize what questions need to be asked about improving pediatric clinical processes (such as pediatric ambulatory medication ordering), to ask how an intervention (such as ACPOE) impacts (positively and negatively) on the process and how to get information that answers these questions (what types of studies or measures are needed). As users affected by implementations of HIT, pediatricians must have some understanding of why and how systems are developed, and more importantly, how to guide that development to improve care and safety.

Examples of questions that pediatricians may need to ask about ambulatory prescribing and ACPOE include:

1. What types of medication ordering, dispensing, and administration errors occur within the local clinic and how frequently? How can that information be captured?
2. How can ACPOE reduce identified errors? How can its impact on errors be measured?
3. How are laboratory tests ordered by and returned to a practitioner within the local clinic?
4. Is there a way that ACPOE systems can help pharmacists with compounded formulations of medications?
5. How do we design, implement, and manage computerized pediatric dosing rules for off-label (but locally sanctioned) use of medications currently not based on FDA-based evidence?

19.6   The Future of ACPOE

ACPOE/eRx is leading health information technology in terms of likelihood of widespread adoption. The Centers for Medicare and Medicaid is quickly moving forward to push the adoption of e-Prescribing with the establishment of the Final Rule on e-Prescribing outlining regulations, incentives, and exemptions.[38] At this time, use of e-Prescribing is not required for participation in Medicare (or Medicaid).

Widespread adoption must also anticipate pushback from practitioners and unanticipated problems that may result in high-cost, high-profile failures due to underlying workflow issues.[39,40] Fitting technical solutions to regulatory constraints and mandates presents challenges that go beyond implementation, and so pediatric health care providers, in addition to their roles as liaisons and facilitators, must also be advocates for pediatric practices in legislation.

19.7   Case Studies: Ordering Scenarios

19.7.1   Scenario 1: Single Visit-Centric ACPOE

This is the simplest use of ACPOE. A medication (such as a aerosolized bronchodilator or immunization) or point-of-care test (such as a hematocrit) is ordered during a single ambulatory visit. These systems are similar to inpatient CPOE (where the patient is present during the entire ordering-fulfillment cycle) (Chapter 26). This model fits many cases of well-child care. In environments in which there are few desktop workstations, personal digital assistants (PDAs) may be useful in promoting safe prescribing (eRx) practices.[41]

19.7.2   Scenario 2: ACPOE Over Multiple Visits

When orders affect more than one visit, more sophisticated functions are needed to assure fulfillment and proper coordination of the order. In the case where a patient requires a test/procedure (such as an imaging study) at a certain time interval prior to a future visit (such as a pre-operative examination), the order for the test/procedure must be scheduled and linked to the future visit. The system should support coordination of the order, the appointments (imaging appointment and pre-op/follow-up visit) and availability of the results at the follow-up. This model fits most cases of referrals and complex care, such as chemotherapy regimens.

19.7.3   Scenario 3: ACPOE Unlinked to Visits

19.7.3.1   Order Execution

When orders are executed between visits, provider workflow and system requirements are simplified. In the previous scenario, the provider could simply order today for the imaging study to be done in 2 months, and the order would be readily apparent to the radiology technologist when the patient is ready to be scheduled.

19.7.3.2 Results Reporting

Some ACPOE system interfaces have adapted the metaphor of an "inbox" for results (Fig. 19.5). In clinic workflow, test results and prescription requests may be initially screened by a nurse (who handles the bulk of routine tasks according to office protocols), passing specific results (panic values, abnormals, etc.) and requests (new prescriptions without an appointment) to the appropriate practice physician. At any stage, a change in availability of one person might dictate a rerouting of the result, and an especially important result might warrant the use of a system of escalation to ensure timely communication with the patient or guardian.

The electronic inbox offers opportunities for added functionality not possible in the paper-based system. For example, certain results may be broadcast to several providers (such as a primary care provider and a specialist) for review or discussion or for team coverage, where the result is requires only one team member to respond to or acknowledge the result. Another example is a result that is part of a series of results that form a trend, in which case a result would be linked to other results as an embellishment on the original result or as an additional message to a different provider altogether. Some sophistication of result transmission is required when inpatient and outpatient care is recorded in the same electronic health record, so that, for example, the hourly blood gas test results for a current ICU patient do not overwhelm the in-box for her cardiologist in the clinic.

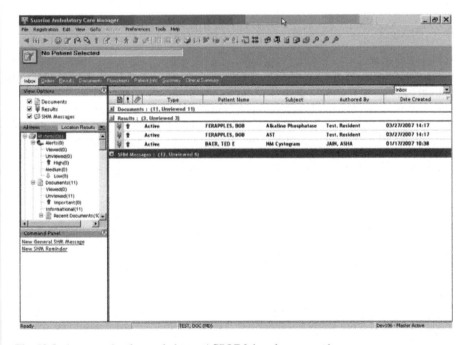

Fig. 19.5 An example of an ambulatory ACPOE Inbox for test results

When a test is performed at a remote site with no ability to send the results across an interface engine into the local ACPOE system, then the results will come back in any of three forms: paper, scanned images or tagged and interoperable results. Any of these forms may then be entered into the ACPOE system, where they are available for analysis by the provider.

References

1. Cabana MD, Rand CS, Powe NR, et al. Why don't physicians follow clinical practice guidelines? A framework for improvement. *JAMA*. 1999;282(15):1458–1465.
2. Cabana MD, Medzihradsky OF, Rubin HR, Freed GL. Applying clinical guidelines to pediatric practice. *Pediatr Ann*. 2001;30(5):274–282.
3. Aiken KD, Clark SJ, Cabana MD. Reasons hospitals give for not offering hepatitis B vaccine to low-risk newborns. *Clin Pediatr (Phila)*. 2002;41(9):681–686.
4. Tierney WM, McDonald CJ, Martin DK, Rogers MP. Computerized display of past test results. Effect on outpatient testing. *Ann Int Med*. 1987;107(4):569–574.
5. Tierney WM, Miller ME, Overhage JM, McDonald CJ. Physician inpatient order writing on microcomputer workstations. Effects on resource utilization. *JAMA*. 1993;269(3):379–383.
6. Tierney WM, Overhage JM, McDonald CJ, Wolinsky FD. Medical students' and housestaff's opinions of computerized order-writing. *Acad Med*. 1994;69(5):386–389.
7. McDonald CJ, Overhage JM, Tierney WM, et al. The Regenstrief Medical Record System: a quarter century experience. *Int J Med Inform*. 1999;54(3):225–253.
8. Dexter PR, Perkins S, Overhage JM, Maharry K, Kohler RB, McDonald CJ. A computerized reminder system to increase the use of preventive care for hospitalized patients. *N Engl J Med*. 2001;345(13):965–970.
9. Overhage JM, Dexter PR, Perkins SM, et al. A randomized, controlled trial of clinical information shared from another institution. *Ann Emerg Med*. 2002;39(1):14–23.
10. Dexter PR, Perkins SM, Maharry KS, Jones K, McDonald CJ. Inpatient computer-based standing orders vs physician reminders to increase influenza and pneumococcal vaccination rates: a randomized trial. *JAMA*. 2004;292(19):2366–2371.
11. Kim GR, Chen AR, Arceci RJ, et al. Error reduction in pediatric chemotherapy: computerized order entry and failure modes and effects analysis. *Arch Pediatr Adolesc Med*. 2006;160(5):495–498.
12. Scavuzzo J, Gamba N. Bridging the gap: the Virtual Chemotherapy Unit. *J Pediatr Oncol Nurs*. 2004;21(1):27–32.
13. Waitman LR, Pearson D, Hargrove FR, et al. Enhancing Computerized Provider Order Entry (CPOE) for neonatal intensive care. *AMIA Annu Symp Proc*. 2003;1078.
14. Leapfrog Group. Computerized Physician Order Entry Fact Sheet; 2009, revised. Available at: http://www.leapfroggroup.org/media/file/Leapfrog-Computer_Physician_Order_Entry_Fact_Sheet.pdf. Accessed December 21, 2008.
15. Center for Information Technology Leadership. CPOE in Ambulatory Environments. Available at: http://69.84.158.158/research/ACPOE.htm. Accessed July 28, 2008.
16. Conn J. More moving to entry level. CPOE adoption slowly gains ground, with larger number expecting installations. *Mod Healthcare*. 2007;37(9):41–42, 44.
17. Simon JS, Rundall TG, Shortell SM. Adoption of order entry with decision support for chronic care by physician organizations. *J Am Med Inform Assoc*. 2007;14(4):432–439.
18. Jha AK, Ferris TG, Donelan K, et al. How common are electronic health records in the United States? A summary of the evidence. *Health Aff (Millwood)*. 2006;25(6):w496–507.
19. Centers for Medicare and Medicaid Services. Physician self-referral exceptions for electronic prescribing and electronic health records technology; 2006, updated 2007. Available at: http://www.cms.hhs.gov/apps/media/press/release.asp?Counter=1920. Accessed July 28, 2008.

20. The Lewin Group. Health Information Technology Leadership Panel, Final Report; 2005. Available at: http://www.hhs.gov/healthit/HITFinalReport.pdf. Accessed July 28, 2008.
21. Committee on Identifying and Preventing Medication Errors, Aspden P, Wolcott J, Bootman JL, Cronenwett LR, eds. *Preventing Medication Errors: Quality Chasm Series.* Washington, DC: National Academy of Sciences; 2007.
22. Valenstein P, Meier F. (1999) Outpatient order accuracy. A College of American Pathologists Q-Probes study of requisition order entry accuracy in 660 institutions. *Arch Pathol Lab Med.* 1999;123(12):1145–1150.
23. Smith PC, Araya-Guerra R, Bublitz C, et al. Missing clinical information during primary care visits. *JAMA.* 2005;293(5):565–571.
24. Halamka J, Aranow M, Ascenzo C, et al. E-prescribing collaboration in Massachusetts: early experiences from regional prescribing projects. *J Am Med Inform Assoc.* 2006;13(3):239–244.
25. Johnson KB. Barriers that impede the adoption of pediatric information technology. *Arch Pediatr Adolesc Med.* 2001;155(12):1374–1379.
26. Spooner SA, American Academy of Pediatrics. Council on Clinical Information Technology. Special requirements of electronic health record systems in pediatrics. *Pediatrics.* 2007;119(3): 631–637.
27. Ash JS, Chin HL, Sittig DF, Dykstra RH. Ambulatory computerized physician order entry implementation. *AMIA Annu Symp Proc.* 2005:11–15.
28. Han YY, Carcillo JA, Venkataraman ST, et al. Unexpected increased mortality after implementation of a commercially sold computerized physician order entry system. *Pediatrics.* 2005;116(6):1506–1512.
29. Sittig DF, Ash JS, Zhang J, Osheroff JA, Shabot MM. Lessons from 'Unexpected increased mortality after implementation of a commercially sold computerized physician order entry system'. *Pediatrics.* 2006;118(2):797–801.
30. Rosenbloom ST, Harrell FE, Jr., Lehmann CU, Schneider JH, Spooner SA, Johnson KB. Perceived increase in mortality after process and policy changes implemented with computerized physician order entry. *Pediatrics.* 2006;117(4):1452–1455; author reply 1455–1456.
31. Kaushal R, Blumenthal D, Poon EG, et al. The costs of a national health information network. *Ann Intern Med.* 2005;143(3):165–173.
32. Carayon P, Schoofs HA, Karsh BT, et al. Work system design for patient safety: the SEIPS model. *Qual Saf Healthcare.* 2006;1(suppl):i50–58.
33. Ash JS, Bates DW. Factors and forces affecting EHR system adoption: report of a 2004 ACMI discussion. *J Am Med Inform Assoc.* 2005;12(1):8–12.
34. Lorenzi NM, Riley RT. Organizational issues = change. *Int J Med Inf.* 2003;69(2–3):197–203.
35. Lorenzi NM, Smith JB, Conner SR, Campion TR. The success factor profile for clinical computer innovation. *Medinfo.* 2004;11(Pt 2):1077–1080.
36. Levine SR, Conen MR, Blanchod NR, et al., Guidelines for preventing medication errors in pediatrics. J Pediatr Pharmacol Ther, 2001;6:427–443
37. Kemper AR, Uren RL, Clark SJ. Adoption of electronic health records in primary care pediatric practices. *Pediatrics.* 2006;118(1):e20–24.
38. Centers for Medicare and Medicaid. E-prescribing; 2008. Available at: http://www.cms.hhs.gov/eprescribing. Accessed December 21, 2008.
39. Massaro TA. Introducing physician order entry at a major academic medical center: II. Impact on medical education. *Acad Med.* 1993;68(1):25–30.
40. Massaro TA. Introducing physician order entry at a major academic medical center: I. Impact on organizational culture and behavior. *Acad Med.* 1993;68(1):20–25.
41. Johnson KB. Pediatric e-prescribing: is the PDA a prescription for safety?: The PedStep Project. Presentation to the Agency for Healthcare Research and Quality; 2008. Available at: http://healthit.ahrq.gov/portal/server.pt/gateway/PTARGS_0_3048_40584_0_0_18/Kevin% 20Johnson-quis%20talk.ppt. Accessed July 28, 2008.

Chapter 20
Telemedicine Applications in Pediatrics

Craig Sable, Molly Reyna and Peter R. Holbrook

Objectives

- To define telemedicine and the structure of a telemedicine program
- To compare and contrast common applications of pediatric telemedicine
- To compare and contrast synchronous and asynchronous telemedicine and distance education
- To discuss barriers to widespread implementation and acceptance of telemedicine

20.1   Introduction: What is Telemedicine?

The roots of telemedicine began in the 1920s when physicians answered questions via radio, with the first video transmission of medical information occurring a few years later. In 1952, video transmission of an x-ray occurred between two sites in Pennsylvania 24 miles apart. In 1965, surgeons in Geneva watched and asked questions of Dr. Michael DeBakey, while he performed heart surgery in Houston. In 1968, Massachusetts General Hospital established a microwave video link between its emergency department and a nurse-staffed medical station at Logan Airport. Within the last 5 years, utilization of telemedicine has increased significantly for radiology, cardiology, and orthopedic surgery services.

Telemedicine is "practicing medicine at a distance",[1] but this simple definition does not capture the complexity of the discipline. Telemedicine is also utilizing technology to improve access to high quality health care, to provide distance education and to compile and maintain health information across the continuum of health care.[2] Telemedicine spans the spectrum of health care environments: the patient's home, rural health centers, community physicians, and hospitals and tertiary care centers.

The two primary modes of telemedicine are asynchronous (store and forward) and synchronous (live or real time).[3] In a "store and forward" model, a technician or physician at one site acquires and stores data on a dedicated local telemedicine computer. The data is transmitted via a specialized connection and copied to a similar remote

C.U. Lehmann et al. (eds.), *Pediatric Informatics: Computer Applications in Child Health*, Health Informatics,
© Springer Science + Business Media, LLC 2011

computer for later review. The most rapidly growing example of asynchronous telemedicine is in radiology picture archiving and communication systems (PACS).[4] In a "live or real-time" model, both sender and receiver view data simultaneously. A common example of synchronous telemedicine is videoconferencing. Each modality has advantages and disadvantages, which are listed in Tables 20.1 and 20.2.

Telemedicine can augment conventional health care delivery. It can reduce geographic barriers to access to care and expertise for patients, physicians, and other health professionals.[5] It can reduce time barriers to appropriate attention and care. Telemedicine-enhanced care can connect community and tertiary care hospitals, patient homes and practitioners and offices and mobile physician. Emergency and critical cases can receive timely attention from providers with appropriate expertise,

Table 20.1 Comparison of real time and store-and-forward telemedicine modalities

	Real time	Store and forward
Live interaction: feedback and physician/family interaction	Yes	No
Cost	Inexpensive $8,000–$25,000 per site	Moderately expensive $20,000–$100,000 per site
Image quality	Acceptable/diagnostic	Optimal (equiv to sending end)
Hard copy at receiving end	No	Yes
Required bandwidth	At least 384 Kbps: For acceptable frame rate	No minimum: Higher bandwidth decreased transmission time
Reliance on intelligent compression	No	Yes
Electronic compression algorithm	H.320 or H.323 videoconferencing	Lossless, JPEG, or MPEG
Time commitment by physician at receiving end	Availability at time of transmission required	Can review study any time
Limited by location at sending site	Yes	No

Table 20.2 Comparison of synchronous and asynchronous distance education

	Synchronous	Asynchronous
Benefits	Live interaction	Individual choice of time and place
	Experience/lecturing skills of presenter	Interactive for varying levels of expertise
	Case discussions with questions	Immediate individualized feedback
	Individually focused learning experience	Evaluation tools
		Easier to link to CME
Challenges	Delivery system and technical issues	No face to face instructor interaction
	Scheduling from both sides	Loose skills of a dynamic lecturer
	Different levels of audience expertise	Not individualized for specific questions
	Program/learner evaluation	Hardware/software requirements
		Comfort with computer based tools

allowing for appropriate triage of patients to tertiary care facilities, especially in disasters, to optimize resource utilization and reduce costs.[6]

Telemedicine can also improve other aspects of health care. Discussion of complex cases by remote experts can improve quality of care and educate local providers, as well as integrate care delivery by guiding patients to centers of expertise and excellence. Conversely centers may use telemedicine as part of business strategies to improve market shares and to promote leading edge academic endeavors, including research and data collection.[7]

20.2 Essential Components of a Telemedicine System

A telemedicine network consists of four basic components: the computer tools (including patient data/medical record, audio, video, and educational content), the transmitter tools, the receiver tools and the connection between the sending and receiving sites. Despite the obvious dependence on technology, the ultimate success or failure of telemedicine is based on building collaborative relationships. People with a variety of skills and backgrounds who may work in different countries and cultures and who may speak different languages must be motivated to work together to build a successful program. The most technically advanced project is a failure if end users are not willing to take advantage of the technology.

Standard desktop, laptop, or handheld computers can be converted to functional telemedicine systems by the addition of hardware and software that allows collection of video and audio data from medical and nonmedical recording devices for transmission via telephone/Internet connections or wireless for asynchronous or synchronous use. Capacity for storing and forwarding files requires additional hardware, software, and memory than videoconferencing, and many systems can be configured for both functions. Costs vary: larger systems with "store and forward" capabilities can cost over $50,000, while a desktop videoconferencing computer can cost less than $5,000.

A basic conferencing input system consists of a video camera and microphone that can collect and transmit data simultaneously ("real-time"). Other telemedicine-compatible medical inputs on the market include radiology scanners (less important as PACS become more prevalent), high-quality dermatology video cameras, stethoscopes, endoscopes, ophthalmoscopes, and otoscopes (costing between $1,000 and $15,000). Input from echocardiography or ultrasound units (S-Video and RGB-Video) can be connected into a standard telemedicine system for the additional cost of a cable (under $10) to connect the unit to the computer, making echocardiography and ultrasound ideal for telemedicine.

The output of a telemedicine transmission, from a local input device or a remote source (desktop or laptop computer, hospital, or physician office network or storage device), must be rendered from the digital form into an audio/video or photographic format that can be used for interpretation and diagnosis. Quality of output may be determined from the source (sufficient signal and information) and at the reception point (sufficient resources to create visual or auditory presentation

Table 20.3 Telemedicine bandwidth options

	Bandwidth	Cost	Availability
POTS Plain Old Telephone Systems	14.4 Kbps	Low	Universal
ISDN Integrated service Digital Network	128 Kbps (three lines commonly bonded)	Low	Wide
T1 Terrestrial 1	1.54 Mbps	Low to Moderate	Wide
SDSL/ADSL Synchronous/ Asynchronous Digital Subscriber Lines	Variable (128 Kbps to 1 Mbps)	Low	Variable Increasing
ATM Asynchronous Transfer Mode	Very high	High	Variable
Satellite	Very high	High	Variable
Internet	Variable	Low	Universal Software/ bandwidth/ security limitations
Wireless	Low	Unknown	Limited/increasing

and/or interaction that can be perceived and used by a user for clinical purposes). The former may be improved by reducing noise or repeating the signal along the transmission path, and the latter may be improved through better rendering tools (higher amplitude, resolution, and contrast).

Many options for connectivity are available, including low and high speed telephone lines, cable, digital subscriber lines (DSL) and wireless (Table 20.3). The rate of data transmission (bandwidth) affects the time required for a "store and forward" file to be sent (hours on a phone connective vs seconds for a high-speed connection. Bandwidth clearly impacts the quality of live videoconferencing because of the required interactivity. Bandwidths of 384 Kbps and higher provide acceptable frame rates (20–30/s) for live videoconferencing, while Internet-based connections may require slightly higher bandwidth for the same quality. Routers that allow transmission of data to multiple destinations simultaneously are available and can bridge alternative types of connections between a sender and receiver.

There are myriad vendors and choices for each component. Some technical expertise is required from in-house engineers or telemedicine consultants to ensure the computers, inputs, and telephone lines work together properly. This requires coordination between computer hardware and software manufacturers, local and long distance telephone companies, and input device vendors.

20.3   Telemedicine Personnel and Organization

Personnel support for installation, use and maintenance is essential, including a telemedicine coordinator who understands telemedicine technology, connectivity options, and how medical practices and hospital administrations work.

For telemedicine systems that are in regular use, on-site technical support is required and must be able to work closely with clinicians, equipment vendors, telephone companies, and connection providers. Ideal services customize telemedicine solutions that successfully combine real-time videoconferencing, digital reporting, image storage and management, data base integration, prompt technical support, and easy implementation of software updates.

Physician champions and administrative leaders are necessary to promote use of this technology to physicians who may be resistant to change. Advocacy for any telemedicine initiative must be active on both sides of the connection. Leadership roles in overcoming barriers to acceptance include removal of technical, organizational and legal blocks and administrative simplification of legal issues surrounding telemedicine.

Medical education support is helpful in increasing adoption. The inclusion of facilitated continuing medical education credits will improve the attractiveness of telemedicine programs that include distance education. Additional added-value tools will allow users to acquire and to create content, to incorporate multimedia and to access evidence easily.

A challenge for a telemedicine practice is to generate sufficient revenue to be self-sustaining. However, significant funding opportunities are available (principally through federal sources), especially for programs that provide support for underserved rural and international areas. A sustainable plan for telemedicine must include funding for maintenance, user support and upgrading (hardware, software, connectivity, and education content).

20.4   Pediatric Telemedicine Applications

Clinical pediatric telemedicine applications can be found in almost every subspecialty,[8] including cardiology,[9] radiology, neurology,[10,11] neonatal care, genetics, emergency medicine, pathology,[12] mental health,[13] hematology, oncology,[14] dermatology, otolaryngology, ophthalmology, orthopedic surgery, urology, and general surgery. Telemedicine applications have also been developed for distance learning, home care, correctional care, international collaboration, humanitarian assistance, rural health,[15] military health, Native American health, pharmacy, and consumer health.

20.4.1   Cardiology

The earliest clinical publications on tele-cardiology were reported in pediatric populations in 1989 and 1993.[16] Live transmission of neonatal echocardiograms is accurate and impacts positively on patient management including: facilitating timely transport of critically ill children with heart disease, preventing unnecessary transport (patients diagnosed not to have heart disease), improving cost-effectiveness without increased echocardiography utilization and reducing length of stay.[17] Live transmission of fetal echocardiograms has also been shown to be diagnostic at bandwidths of 384 Kbps.[18] Use of "store and forward" telemedicine for emergency echocardiography consultation during weekend, evening, and overnight hours to assess ventricular function, ischemia, pericardial effusions, valvular disease, and heart donor status in adult patients was reported in 1996.[19]

One percent of all newborns have a congenital heart defect and a significant number require urgent medication and surgery.[20] It may take 3–5 days for the circulation to transition from the fetal pattern to the newborn pattern, which can mask a potentially life threatening heart condition. Symptoms may not occur until after the baby has left the hospital. Most community hospitals have access to echocardiography, but no immediate access to a pediatric cardiologist who can make an expedient interpretation. In 10 percent of cases of a newborn with an audible murmur does the child require urgent intervention. Prior to telemedicine, in community hospitals without pediatric cardiologists, echocardiograms could be performed, but needed to be sent by courier for interpretation. Problems with this approach include: suboptimal quality of the echocardiogram, delays in timely diagnosis and intervention and unnecessary transports (resulting in higher costs and emotional stress to the family) in the case of a benign condition.

Telemedicine has streamlined the approach to newborns with suspected heart disease. Real-time transmission of echocardiograms to a pediatric cardiologist provides an immediate interpretation and recommendations. Benefits of this approach include:

- Increased echocardiography quality and sonographer proficiency and efficiency through the interactions between remote pediatric cardiologists and local technicians
- Reduced unnecessary transports, resulting in decreased morbidity and direct financial savings from prevention from timely diagnosis and management
- Shorter hospital stays, and avoidance of the burdens of travel and lost wages on the patient's family

A multicenter study, supported by an American Society of Echocardiography grant (Table 20.4), found that patients with access to telemedicine were transported less often, had shorter hospital stays, and were less likely to receive unnecessary invasive management than diagnosed-matched control patients.[21]

At the Children's National Medical Center (CNMC) in Washington, DC, the pediatric tele-cardiology program uses live videoconferencing over three bonded

Table 20.4 American society of echocardiography multicenter study: patients with mild or no heart disease

	Telemedicine (n = 338)	Control (n = 338)	p value
Transported to tertiary care hospital	5% (n = 15)	10% (n = 32)	0.01
Total length of stay	1.0±6.8 days Range: 0–102 days	2.6 ± 11 days Range: 0–96 days	0.005

a

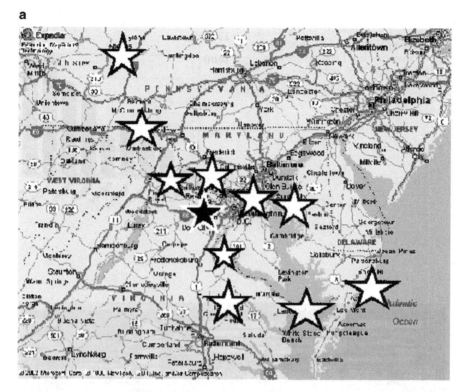

Fig. 20.1a Washington, DC Pediatric Telemedicine Community Hospital Network—Map of Washington, DC metropolitan area showing our tertiary care hospital (Black star) and ten community hospitals in Maryland where telemedicine (cardiology and/or neurology) is performed. These sites are Annapolis, Cheverly, Clinton, Frederick, Hagerstown, Leonardtown, Prince Frederick, Rockville Salisbury, and Silver Spring

ISDN lines (384 Kbps). Over 6,000 studies have been performed from nine hospitals since our telemedicine program began in 1998 (Fig. 20.1a and b). The average time from request of a study to having a faxed report at the referring site is under 30 min. Telemedicine has had a significant benefit to our pediatric cardiology practice including an average saving of 4.2 person–hours each week from avoidance of unnecessary consultations. The pediatric cardiologist also records a digitized version of the study on the telemedicine computer (Fig. 20.2) using MPEG technology that is of diagnostic quality and allows for "bookmarking" of images and offline measurements. Reports can be transmitted or faxed immediately to the referring physician and form a digital medical record and database.

Telemedicine is also used for patient discussions during weekly surgical case management conference. Multiple forms of digital data (echocardiography, angiography, x-rays, and MRIs), videotape displays, and audio and video of audience members can be shared among CNMC, two satellite clinics, the local referral

Fig. 20.1b Washington, DC Pediatric
Telemedicine Community Hospital Network—
Graph showing annual teleechocardiography
volume; approximately 1,000 studies were
transmitted in both 2005 and 2006

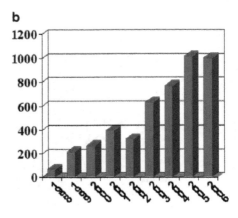

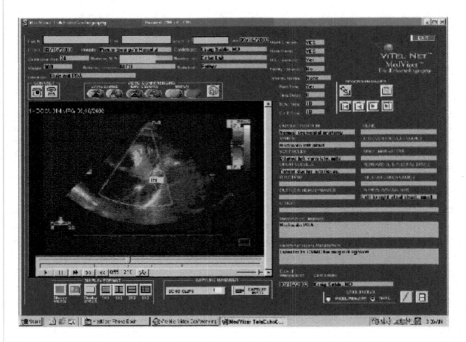

Fig. 20.2 MPEG Digitization and Medical Record—Screen shot of telecardiology application
(developed by collaboration between Children's National Medical Center and VitelNet, Inc,
McLean, VA). The incoming live echocardiogram is reviewed and can be digitized with allowance
for bookmarks and measurements. A patient database is built with demographic information and
a report is created on the same screen. The report can be faxed or transmitted via telemedicine.
A permanent digital medical record is immediately created

hospital 5 mi away and a remote referral hospital in Germany. Patients scheduled for surgery and those who are candidates for surgery are discussed, with all sites being able to see the same data simultaneously.

A new tele-cardiology application is being piloted involving home health care.[22] The most complex congenital heart defects: hypoplastic left heart, hypoplastic right heart (tricuspid atresia and pulmonary atresia) and other complex single ventricle hearts require staged surgeries including: an initial surgical procedure in the first 2 weeks of life (Norwood procedure), a second surgical procedure between 3 and 8 months of life (Glenn procedure) and a third surgical procedure between 18 months and 3 years of life (Fontan procedure). Improved surgical techniques along with better preoperative, intraoperative, and postoperative care have led to survival to hospital discharge approaching 90% for the most complex of these conditions (hypoplastic left heart) and even higher for other defects. Well over 95% of patients who reach the second operation survive into adulthood and have excellent quality of life. This makes it imperative that considerable focus is put upon this vulnerable period in the first 6 months of life.

Despite vastly improved outcomes, children with single ventricles remain at high risk during the vulnerable period between hospital discharge and the second operation with a risk of death up to 15% during this period. They are much more susceptible to normal child illnesses that cause fever, dehydration, and low oxygen. Close daily monitoring of simple parameters (formula intake, weight gain, pulse oximetry) has been shown to almost eliminate this mortality. We are in the process of instituting a simple home device that will electronically measure these parameters in this patient population and transmit them to a centralized computer over regular telephone lines for daily review.

20.4.2 Neurology

Seizure disorders are common in children, especially premature babies. At CNMC, the remote interpretation of electroencephalograms (EEG) began in 2002, and we are now connected to three community hospitals. These hospitals have the ability to perform EEGs on infants and children but not the pediatric neurology expertise to interpret them. EEGs are now acquired in a digital format and stored on a server at the remote hospital or transmitted to CNMC. Pediatric neurologists may connect via a Web client to the server, interpret the EEG and submit the final report online. Over 500 studies have been interpreted in this manner, with a next business day turnaround, and the option for stat studies. EEG interpretation lends itself nicely to a "store and forward" model because the quality of the test has very little dependence on the interaction between physician and technician.

Telepathology is another tele-neurology application, offered in both "live" and "store and forward" modes. A formal collaboration between CNMC and hospitals in Cincinnati and Chicago permits referral of brain tumor pathology cases for second opinions. Slides of pathology specimens are digitized and send for review prior to case discussions and live review using tele-microscopy is available. CNMC has provided second opinions in this manner for a hospital in Saudi Arabia.

20.4.3 Radiology

Picture Archiving and Communication Systems (PACS) provide access to imaging studies throughout many hospitals in a "store and forward" format. Physicians can review and interpret studies remotely through virtual private network (VPN) connections. Many physicians worldwide now practice radiology exclusively in this manner and some practices and hospitals are outsourcing official interpretation (and billing) of imaging studies to physicians in other countries half way around the world. At CNMC, radiology is one of the largest users of telemedicine technology and will continue to increase with the vast increase in use of digital radiology.

20.4.4 Multispecialty Pediatrics

Interpretation of echocardiograms, EEGs, and x-rays have been very successful telemedicine models, in part because they are based on tests that lend themselves to telemedicine and are directly reimbursable. However, the need for subspecialty consultation for infants and children at community hospitals extends to other subspecialties by teleconsultation.[23] CNMC has established a multispecialty tele-consultation program with one hospital in suburban Maryland. Digital x-rays, photographs, video clips, along with a digital medical record that includes history, physician notes and laboratory tests can be stored and forwarded from a telemedicine unit at the remote site to a unit at CNMC. A telemedicine consult coordinator then contacts the appropriate physician to review the case and create an electronic opinion. A digital medical record is created and can be accessed if the patient is transferred or returns for outpatient evaluation.

Several specialties including genetics, general surgery, urology, neurosurgery, and orthopedic surgery are available. Store and forward is ideal for most of these cases, but live consultation to talk with the family and look at the patient can be useful, especially for genetic syndromes. Reimbursement for second opinion consultations are much more difficult to obtain from insurance providers. To sustain this type of program a contractual agreement with annual fees per specialty service exists between the two hospitals.

20.5 International Programs

Telemedicine has had a major impact on CNMC's ability to provide support for our international partners. CNMC has international partner hospitals in three categories: charity programs (Morocco, Uganda, Iraq, Serbia/Kosovo), military programs

(Germany, Italy), and reimbursement programs (United Arab Emirates, Qatar, Kuwait, Saudi Arabia). Telemedicine use models vary from country to country and include "store and forward" and "live" consultation in: cardiology, gastroenterology and nutrition, infectious disease, nephrology, oncology, and trauma. In most cases, telemedicine is used to assist with patient management at the referring center. In some cases, telemedicine is used to discuss cardiology patients and the need to refer to CNMC for catheterization and/or surgery. Many international partners are in distant time zones, have different work weeks (e.g., the weekend in Saudi Arabia is Saturday through Wednesday) and do not speak English as their primary language.

CNMC, funded by a grant from the Mosaic Foundation, provides telemedicine and distance education services in Morocco. Three components of this program include: tele-consultation, live distance education and case discussions and stored educational content. The tele-consultation component includes a remote telemedicine workstation that acquires digital medical data (photos, xray images, lab data, etc.) and forwards it to CNMC for review. The distance education program is described below. A future application of this program will be to allow tertiary care hospitals in Morocco to provide support for more rural health care workers in remote villages through telemedicine technology to address such medical problems as maternal and newborn care, malnutrition, and infectious disease prevention.

20.6   Distance Education

Distance education is one of the most common applications of telemedicine. CNMC offers synchronous and asynchronous distance education programs in several topics and formats, with physician-led live videoconferences, including presentations to local, national, and international audiences, and weekly hospital grand rounds to regional hospitals. In 2006, CNMC conducted a lecture series with physicians in Iraq, supported by Wired International (a nonprofit organization that supports distance education for several third world countries). Despite the challenges of living and practicing in war time, we found that Iraqi physicians still craved collegiality and ongoing educational support.

CNMC also has a program for creating asynchronous distance education content from digitally recorded pediatric lectures, accessible to medical students from a secure Web site. This program was grant funded by the Mosaic Foundation and is being extended to Morocco, and required translation of the content into French for use in the largest Moroccan medical school in Rabat. New content is made available via Internet as it becomes available.

20.7   Challenges and Obstacles

There are many obstacles to more routine telemedicine implementations: resistance from primary care providers and specialists, lack of standardized telemedicine practice protocols and concern that telemedicine may decrease the bedside presence of consulting physicians in local hospitals. Technical challenges include the complexity of many different software, hardware, and telephone line options in different locations (all of which may function normally in isolation but not in concert) which may pose difficulties in locating system malfunctions. Essential to any effort is planning for "down time" and for disaster recovery.

The legal ramifications and licensure requirements of using telemedicine are still evolving.[24] There have been no telemedicine lawsuits to date, but as the field grows, this likely to change. Patient confidentiality must be secured as data is transmitted across various types of telecommunications tools. Legal questions may also arise when a tertiary care center provides equipment or support to a referring hospital or practice. The legality of such arrangements depends on the details of the arrangement; it is advisable to seek legal counsel when developing a telemedicine program and contractual agreements with telemedicine partners. Licensure requirements for telemedicine vary by state and may also pose limitations.

Reimbursement for telemedicine consultation is limited in the United States and may discourage many physicians from participating.[25] Tele-cardiology and tele-radiology are often profitable due to professional interpretation fees and downstream revenue from patient referrals, especially those requiring invasive procedures. However, reimbursement for telemedicine consultation in most other fields is limited and may discourage many physicians to participate. Not all states in the United States provide Medicaid reimbursement for telemedicine services, and those that do only provide reimbursement for a limited number of procedures. Medicare reimbursement for telemedicine has been limited to live interactive consultations in rural health professional shortage areas. Telemedicine advocates are seeking legislation that would broaden the coverage to include any type service and include "store and forward" technology.

20.8   Vision for the Future

Moore's law states that technological capability will double approximately every 18 months. The implications of this for the exponential growth and widespread acceptance of telemedicine are tremendous. The line between traditional health care and telemedicine will continue to blur as computing speed becomes greater, storage space becomes less expensive, and options for high speed bandwidth become more universal. The vision of being able to open up a computer (or hand held device) at anytime in anyplace and have full access to any type of medical test (including full motion video) and any education content with wireless technology at acceptable speed is not far off. Of course the ability to maintain confidentiality and security will need to expand at the same time.

Virtual diagnostic and therapeutic health care centers could be established in community hospitals without access to subspecialists, rural areas, and third world countries. These centers could also serve as education hubs for nurses, physicians, and the public. A parent could take their child to one of these centers and receive almost any type of medical test through on site personnel who are guided by physicians at tertiary care sites. As long as high quality care is maintained, the conveniences of this type of program will likely lead to equivalent or greater satisfaction than traditional office visits.

Telemedicine is an answer to many of the global health care and medical education needs. Yet, many obstacles remain and telemedicine is nowhere near its potential. As health care costs continue to spiral out of control and the variability in health care among socioeconomic groups widens, it is critical for physicians, hospital administrators, lawmakers, and the public to be forward thinking and take advantage of the great potential telemedicine affords.

References

1. Wooten R, Craig J, Patterson V. *Introduction to telemedicine*. Rittenhouse Book Distributors. Royal Society of Medicine Press Ltd, London, England. 2nd ed. 2006
2. Pushkin D, Johnston B, Speedie S. American Telemedicine Association White Paper: Telemedicine, Telehealth, and Health Information Technology; 2006. Available at: http://www.americantelemed.org/files/public/policy/HIT_Paper.pdf. Accessed December 21, 2008.
3. Norris A. *Essentials of Telemedicine and Telecare*. John Wiley and Sons, New York, NY; 2002.
4. Allen A, Alvarez D. Cutting edge Internet teleradiology from nine leading vendors. *Telemed Today* 1998;6(3):15–17.
5. Marcin J, Ellis J, Mawis R, et al. Using telemedicine to provide pediatric subspecialty care to children with special health care needs in an underserved rural community. *Pediatrics*. 2004;113:1–6.
6. Marcin J, Schepps D, Page K, et al. The use of telemedicine to provide pediatric critical care consultations to pediatric trauma patients admitted to a remote trauma intensive care unit: a preliminary report. *Pediatr Crit Care Med*. 2004;5:251–256.
7. Sable CA, Cummings SD, Pearson GD, et al. Impact of telemedicine on the practice of pediatric cardiology in community hospitals. *Pediatrics*. 2002;109:131–132. Available at: http://www.pediatrics.org/cgi/content/full/109/1/e3. Accessed December 21, 2008.
8. Spooner SA, Gotlieb EM, Committee on Clinical Information Technology; Committee on Medical Liability. Telemedicine: pediatric applications. *Pediatrics*. 2004;113(6):e639–643.
9. Sable C. Telemedicine applications in pediatric cardiology. *Minerva Pediatrica*. 2003;55:1–13.
10. Ganapathy K. Telemedicine and neurosciences. *J Clin Neurosci*. 2005;12:851–862.
11. Kuhle S, Mitchell L, Andrew M, et al. Urgent clinical challenges in children with ischemic stroke: analysis of 1065 patients from the 1-800-NOCLOTS pediatric stroke telephone consultation service. *Stroke*. 2006;37:116–122.
12. Piccolo D, Soyer P, Burgdorf W, et al. Concordance between telepathologic diagnosis and conventional histopathologic diagnosis: a multiobserver store-and-forward study on 20 skin specimens. *Arch Dermatol*. 2002;138:53–58.
13. Pesamaa L, Ebeling H, Kuusimaki ML,et al. Videoconferencing in child and adolescent telepsychiatry: a systematic review of the literature. *J Telemed Telecare*. 2004;10:187–192.
14. Wilimas J, Ribeiro R. Pediatric hematology-oncology outreach for developing countries. *Hematol Oncol Clin North Am*. 2001;15(4):775–787.
15. McConnochie KM. Potential of telemedicine in pediatric primary care. *Pediatr Rev*. 2006;27:e58–65.
16. Finley JP, Human DG, Nanton MA, et al. Echocardiography by telephone—evaluation of pediatric disease at a distance. *Am J Cardiol*. 1989;63:1475–1477.

17. Sable C, Roca T, Gold J, Gutierrez A, Gulotta E, Culpepper W. Live transmission of neonatal echocardiograms from underserved areas: accuracy, patient care, and cost. *Telemed J.* 1999;5:339–347.
18. Sharma S, Parness IA, Kamenir SA, Ko H, Haddow S, Steinberg LG, et al. Screening fetal echocardiography by telemedicine: efficacy and community acceptance. *J Am Soc Echocardiogr.* 2003;16(3): 202–208.
19. Trippi JA, Lee KS, Kopp G, Nelson D, Kovacs R. Emergency echocardiography telemedicine: an efficient method to provide 24-hour consultative echocardiography. *J Am Coll Cardiol.* 1996;27:1748–1752.
20. Stevenson JG. Evolution of echocardiography in neonatal diagnosis. *Acta Paediatr Suppl.* 1995;410:8–14.
21. Webb CL, Sable CA, Waugh CL, Grigsby J, Berdussis DJ. Impact of Telemedicine on Medical and Financial Outcomes in Infants with Suspected Heart Disease. Presented at the Twelfth Annual Scientific Sessions American Society of Echocardiography, Seattle WA, June 2001.
22. American Telemedicine Association. White paper: federal policy recommendations for home telehealth and remote monitoring; 2006. Available at: http://www.americantelemed.org/files/public/policy/Home_Telehealth_Policy_ver3_5.pdf. Accessed December 21, 2008.
23. Marcin J, Ellis J, Mawis R, et al. Using telemedicine to provide pediatric subspecialty care to children with special health care needs in an underserved rural community. *Pediatrics.* 2004;113:1–6.
24. Fleisher L, Dechene J. *Telemedicine and E-Health Law (Healthcare Law Series).* New York: Law Journal Press; Ringbound (ed); 2004.
25. Whiten P, Duis L. American Telemedicine Association White Paper: Private Payer Reimbursement for Telemedicine Services in the United States; 2006. Available at: http://www.americantelemed.org/files/public/policy/Private_Payer_Report.pdf. Accessed December 21, 2008.

Chapter 21
Personal Health Records

Alan E. Zuckerman and George R. Kim

Objectives

- To provide motivation and definitions for personal health records (PHRs)
- To summarize current progress in development and adoption of PHRs
- To project the use and challenges of PHRs in pediatrics

21.1 Introduction

A personal health record (PHR, also known as a personally controlled health record or PCHR) is "an electronic application through which individuals can access, manage and share their health information, and that of others for whom they are authorized, in a private, secure, and confidential environment."[1] PHRs are life-long summaries of key information from all providers and include data gathered between encounters, and although they may be linked to and share information with electronic health records (EHRs), PHRs are distinct in that the locus of control of information is the patient[2] (and in the case of pediatrics, the parent or guardian) instead of a clinician or health care institution.

While specific definitions are still evolving (including the HL7 PHR-S functional model[3]) the goals of PHR development and adoption include: education and empowerment of health consumers, improvement of patient safety, health quality, and reduction of costs through information access (to improve efficiency and reduce duplication of services). Interest in development and adoption of PHRs has increased among employers,[4] professional health groups[5] and government agencies,[6] and a list of 20 recommendations on privacy, security requirements, interoperability, research and evaluation and federal roles in PHR and PHR system development has been published.[7]

C.U. Lehmann et al. (eds.), *Pediatric Informatics: Computer Applications in Child Health,* Health Informatics,
© Springer Science + Business Media, LLC 2011

21.2   Technical Perspectives

21.2.1   Hardware and Connectivity

Technical specifications of PHRs include their storage, distribution and connectivity:

- Storage forms include paper, personal computer disk, Internet, and portable media (such as USB drive)
- Distribution may be controlled by the patient (as in paper and personal computer based PHRs), patient-related sponsor (employer, hospital, payer) or third-party contractors (service provider to sponsor or patient)
- Connectivity may be: standalone (unconnected to a network), tethered or view (offering views (or access) to selected data from a specific EHR) or networked (providing patient controls for access and exchange of personal health information)[2,8,9]

Interoperablity of PHRs is essential to assuring data integrity and availability. General consensus of a group of national leaders in medical informatics was that PHRs integrated with EHRs, either through tether or network, provide greater benefits than stand-alone PHRs, including conveyance of relevant and current data to patients, more robust backup in the case of system failures and an easier business case.[2] A Common Framework has been proposed for PHRs in the contexts of a National Health Information Network (NHIN), regional health information organizations (RHIOs) and subnetwork organizations (SNOs)[10] and information technology platforms[11,12] to support PHRs are being made available for development and production.

21.2.2   Software and Content

Technical specifications of PHRs also include user functionality, access control, and content/structure standards:

- User functions should allow patients to: retrieve information retrieval and generate reports based on data contained in the PHR, enter and correct data (with audit trails), request correction of errors provider records, access current clinical data from laboratory reports and other data sources (such as immunization registries) and make informed decisions (using decision support and communication tools).
- Access controls should allow patients (and families) to authorize who may see their records and under what circumstances and to see who has accessed their records. Included in access controls should be emergency access procedures for extreme circumstances.
- Content/structure standards include: core data fields on demographics, administrative and clinical items (problem lists, immunization status, laboratory tests, encounter notes, etc.).

Basic user functionality and access control issues have been articulated but not standardized to date. A single standard for content and structure, the Continuity of Care Document (CCD),[13] has resulted from the harmonization of two published standards (ASTM's continuity of care record (CCR) and HL7's clinical document architecture (CDA)[14]) for universal electronic health information exchange for PHRs.

21.3 The Pediatric Perspective

The American Academy of Pediatrics (AAP) has made *The Child Health Record*, a book for tracking and recording health information, including birth and growth data by age, immunizations, illnesses, and health maintenance details[15] available for distribution by hospitals and practices. In addition, an *Emergency Information Form* (EIF) has been articulated and advocated by the AAP and the American College of Emergency Physicians (ACEP)[16] for children with special health care needs (CSHCN) in emergency or disaster situations. Both are currently available only in paper format.

Electronic formats for pediatric PHRs have been explored. The EIF has been piloted as a patient-carried USB drive in conjunction with a nationwide emergency call center,[17,18] and "shuttle sheets" have also been explored for use by pediatric oncology patients.[19] Access to external information sources such as laboratory reporting systems and immunization and newborn screening registries has been explored but are not widely implemented to date[20] to PHRs or EHRs.[24]

Two recent investigative PHR projects that have been aimed to empower youth in the areas of medication management in chronic disease (cystic fibrosis)[21] and in the care transition from pediatric to adult care[22] have been sponsored by the Robert Wood Johnson Foundation (RWJF) Project HealthDesign. Each uses a combination of Web applications and mobile devices to empower an already technology-knowledgeable population.

Recommendations on pediatric PHRs include:

- All children should have access to a PHR, as an essential component of a Medical Home regardless of income. Medicaid and SCHIP programs should provide PHRs that are on par with those offered by private insurers and Medicare.
- PHR data must be owned and controlled by the patient or the patient's parent/ guardian, including authorization for access and emergency access. Data provided by health professionals and institutions should be subject to comment and review by the patient, but should not be modifiable. Data must be protected, technically and legally, from abuse and unauthorized secondary or commercial use.
- PHR content must include:
  ○ Demographic and insurance information
  ○ Contact information for family members, other support providers and health care providers

- ○ Advance Directives
- ○ Clinical information
  - ▪ Problems lists, encounters, procedures, chronic conditions
  - ▪ Medications, immunizations, and allergies
  - ▪ Vital signs including weight, length/height, and body mass index
  - ▪ Laboratory Results
  - ▪ Family History
  - ▪ Birth History
  - ▪ Durable Medical Equipment and Supplies
- Data integrity protection and clear identification of the source of all data.
- PHR standards should align with the special requirements for pediatric EHRs[23].
- PHRs should adhere to privacy standards, including special privacy requirements[24] and concerns for adolescents and children in foster care.
- PHR functionality should include:
  - ○ Data entry by patients or parents/guardians that is easily identifiable and provisions for providers who do not use an EHR to enter data efficiently.
  - ○ Extensibility tools that include clinical decision support (such as vaccination reminders), growth chart visualization, report generation and linkages to immunization and newborn screening information registries.
- Pediatricians should incorporate PHRs in ALL encounters to maintain continuity of the PHR with the EHR.

21.4   Current and Future Challenges

Many of the aforementioned issues are still in the development stage. A report of early experiences with three different PHR implementations[25] has produced a number of challenges and questions for future developments, including:

- Sharing of certain parts of the medical record that may reveal diagnoses, including problem lists, medication and allergy lists and laboratory and diagnostic test results, be shared
- Mechanisms by which patients and caregivers are to be authenticated and authorized to access the PHR
- Privacy issues re: minors and sharing of information via proxies
- Inclusion of functionalities such as secure messaging, integration of external knowledge sources (such as school-based health records), connection to online communities of support with others of similar diagnoses, surveillance and participation in clinical trials
- Interoperability of institution-based PHRs

In addition to these are individual barriers that vary according to population,[26] including: access to computers (and associated devices) and PHR systems, physical and cognitive disabilities, language barriers, low computer or reading literacy and low health literacy.

PHR adoption is at an early stage in pediatrics, with current challenges of establishing standards for content, information assurance and exchange as well as overcoming many of the barriers to adoption of the technology.

21.5 Conclusion

Personal health records present a great opportunity for patient empowerment and control of health information. Much attention has been given to their definition, research and development, inclusive of child health, and standards for pediatric use are still in development.

21.6 Case Studies: Examples of PHRS Planned or Currently in Use (2007)

21.6.1 PHR in a Pediatric Office Practice

Pediatric Health Care at Newton Wellesley, Massachusetts[27]

This small private group practice offers a PHR to families in their practice based on a patient-carried USB drive. The practice uses the NextGen EHR[28] for medical records and the CapMed PHR[29] with a special interface to transfer data between the two systems. A single USB disk carries information about multiple family members with the software that allows the system to be used on home computers or on computers in hospitals and other physician offices. Information may be printed prior to use when a computer will not be available. The system pre-populates the PHR with information from the EHR and automatically updates it at each visit. The PHR includes well child care patient education materials on the disk.

Benefits of this approach include: accurate and timely information from the provider's EHR, a single device for multiple children, encryption of data to prevent exposure and easy recovery in the case of device loss and facilitated data collection from home and office. An interface that allows capture of electronic prescribing data facilitates medication reconciliation. Use of the technology is also perceived as a marketing tool to build patient loyalty, especially for patients with complex problems.

Challenges created by this approach include: the need for patients to bring their USB device with them to each visit, problems with permissions and workflow when providers new to the system first provide care for the patient, the costs associated with the hardware and software. The system may not be appropriate for all patients in the practice, but is popular with many.

21.6.2   PHR in a Children's Hospital

Children's Hospitals and Clinics of Minnesota/St. Paul[30]
This children's hospital offers a PHR called the Children's Medical Organizer as a free service to their patients and families. This is a patient-controlled PHR that is advertised on the institutional Website, with the purpose of helping patients to track visits and important medical data. Much of the data in the PHR is entered by the patient, and the system helps coordinate visits to multiple specialists.

Some patients in a children's hospital use it as the main source of both primary and specialty care that will require integrating both inpatient and ambulatory data. In many cases, children's hospitals are central community health resources that serve many patients. As with the private practice model, PHRs may serve as marketing tools that build loyalty from patients and from community practitioners.

21.6.3   PHR Sponsored by Employers

Dossia[31]
This nonprofit consortium of major US employers, including Applied Materials, BP America Inc., Cardinal Health, Intel Corporation, Pitney Bowes Inc., Wal-Mart, AT&T Inc., and sanofi-aventis, has partnered with the Children's Hospital Informatics Program (CHIP) from the Children's Hospital Boston, to use technology used to develop the first personally controlled health record.[11,32] The purpose of the consortium is to provide a Web-based, employer-sponsored PHR to employees of the constituent companies.

According to the Dossia press release: "Based on the Indivo system, and with the individual's consent, the Dossia framework will gather health information from various sources and store it within secured databases. Dossia's use of the Indivo open architecture will support multiple personal health applications, allowing users to organize and summarize their information in ways that are most useful to them. Health records will be secure and private, accessible only by the individual or others to whom the individual has granted permission. Records also will be portable, enabling individuals to continue using the records even if they change employers, health plans or doctors. Participation by employees will be voluntary."[33]

21.6.4   PHR by an Individual Vendor

HealthVault[34]
HealthVault, which was announced by the Microsoft Corporation in October 2007, is an online platform for storing personal health records. It provides a Web-based interface where consumers can upload or share health documents from their providers (such as letters, reports, and discharge summaries). Information from

stored documents (or entered directly by the patient/user) is stored in a secure, encrypted database with privacy set by the user. In addition, the platform allows anonymous Internet searches for health topics as well as interfaces to and from a number of health and communications devices and data sources, including fax, physiologic monitoring tools, and laboratory and encounter reports.

Still in development, a number of vendor organizations, including the American Heart Association, Johnson & Johnson LifeScan, NewYork-Presbyterian Hospital, the Mayo Clinic, and MedStar Health are partnering with HealthVault to build applications and infrastructures that support and use PHR data.[35]

References

1. Connecting for Health. The personal health working group final report. Markle Foundation; 2003. Available at: http://www.connectingforhealth.org/resources/final_phwg_report1.pdf. Accessed December 21, 2008.
2. Tang PC, Ash JS, Bates DW, Overhage JM, Sands DZ. Personal health records: definitions, benefits, and strategies for overcoming barriers to adoption. *J Am Med Inform Assoc.* 2006;13(2):121–126.
3. Health Data Management. Draft PHR Standard Model Approved; 2007. Available at: http://www.healthdatamanagement.com/news/standards_PHR25313-1.html. Accessed December 20, 2008.
4. Walton CG. Written testimony before the Secretary of HHS's Public Advisory Body, the National Committee on Vital Health Statistics and the Subcommittee on Privacy and Confidentiality. January 23, 2007. Available at: http://www.ncvhs.hhs.gov/070123p1a.htm. Accessed December 21, 2008.
5. Endsley S, Kibbe DC, Linares A, Colorafi K. An introduction to personal health records. *Fam Pract Manage.* May 2006;57–65.
6. Centers for Medicare and Medicaid Services. Medicare Testing Personal Health Records to Health Beneficiaries Better Manage Own Health Care. Press release; 2007. Available at: http://www.cms.hhs.gov/apps/media/press/release.asp?Counter=2217. Accessed November 23, 2007.
7. National Committee on Vital and Health Statistics. Personal Health Records and Personal Health Record Systems: A Report and Recommendations from the National Committee on Vital and Health Statistics. U.S. Department of Health and Human Services, Washington, DC; 2006. Available at: http://www.ncvhs.hhs.gov/0602nhiirpt.pdf. Accessed November 23, 2007.
8. Esterhay RJ. Opportunities and Challenges with PHRs: Discussion. Panel on Opportunities and Challenges Facing PHI and PHR Initiatives, 2007 AMIA Spring Congress; 2007.
9. Blechman EA. Testimony to American Health Information Community Consumer Empowerment Workgroup Hearing on Personal Health Records; 2006. Available at: http://www.hhs.gov/healthit/ahic/materials/meeting07/cemp/testimony/3-blechman.doc. Accessed November 23, 2007.
10. Markle Foundation. Connecting for Health. Connecting Americans To Their Health Care: A Common Framework for Networked Personal Health Information; 2006. Available at: http://www.connectingforhealth.org/commonframework/docs/P9_NetworkedPHRs.pdf. Accessed November 23, 2007.
11. The Children's Hospital Informatics Program. IndivoHealth Boston, MA. Available at: http://www.indivohealth.org. Accessed December 21, 2008.

12. Microsoft Corporation. HealthVault Redmond, WA; 2008. Available at: http://www.healthvault.com. Accessed December 21, 2008.
13. Health Information Technology Standards Panel. Available at: http://www.hitsp.org. Accessed December 21, 2008.
14. Ferranti JM, Musser RC, Kawamoto K, Hammond WE. The clinical document architecture and the continuity of care record: a critical analysis. *J Am Med Inform Assoc.* 2006;13(3): 245–252.
15. American Academy of Pediatrics. Child Health Record. Commercially available from the AAP Website; 2008. Available at: https://www.nfaap.org/netforum/eweb/dynamicpage. aspx?webcode=aapbks_productdetail&key=e384de72-0f58-4a15-9e21-cf2cebfb52cb. Accessed December 21, 2008.
16. American Academy of Pediatrics Committee on Emergency Medicine. Emergency preparedness for children with special health care needs. Committee on Pediatric Emergency Medicine. American Academy of Pediatrics. *Pediatrics.* 1999;104 (4):e53.
17. MedicAlert Foundation. Personal Health Record. Commercially available through MedicAlert; 2008. Available at: http://www.medicalert.org/Main/PersonalHealthRecords.aspx. Accessed December 21, 2008.
18. American Academy of Pediatrics. Emergency Preparedness for Children with Special Health Care Needs. Commonly asked questions and answers regarding the American Academy of Pediatrics/American College of Emergency Physicians Emergency Information Form (EIF); 2007. Available at: http://www.aap.org/advocacy/epquesansw.htm. Accessed December 21, 2008.
19. Stevens MM. 'Shuttle sheet': a patient-held medical record for pediatric oncology families. *Med Pediatr Oncol.* 1992;20(4):330–335.
20. Rocha RA, Romeo AN, Norlin C. Core features of a parent-controlled pediatric medical home record. *Medinfo.* 2007;12(Pt 2):997–1001.
21. Johnson K. My-Medi-Health: A Vision for a Child-focused Personal Medication Management System. Project HealthDesign. Robert Wood Johnson Foundation; 2007. Available at: http://www.projecthealthdesign.org/projects/190928. Accessed December 21, 2008.
22. Sandborg C. Living Profiles: Transmedia Personal Health Record Systems for Young Adults. Project HealthDesign, Robert Wood Johnson Foundation; 2007. Available at: http://www.projecthealthdesign.org/projects/191096. Accessed December 21, 2008.
23. Spooner SA, Council on Clinical Information Technology. American Academy of Pediatrics. Special requirements of electronic health record systems in pediatrics. *Pediatrics.* 2007;119(3):631–637.
24. Chilton L, et al. American Academy of Pediatrics. Pediatric Practice Action Group and Task Force on Medical Informatics. Privacy protection and health information: patient rights and pediatrician responsibilities. *Pediatrics.* 1999;104(4 Pt 1):973–977.
25. Halamka J, Mandl KD, Tang P. Early experiences with personal health records. *J Am Med Inform Assoc.* 2007;15:1–7.
26. Lober WB, Zieler B, Herbaugh A, Shinstrom,SE, Stolyar A, Kim EH, Kim Y. Barriers to the use of a personal health record by an elderly population. *AMIA Annu Symp Proc.* 2006;514–518.
27. Pediatric Health Care at Wellesley-Newton, PC. Practice Website; 2008. Available at: http://www.pediatrichealthcare.com/. Accessed December 21, 2008.
28. NextGen. Corporate Website; 2008. Available at: http://www.nextgen.com/. Accessed December 21, 2008.
29. CapMed. Capmed Personal Health Record; 2008. Available at: http://www.capmed.com/. Accessed December 21, 2008.
30. Children's Hospitals and Clinics of Minnesota/St. Paul. Children's Medical Organizer; 2008. Available at: http://www.childrensmn.org/cmo/. Accessed December 21, 2008.
31. Dossia. Corporate Website; 2008. Available at: http://www.dossia.org. Accessed December 21, 2008.

32. Mandl KD, Simons WW, Crawford WC, Abbett JM. Indivo: a personally controlled health record for health information exchange and communication. *BMC Med Inform Decis Mak.* 2007;12;7:25.
33. Dossia. Dossia gains momentum toward providing employees with personal, private, portable and secure health records. Dossia press release; September 17, 2007. Available at: http://www.dossia.org/news-events-media/media-center/doc_download/16-dossia-gains-momentum. Accessed December 21, 2008.
34. Microsoft Corporation. HealthVault; 2008. Available at: http://www.healthvault.com/. Accessed December 21, 2008.
35. Lohr S. *Microsoft Rolls Out Personal Health Records.* New York Times; October 4, 2007. Available at http://www.NYTimes.com/.Accessed March 20, 2009.

Chapter 22
Privacy Issues

David M.N. Paperny

Objectives

- To outline the nature of privacy requirements for pediatric health information systems
- To define Protected Health Information (PHI), its inappropriate access and release
- To describe information assurance (IA), workflows, and systems that are able to distinguish IA requirements for different pediatric diagnoses and populations

22.1 Introduction

Pediatric privacy issues are distinct from those of adult patients because the details of confidentiality and access to child health information vary across social and legal situations and across the age ranges from infancy to young adulthood. Health information technology tools must be able to adapt to those needs and to allow easy access to the personal health information of children in medical care while protecting their rights and privacy.

22.2 Basics

22.2.1 Information Assurance

Information assurance (IA) is the management of data-related risks. The processing and communication of data creates three categories: data at rest (stored), data in

C.U. Lehmann et al. (eds.), *Pediatric Informatics: Computer Applications in Child Health*, Health Informatics,
© Springer Science+Business Media, LLC 2011

transit (transmitted or received) and data in use (created, read, updated, deleted, or altered). Key points of information assurance include:

- Confidentiality: Can **users/nonusers** be trusted?
  - Authentication: How is the user identified?
    - "Something the user is" (intrinsic to the user): biometrics
    - "Something the user has" (an object): keys
    - "Something the user knows": passwords
  - Authority: What is a user allowed to do?
    - Read (and copy) records
    - Alter (create, update, delete) records
- Integrity: Can the **information** be trusted?
  - Content integrity: Can the content be trusted?
    - Audit trails of alterations
  - Source integrity: Can the source be trusted?
    - Includes non-repudiation, the inability to deny that a transaction has occurred
- Availability: Can the **system** be trusted?
  - Physical accessibility: includes access by hardware, software, and communications networks
  - Functional accessibility: includes downtime and denials of service

IA also consists of processes to assess and mitigate risks, including establishment of procedures, training of personnel and certification of hardware, software, and communication tools to achieve that. Included in IA processes are downtime procedures and recovery from breaches.

22.2.2   The Health Information Portability and Accountability Act (1996)

The Health Information Portability and Accountability Act (HIPAA)[1] of 1996 defines the floor for health care requirements to maintain privacy. These include:

- Privacy regulations, which define protected health information (PHI, specific health information that can link a record to a specific patient) and establishes rules for their use and disclosures of PHI use by "covered entities." PHI may be shared for the purposes of transactions, payments and operations, with the quality improvement initiatives (as part of operations) coming under closer scrutiny by regulators.
- Security regulations, which specify and set standards for physical, technical, and administrative safeguards for covered entities.
- Specific exceptions to the consent and authorization requirements.
- Rights of patients to access their own records.

22.3   Pediatric Privacy and Confidentiality Issues

22.3.1   Infants and Children

For infants and children younger than the age of majority (depending on the jurisdiction), privacy of health information is managed through parents or guardians. Problems with privacy and security of health information may occur with:

- Assignment of authentication, authority (and for which functions), and availability of a child's health information:
  ○ For multiple individuals (such as both parents or shared guardianship)
  ○ When parental or guardianship roles exist but are not recognized by the law
  ○ When families are undergoing separation, divorce or other legal processes
  ○ When children have statutory right to consent for confidential treatment
  ○ When children reach the age of majority
  ○ For children in foster care or emergent guardianship
- Breaches of confidentiality and integrity of health information in children:
  ○ With specific diagnoses that may not be openly shared (such as HIV)
  ○ With legal issues that are not known by family members (adoption, foster care)
  ○ With families who have high-profile relatives (politicians, etc.) or members who work in health care ("within the system")

22.3.2   Adolescents

Confidentiality in adolescent care is covered in Chapter 5. In adolescent health, confidentiality in communications is a *sine qua non* between provider and patient.[2] Teens are legally allowed to consent for certain confidential health care and have the right of "privileged communication" by rules of professional privilege. This mandate also applies to nonprofessionals working under or supporting the clinician, including the IT staff, system, and the EMR. Information assurance processes for this population must be comprehensive, as inappropriate notification of health issues may be communicated to parents and guardians through unintentional data releases and insurance notifications. This is often closely bound to practice workflows and reimbursement.

22.4   Common Issues and Scenarios

22.4.1   Consenting to Treatment

Only a legal parent or guardian can consent to treatment of a minor (except in documented emergencies and by specific statute):

Aunt Lisa transports her 6 month old niece to the doctor at the mother's request for a fever. She hand carries a note signed by mother giving Aunt Lisa permission to consent for treatment. The pediatrician assesses that a lumbar puncture is necessary. The mother is unavailable by phone.

The pediatrician may: 1) accept the note in good faith if it appears to be valid, 2) ask a MD colleague to co-sign consent with him as an emergency, or 3) look in the scanned document portion of the EMR for aunt's name or others who can consent.

22.4.2   Releasing Information

Only the person who can CONSENT for treatment can release EMR information related to that treatment:[3]

A teenager consents for family planning, including a pelvic examination. Only she is allowed direct access to release the portion of the medical record regarding that procedure/ treatment.

When custody issues are present, documentation that establishes legal guardianship including but not limited to court orders and Durable Power of Attorney for Health Care are required.

22.4.3   Restricting Access to PHI According to Role

"The information belongs to the patient, but the actual record belongs to the physician."[4] To control PHI to the level of detail needed to assure confidentiality, restricted access to specific data according to role is required (adolescent patient: all records; parent: all records up to age 13; physician and case manager: all; nurse: vital signs and immunizations; pharmacist: medications/allergies; receptionist: demographics/billing):

A medical assistant mother looks into an EMR to see if her teenager's antihistamine is refillable, and notices her daughter is also on birth control pills.

Organizational and employee agreements in health systems must include and specify precise restrictions on access and use of PHI as well as disciplinary actions in the case of violations.

22.4.4   Restricting Access to Psychiatric PHI

Psychiatry notes are frequently separated physically from other parts of the medical record. In EMRs, mental health diagnoses and progress notes may be restricted electronically to Psychiatry staff, but psychotropic medications prescribed for the patient must be visible (or restricted) to all clinicians. Similar restrictions may be created for Adolescent Medicine and Obstetrics/Gynecology issues:

> *A locum tenens physician is covering a clinic for a medical group. Review of a sick 14 year old female's EMR by the physician reveals an SSRI and an oral contraceptive on the medication list. There is a record for a previous visit to the groups' family practitioner who prescribed the oral contraceptive. The SSRI was prescribed by the group's psychiatrist, for which there is no progress note or diagnosis available in the EMR.*

22.4.5 Restricting Access to Diagnosis and Problem Lists

The personal, legal and economic impact of certain diagnoses (especially when generated by templates) on liability, job qualifications, medical and life insurance and security clearances[5-6] make control over active problem lists and diagnoses essential from a privacy viewpoint. Psychiatric issues and other medical diagnoses such as drug abuse, malingering, poor parenting, prenatal drug abuse on newborn lab screening, gender identity issues,[7] HIV, and Munchausen's Syndrome (including by proxy) have potential consequences and must be verified with valid medical findings and facts beyond a simple notation:

> *A mother completes an application to add life insurance for her 22 year old daughter to her policy. An EMR report is automatically released to the insurance company as part of the application process. The daughter is denied coverage based on a diagnosis of suicidal thoughts 5 years prior, although no diagnosis of depression is currently on the problem list.*

> *A 21 year old works for a company contracting to the federal government, which requires all employees to pass security clearance. The employee fails the security clearance based on a positive drug test discovered in the EMR for marijuana at age 17.*

22.4.6 Documenting and Releasing Information on Alleged Abuse

Documentation standards for interviews and examinations of minors for sexual abuse and physical abuse must meet defined legal standards and be available to legal and protective services. Documentation and evidence must be passed through an auditable chain of custody and is confidential, unless there is a concern that a child or teen is in imminent danger by a caretaker or parent:

> *A mother requests a clinic nurse to review the EMR of a developmentally delayed 4 year old evaluated 2 weeks previously for bruises (with digital photos that are in the EMR). The mother alleges that the father (who has joint custody of the child and who has the child for the weekend) inflicted the bruises and requests the nurse to file a protective services report to get the child back. Upon review of the record with the physician, the nurse finds the physician remembers numerous contacts in the past, previously cleared by CPS (but documented only in the archived paper chart) and evidence of a custody battle with a restraining order against the mother.*

22.4.7 Maintaining Confidentiality in Workflow

An appropriate workflow for *confidential (nonpsychiatric) medical visits* must alert staff to the needs for confidentiality of visits:

- Use confidential *appointment codes* to suppress home mailers (results, bills, and quality of service surveys) and *coverage codes* (used when the patient is unable to pay on date of service)
- Create two encounters, one for the confidential component of a visit (i.e., a routine physical and a confidential visit), with one registration fee
- Assign a temporary private billing address for the confidential visit (primarily if the patient is paying out-of-pocket)
- Note sensitive diagnoses in the problem list and laboratory test results as "confidential"
- Do not release information for the confidential portion of the visit without patient consent
- Maintain information assurance standards during the visit

  A family practice physician seeing a mother and her teenage daughter in the exam room was charting in the EMR and was called out of the room by the nurse for an urgent call. He neglected to lock the workstation screen and the mother was able to read the following diagnosis from her daughter's record problem list: "CONTRACEPTIVE MANAGEMENT – "confidential"

  A 16 year old girl seen in a hospital emergency department (ED) with gastritis was surprised to find she was pregnant (on routine ED screening), and she asked the ED physician not to tell her mother who accompanied her. When the hospital ED bill was sent to the home 3 weeks later, her father, the hospital custodian, noticed the pregnancy test on the bill. The next day at work he was able to access the positive result in the unprotected lab computer system by simply typing in her medical record number.

22.4.8 Using Communications Practices That Assure Privacy

Appropriate "good practice" communication policies should be made clear for patients and staff. Appropriate telephone and fax practices include:

- Contact patients directly when possible for telephone messages or leave a message for a call back
- Educate patients, families, and staff of inappropriateness of leaving messages about sensitive issues
- Use alternative forms of communication if there is no reply to a message
- Document all communications, attempts, and discussions in the patient record with date/times.

For fax, include sender telephone number for contact in the case of mis-delivery. Double-check with recipients regarding the secure location of the receiving machine and receipt of the fax. Include standard fax privacy and intended addressee notices on all fax communications, and disclose (and document) any errors in delivery.

22.4.9   Sharing Local Adolescent Health Privacy Laws with Patients and Staff

Although adolescents under age 18 are legally minors (depending on the jurisdiction), there are precedents which permit them to consent to health services:

- Specific statutes empower minors to consent for pregnancy care as well as confidential contraception, STI/HIV testing and treatment, alcohol and drug abuse treatment, and mental health counseling and treatment.
- Legally *emancipated minors* are those: (a) serving in the armed forces, (b) living away from home and managing their own financial affairs, or (c) who are or have been pregnant or are parents.
- By common law doctrine, *mature minors* demonstrate sufficient cognitive maturity to understand the risks and benefits of proposed medical treatments and alternatives, and can thereby voluntarily and responsibly consent.
- Exceptions to confidentiality may include situations where an adolescent patient:
  - Is suicidal/homicidal or poses a danger to self or others
  - Is a victim of sexual or physical abuse

22.5   Conclusion: The Place of IT in Information Assurance

The protection of child and adolescent privacy and of PHI security is complex in pediatric care because of the different and changing patterns of authorization that occur over the lifetime of the child. In assuring these protections, the design and implementation of health IT must incorporate and enforce the basic premises of information assurance and HIPAA while taking into account developmental and chronological differences.

References

1. Gostin LO. National health information privacy: regulations under the Health Insurance Portability and Accountability Act. *JAMA*. 2001;285(23):3015–3021.
2. Hoffmann AD, Greydanus DE. Chapter 6: consent and confidentiality. In: *Adolescent Medicine*. 3rd ed. Stamford, CT: Appleton & Lange; 1997.
3. American Academy of Pediatrics Committee on Adolescence. Achieving quality health services for adolescents. *Pediatrics*. 2008;121:1263–1270.

4. Zurhellen WM. The computerization of ambulatory pediatric practice. *Pediatrics*. 1995;96 (4 Pt 2):835–842; discussion 842–844.
5. American Academy of Pediatrics Committee on Substance Abuse and Council on School Health. Testing for drugs of abuse in children and adolescents: addendum—testing in schools and at home. *Pediatrics*. 2007;119 (3):627–630.
6. Bukstein OG, Bernet W, Arnold V, et al. Practice parameter for the assessment and treatment of children and adolescents with substance use disorders. *J Am Acad Child Adolesc Psychiat*. 2005;44(6):609–621.
7. Parents, Families and Friends of Lesbians And Gays (PFLAG). 1726 M Street, NW, Suite 400, Washington, DC 20036. Available at: http://community.pflag.org. Accessed December 21, 2008.

Chapter 23
Electronic Mail in Pediatric Practice

Robert S. Gerstle

Objectives

- To be able to integrate e-mail effectively and efficiently into a medical practice
- To be able to limit potential e-mail liability issues by being aware of best practices and legislation that impacts the use of email in medical practice
- To recognize that e-mail is a patient satisfier and its use in practice may help to build a successful practice

23.1 Introduction

E-mail is an important component of the revolution in the delivery of health care.[1] "Just as the telephone transformed American society and the practice of medicine, electronic communication is having a similar impact and will become an integral part of pediatrics."[2] E-mail use has benefits to the patient and the physician. It can reduce unnecessary office visits, increase practice efficiency, make office visits more productive; improve access to care, improve physician–patient communication and improve chronic disease management.[3,4]

Of non-face-to-face patient–physician communications (telephone/fax, electronic mail, short message service (SMS or texting), videoconference), e-mail is the most ubiquitous. However, barriers to its adoption in practice are: (a) lack of physician reimbursement for adopting such technology for patient-centered work (that can be time-consuming), (b) uncovered liabilities incurred during such transactions, and (c) fear of breaches of security and privacy.

C.U. Lehmann et al. (eds.), *Pediatric Informatics: Computer Applications in Child Health,* Health Informatics,
© Springer Science+Business Media, LLC 2011

23.2 Issues in Patient–Physician Electronic Communication[1-2]

23.2.1 Reimbursement

Recently, the value of e-mail encounters has been recognized by selected insurers by their willingness to allow billing for e-mail consultations with established patients, subject to individual contract negotiation with the insurer. Interestingly, insurers seem more amenable to reimburse pediatricians for e-mail "visits" then for telephone care (which has long been a part of pediatric practice), perhaps because of the inherent ability to "capture" documentation. Typically insurers have allowed charges that typically reflect the patient's office co-pay, usually resulting in little or no actual cost to the insurer itself. Recently Current Procedural Terminology (CPT 2008)[8] was updated to include a code specifically referencing direct e-mail care or consultations.

> 99444 Online evaluation and management service provided by a physician to an established patient, guardian, or health care provider not originating from a related E/M service provided within the previous 7 days, using the Internet or similar electronic communications network.

However, recognize that the availability of a CPT code for a procedure does not automatically guarantee insurer payment for the procedure.

Secure messaging and charge capture

- Some physician office portals allow capture of and charging for e-mail services through online prepayment.
- Charges for such online queries that require or result in a face-to-face visit can be credited back to patients.

23.2.2 Liability and Appropriate Use of E-Mail

The appropriateness and limitations of e-mail use must be clearly communicated and reiterated to patients. Suggestions to implement this include:

Using secured sites and portals

- Require full identification of patients registered to the practice in all transactions
- Post policies and limitations of e-mail services
- Use structured messages for a set of specific information or procedures: prescription refills, referrals, school forms, etc

Posting specific information ("auto-reply") on all outgoing messages

- Note expected time of reply, including unavailability of personnel.
- Use disclaimers for emergency care ("Call 911").

23.2.3   Breaches of Security and Privacy

The Health Insurance Portability and Accountability Act (HIPAA) sets federal requirements for privacy and security of protected health information (PHI). Though this legislation primarily deals with electronic data transmission and interchange of billing information, it also addresses all electronic health care communications, including e-mail communications.

HIPAA does not prohibit e-mail communications between physicians and patients or between physicians but recognizes that e-mail (and any health information technology) presents risks to privacy and that anyone using e-mail needs to (a) identify risks to the unauthorized access to personal health information and (b) adopt policies and procedures to mitigate those risks. HIPAA also requires that office policies, as they relate to its use of medical information be made known to patients and made available in the practice's Information Privacy Notice.

Practice policies
The HIPAA Security Rule specifies that practices (and other "covered entities") must use physical, technical, and administrative safeguards with PHI. The HIPAA Privacy Rule specifies that safeguards must include auditing and disclosure procedures (for breaches). For e-mail, this includes, but is not limited to:

- Limited physical and password-protected access to practice computer systems (including e-mail)
- Use of secure e-mail (either secure messaging or private service) with backup systems
- Policies to remove access for employees who no longer work for the practice

E-mail practices
Patients and families themselves may be the greatest threat to their e-mail privacy. Poor e-mail practices (by patients and/or practices) that may put privacy at risk include:

- Leaving computers unattended while logged into e-mail or leaving screens or printed messages open and accessible to others; not destroying discarded messages appropriately (shredding documents, emptying "Trash" or "Recycle" bins)
- Sharing e-mail accounts or passwords with others (or using poor password security)
- Handling messages inappropriately: forwarding e-mail messages to others, sending replies to a group of recipients ("reply to all")

23.3   Issues in Physician–Physician and Physician–Staff Electronic Communication

23.3.1   Technical Issues

Secure e-mail communications between physicians (for patient-related matters) may be provided by a shared private network, provided by a common hospital, IPA,

PHO, HMO, or medical society. In such arrangements, connections are protected and messages are encrypted through standard protocols prior to transmission. Thus physician–physician communications for referrals, consults, follow-up, or general questions can be made relatively securely and simply within the confines of that network.

Where e-mail communication between physicians occurs between networks, such as between different medical centers, a Virtual Private Network or VPN (to connect external physicians to those within a network securely) may be established to comply with HIPAA regulations when a sufficiently high volume of information is exchanged between centers.

In addition to encryption, messages may be sent as password-protected e-mail attachments. Passwords may be assigned through standard word and document processing tools or through software designed specifically for such a purpose. Sender and recipient need to have the software tools and knowledge of the password (or key). The method of protection and the strength of the security depend on the sensitivity and importance of the information.

23.3.2   Organization and Personnel Issues

The handling of e-mail containing PHI once it has been received is equally important in security. Defined procedures on handling e-mail: who may access it (physicians only, nurses, clerical personnel), where they may access it (at work only, at home, on mobile tools), what they are prescribed to do with it (print, save, delete, forward via e-mail, file with the record) are needed, with an audit trail for tracking messages. Increasingly, EHR vendors are integrating e-mail modules into their products to improve productivity.

Other organizational issues include handling permissions for employees who leave the practice and adequate training of new employees charged with handling clinical e-mail messages. Periodic review of procedures is needed to assure due diligence in considering security and efficiency of e-mail practice.

23.4   Issues in Improving Access, Quality, and Revenue with E-Mail

23.4.1   Access

Although e-mail is ubiquitous, a "digital divide" may exist between "the haves and the have-nots." Barriers to e-mail accessibility and usability may include lack of access to: computers, Internet access and e-mail, computer and health literacy, adequate language or typing skills, and ability to receive responses. For the poor and underserved, e-mail accessibility issues are compounded by the recognition that for some, their only e-mail access or most convenient access is at work and that using workplace based e-mail systems results in privacy problems.

23.4.2 Quality

In conjunction with good practices, e-mail provides a transcribed record of communications (either patient–physician or physician–physician) with a time-stamp. E-mail can be used to handle nonurgent matters. For adolescents, it may be helpful in initiating discussions on sensitive topics that would otherwise be missed in parent-accompanied office visits.

23.4.3 Revenue

Because e-mail is a fixed expense, there is a large benefit to leveraging its use to improve office processes and patient satisfaction. While none of the possible uses of e-mail are novel, in that they can be accomplished utilizing traditional mail, the fact that e-mail messaging is essentially free, information flow is rapid, and systems exist to automate functions make e-mail communication particularly attractive to patients and physician practices. E-mail messages can be used to educate families through electronic pamphlet attachments or by linkage to practice portals, to send reminders and to send notices (such as practice newsletters).

23.5 Selecting a Practice E-Mail System

In selecting a practice e-mail solution there are many of issues to consider:

- Does the practice want e-mail alone, or as part of a complete web presence, integrating an office Web site, with e-mail accessibility or secure messaging?
- Will messages from anyone be allowed (as a marketing tool) or will e-mail be allowed only for patients registered to the practice? Will patients need to sign a contract on practice e-mail policies prior to participation?
- What type of security should be specified: encrypted connection, passwords, etc.?
- Will e-mail be limited to clinicians or will routing of messages to office staff (such as for appointments and referrals) be allowed?
- Will the practice bill for e-mail rendered services? If so, how will e-mail be integrated into the practice management system for payment?
- How will the e-mail system be protected from external attack, failure or data loss?
- How will e-mail communications be incorporated into the medical record? Will paper copies of communications be printed? Will they be saved electronically?

23.6   E-Mail Scenarios (Hypothetical)

23.6.1   Behavior Problems and Practice Pamphlets

Matilda Rivera, mother to 3 year old Jose, e-mails you that she is having difficulty with his negative behavior, refusing now to sit on the toilet and beginning to have more tantrums when she doesn't let him get his way. What should she do?

You remember that you had a similar question posed to you previously and found a good document on the Internet that you modified. You saved your recommendations as a document (negative behavior in 3 yr-old.doc) for possible future reuse. Reviewing that document, you make some minor edits and personalize it for Jose's situation. You've also included a couple of web site URLs which you re-review to make sure they are still accurate, to provide Jose's mother with additional information about typical 3 yr old behavior problems. You attach the document to the reply to the original e-mail she sent to you, and encourage Jose's mother to try your suggestions, but to come to the office if things don't improve over the next month's time. Your response is saved in Jose's medical record (either by printing out the reply and document, or by saving a copy of the e-mail question and response to the electronic medical record).

This is an example of incorporating e-mail and electronic documents into the office practice. It is a nonemergency problem, and no harm will result from a short delay. For recurring or common issues, recommendations may be "reused." Reference and links to online resources will provide written information that may be consulted or discussed at a later visit.

Patients will use e-mail for a variety of health care matters. A study of e-mail content from two large academic medical practices[9] found the following distribution of e-mail use (Table 23.1):

Table 23.1 Patient e-mail content from two large academic practices

Message content	%
Information updates to the physician	41.4
Prescription renewal requests	24.2
Health questions	13.2
Messages about medical tests	10.9
Referral requests	8.8
Appointment requests	5.4
Information seeking (directions, office hours, etc.)	4.8
Billing questions	0.3
Other (thank you, apologies, non-medical, study related)	8.8

For pediatric practices, 80% of patients in a pediatric practice expressed interest in using email for six functions:[10]

- Schedule an appointment
- Give/get test results
- Refill prescriptions

- Answer/ask questions
- Provide/get additional information
- Discuss symptoms

An analysis of 81 e-mail messages within a pediatric office[11] revealed (Table 23.2):
The response type frequencies **were** (Table 23.3):

Table 23.2 Types of e-mail requests in a pediatric office

Type of request	%
Medical question	53
Medical update	25
Subspecialty follow-up	11
Administrative request	11

Table 23.3 Responses to e-mail from a pediatric office

Type of response	%
Medical guidance	63
Phone call	10
Prescription	16
Subspecialist referral	2
Administrative paperwork	5
Appointment	4

23.6.2   Chronic Disease Management and Privacy

A pediatric office decides to send an e-mail alert (message) all the asthmatic patients in the practice to let them know that the office has influenza vaccine and all patients with asthma should call to come in for their yearly immunization. One e-mail "flier" is sent by e-mail to multiple patients utilizing the office's "asthma group e-mail address list". Patients are happy to get notice – until they recognize that they can see the names and e-mail address of every asthmatic in the practice, and realize that this information about themselves is visible to all the other recipients of the mass e-mail.

Situations, similar to that above, occur commonly. Such errors, including inadvertent transmission of a patient's diagnoses, are a breach of privacy under HIPAA and are subject to regulations on penalties and disclosures. Another privacy issue relates to staff access to patient e-mail messages intended for a physician. In some offices a nurse or clerk may read all incoming e-mail and triage billing questions to the office, appointment requests to front desk and medical questions to the physician. These are part of practice operations, and patients sending medical questions specifically to their physicians should be aware that office personnel may read and act upon their question before or on behalf of the physician. Clear office privacy policies must be in place, and staff must adhere to them as part of their employment contracts. Patients using e-mail must be informed of practice policies and procedures regarding e-mail: HIPAA regulations, "Do's and Don'ts" and expectations before e-mail use with the practice is allowed. The use of secure messaging and/or reimbursed e-mail services[12] may streamline some of these tasks.

References

1. Kassirer JP. The next transformation in the delivery of health care. *N Engl J Med.* 1995;332(1):52–54.
2. Bauchner H, Adams W, Burstin H. 'You've got mail': issues in communicating with patients and their families by e-mail. *Pediatrics.* 2002;109(5):954–956.
3. American College of Physicians. Policy Paper: The Changing Face of Ambulatory Medicine: Reimbursing Physicians for Computer-Based Care; 2003. Available at: http://www.acponline.org/about_acp/special_programs/revitalization/tel_care.pdf. Accessed December 21, 2008.
4. Rosen P, Kwoh CK. Patient-physician e-mail: an opportunity to transform pediatric health care delivery. *Pediatrics.* 2007;120(4):701–706.
5. Gerstle RS. American Academy of Pediatrics Task Force on Medical Informatics. E-mail communication between pediatricians and their patients. *Pediatrics.* 2004, reaffirmed 2008;114(1):317–321.
6. Kane B, Sands DZ. Guidelines for the clinical use of electronic mail with patients. The AMIA Internet Working Group, task force on guidelines for the use of clinic-patient electronic mail. *J Am Med Inform Assoc.* 1998 January–February;5(1):104–111.
7. Spielberg AR. On call and online: sociohistorical, legal, and ethical implications of e-mail for the patient-physician relationship. *JAMA.* 1998;280(15):1353–1359.
8. American Medical Association. Current Procedural Terminology; 2008. Available at: http://www.ama-assn.org/ama/pub/category/3113.html. Accessed July 11, 2008.
9. White CB, Moyer CA, Stern DT, Katz SJ. A content analysis of e-mail communication between patients and their providers: patients get the message. *J Am Med Inform Assoc.* 2004;11:260–267.
10. Kleiner KD, Akers R, Burke BL. Parent and physician attitudes regarding electronic communication in pediatric practices. *Pediatrics.* 2002;109:740–744.
11. Anand SG, Feldman MJ, Geller DS, Bisbee A, Bauchner H. A content Analysis of e-mail Communications between Primary Care Providers and Parents. *Pediatrics.* 2005;115:1283–1288.
12. Freudenheim M. Digital Rx: Take Two Aspirins and E-mail Me in the morning. New York Times; March 2, 2005. Available at: http://query.nytimes.com/gst/fullpage.html?res=940CEEDD133DF931A35750C0A9639C8B63. Accessed December 21, 2008.

Chapter 24
Information Management by Patients and Parents in Health and Disease

Mark M. Simonian

Objectives

- To outline patient and parent information needs and communication in pediatric care
- To describe the evolution of information and communications technology (ICT) and its effect on the relationship between families and pediatricians
- To explore specific ICT tools with current examples and how pediatricians are leveraging them to improve care, communication and patient satisfaction

24.1 Introduction

An effective partnership between a family and a pediatrician depends on good communication. One of the most valuable services a pediatrician can provide a child and family is his/her experience and skills in eliciting a history to diagnose and treat a problem and in sharing health information to educate and empower patients and families. Communication tasks that a practitioner performs may range from explaining a diagnosis or test results to obtaining informed consent from a literacy-challenged parent for a medical procedure to listening to and counseling a distraught teenager.

Information and communication technology (ICT) can provide both benefits and tradeoffs to patients, parents, and pediatricians. For families, telephone, fax, and electronic mail with their health care providers may provide flexibility, speed, and ease in exchange for the reassurance and other nuances of direct contact with a trusted provider. For pediatricians, ICT may increase access, but must be managed to prevent overload and to maintain quality of care and clinical and fiscal productivity.

C.U. Lehmann et al. (eds.), *Pediatric Informatics: Computer Applications in Child Health*, Health Informatics,
© Springer Science+Business Media, LLC 2011

24.2   Communication Modes and Reimbursement

24.2.1   Face to Face Communication and the Office Visit

The traditional relationship between a family and pediatrician is in direct consultation: a face-to-face systematic history to discover symptoms and health problems and a physical examination to assess signs and abnormalities that corroborate or contradict the history, provide clues to diagnoses and direct further tests. In addition to the traditional office or clinic visit, house calls offered the pediatrician additional information about the patient and family within the context of the home environment.

Data collected from a patient encounter is transcribed into the patient's medical record for future reference. The record additionally may store other clinical and administrative information, including written communications: sequential clinic notes, correspondence, prescriptions, consultation reports, test results, procedure summaries, and billing. Extended communications with patients (such as family conferences or discussions about complex care) are usually face-to-face, as third-party reimbursements are linked to specific office and inpatient encounters.

24.2.2   Telephone and Fax: Traditional Communications Tools Facilitating Care

Telephone facilitates communication between families and pediatricians (and their office staff) without a specific face-to-face encounter. In fact, most telephone consultations do not require office visits (or house calls) and may be used to triage those that do. Facsimile, or "fax," extends the electronic power of telephone to written communication between patients and providers (school forms) and between practitioners and other health care professionals, such as pharmacists (prescriptions), consultants and schools (reports) for the cost of the equipment and a telephone line. In most cases, services linked to fax communications (prescriptions, preoperative reports, and school forms) must be linked to a previous face-to-face encounter that documents a history, physical examination with evaluation and management.

In other domains (such as law), fees for telephone consultation are billed directly to clients rather than through insurance. In primary care, telephone and fax services have traditionally been uncompensated, which, in addition to medico-legal requirements for a bona-fide patient–physician relationship (usually linked to a previous direct encounter) and the fact that considerable time is already spent on the telephone, has probably contributed to resistance to promote or extend their use in routine care.[1,2] Third-party payors, however, have begun to recognize the value of telephone care and are beginning to reimburse it (although at rates lower than equivalent office-based services).[3] The increasing prevalence of ICT in patient care (including the use of electronic mail) has prompted professional organizations such as American Academy of Pediatrics (AAP) to consider and publish articles on standards for its use and reimbursement.[4] The AAP has proposed to replace current insurance codes (current procedural terminology (CPT)) for telephone care with a new group of "Non-Face-to-Face Care" codes that include telephone, e-mail, and online services. These codes are still in development and will require assessments for appropriate resource-based relative value scales (RBRVS) that will help determine reimbursements.

24.2.3 Electronic Mail and Secure Messaging: Asynchronous Communication

Electronic mail (also discussed in Chapter 23) use by physicians with their patients is currently low (about one in four physicians), although there has been some increase in the last five years, with rates of increased adoption correlated to practice size (see Fig. 24.1).[5]

Reasons for this trend include non-reimbursement for advice and services rendered through e-mail and other issues about security, medico-legal liability

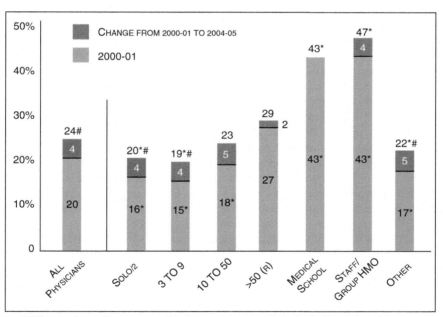

* Difference from reference group (R) within each year is statistically significant at p <.05.

\# Change between 2000-01 and 2004-05 is statistically significant at p <.05.

Source: Community Tracking Study Physician Survey

Fig. 24.1 Patient–physician e-mail use according to practice size[5]

and concerns about the reliability of patient use of e-mail.[6,7] In general, physician resistance to use e-mail with patients has been high, except in individual practice groups and associations.

Advantages of e-mail over telephone include its *asynchronous* nature, which reduces "phone tag" and can be used as appointment reminders (which in conjunction with patient self-scheduling can reduce no show rates) (reference to reduced no show rates). E-mail also allows options for templates for answers for common questions that allow readers to "drill-down" to online information libraries (via embedded hyperlinks).[8] Some EMR vendors are exploring ways to coordinate e-mail messages with clinical content such as lab tests and consultation requests and integrated patient information services (i.e., personal health records) through online practice portals.[9]

One concern in adopting patient care ICT is its conformance to the Health Information Portability and Accountability Act (HIPAA) privacy rules with regard to security and management of protected health information (PHI). Physician groups and IT vendors have collaborated to develop Web and e-mail technologies and standards that conform to HIPAA, and the AAP has recently updated its guidelines on the use of e-mail with patients.[10,11]

An online modality specifically developed to address these concerns is *secure messaging*, an online system for registering and tracking all electronic communications between patient and provider for documentation and reimbursement[12] through secure Web technology that meets HIPAA requirements. Secure messaging allows (and restricts) viewing of an online communication to a specific sender and receiver of a message, a security restriction that is not possible with traditional e-mail. Secure messaging limits access to a message to its sender and intended receiver by encryption (encoding or scrambling a message so that it cannot be read by others) and decryption (decoding or restoring a message for reading). Secure messaging conforms to HIPAA standards for privacy and security and may be used by patients to schedule appointments, to request prescription refills and/or to ask questions to and receive answers from their providers.

In adopting and using secure messaging (or any form of ICT for patient communication), pediatricians (and other health care providers) must ensure that: (1) the recipient of an electronic message has a legitimate right to access the contained information, (2) the message is transmitted only to the intended recipient, and (3) the information is accurately transmitted and received.

Despite the availability of tools and guidelines to circumnavigate the medico-legal aspects of its use and the recommendations of satisfied physician and patient users, there has not been enough incentive to make patient–provider e-mail a widespread practice. Currently, only a limited number of insurers reimburse e-mail consultations. In situations where non-compensation is less of a barrier (such as salaried clinicians or fee-for-service reimbursement), positive return on investment (ROI) and improved quality of care have been noted by those holding responsibility for the costs of care. The federal government's recognition of the great amount of work done outside the office has generated efforts to outline recommendations for payment mechanisms for such services as e-mail consultation and communication.[13]

24.3 Other ICT Tools and Enhancement of Patient Care

24.3.1 Practice Websites

Practice Websites are Internet-based collections of information that are related to a physician, an office or a practitioner group. Over time, Websites have become simpler and faster to create and maintain and can be customized by practitioners to include practice information, current health news, and seasonal information for patients. To standardize this process, a consortium of stakeholders has been formed to provide electronic services, including online tools to facilitate practitioner Website creation and maintenance. The Medem (**MED**ical **EM**powerment) consortium, consisting of more than 80,000 physicians, 47 specialty and state medical societies, a number of health systems, health plans, patient advocacy groups, professional liability carriers, provides a single Web entry point for patients to their physician's Website and online patient information libraries.[14] Practice Websites are branded by practice name and the professional society to which the provider a member (Fig. 24.2).

Practitioners often provide self-written or collected information for patients in the form of pamphlets with frequently asked questions and answers about normal and abnormal conditions. Professional medical societies (such as the AAP) sell pre-pared materials for patients and families as a value-added resource for a practice[15] to educate families and to market practices. Electronic versions of pamphlets have advantages of easy creation, updating and dissemination by e-mail, Web and fax,

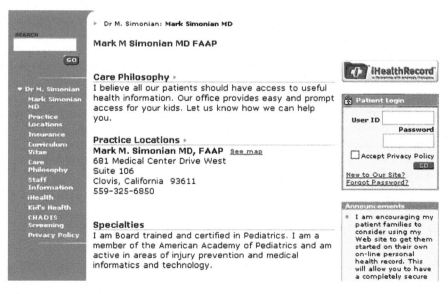

Fig. 24.2 Example of a pediatric practice Website (Vendor: Medem. Practice of Mark M. Simonian MD)

with reduced paper waste. Vetted, unbiased patient information is available from a number of sources: the federal government (from the NIH,[16] CDC[17], and FDA[18]), professional medical societies (such as the AAP), patient advocacy groups and also from insurance and pharmaceutical companies.[19]

Practice Web sites have been driven by several circumstances: the popularity of the Internet, the availability of libraries of published information, the technology to make them widely and easily available at low cost, the opportunity to reuse them to the advantage of member practices (and provide added value to membership). Additionally, practitioners and professional groups have expressed the concern that patients (in the case of pediatrics, both children and families) randomly search the Internet and find erroneous (and possibly harmful) health information. By centralizing and branding sources, patients may access trusted information in the context of their ongoing relationship with a practitioner.

Practice Websites may be customized to include special services to support patient care: secure messaging (described previously), adherence programs and online consultation:

Adherence programs[20] provide customized, automated e-mail messages to patients (from their providers) to remind and reinforce information that is provided in the office. Physicians may program messages that focus on patient-specific medical conditions and provide instructions and about treatment and medication regimens, with linkages to information vetted and approved by the member's society or the Food and Drug Administration (FDA) (or to information from the physician's own library).

Online consultation[TM21] allows established patients or parents to receive individualized medical advice without an office encounter. Using secure messaging technology (described previously), physicians may share information with families about established problems (with new diagnosis and treatment being appropriately initiated through an office encounter). Patients and families eligible for this service must be registered and acknowledged by the physician (thus establishing an ongoing relationship). Parents must agree to a contract of responsibilities for both patients and physicians prior to being allowed to use the service, and are notified by e-mail (with a "Terms of Service" agreement) when the service is activated. A standard fee for online consultations, payable by credit card at the time of service, is established by the physician and posted on the Website, so the patient knows what the consultation will cost. Once activated, Online Consultation[TM] a physician responds to patient requests and questions within a specified time period.

24.3.2   Practice Portals

Practice portals add an additional layer of functionality by linking practice Websites to electronic health records (EHRs) and external services (such as local pharmacies) to facilitate routine health processes (such as electronic prescription).[22-24] Web portals provide a personal, online, secure patient interface to online Web services offered by the practice (secure messaging, self-scheduling of appointments, and prescription refills). Services to streamline and improve care include: online pre-visit forms (that can be completed through in-office kiosks, saving on paper, clipboards and time spent on redundant paperwork), Web-based patient surveys, online health monitoring, and patient teaching that have been shown to be effective. It is believed that physicians can use these tools to increase productivity by reducing redundant data entry.

Web portals empower patients by allowing them to manage their appointments, refills, and referrals. Through portals, patients may: access laboratory and imaging test results as they become available, update their medication lists, drug and food allergies and medical histories and communicate directly with their providers via secure messaging. Patients may also manage and their patient accounts with practices. Many EMR vendors currently provide Web portal services to participating practices, with practitioners show increasing interest.

Example:
The following Web portal example, provided by an electronic medical record vendor, shows a (test) patient's visit dates, immunization history, allergy history and allows the patient/family to schedule an appointment for health maintenance and to request information:

In addition to patient appointment scheduling/cancellation, some portals offer patients online request forms for prescription refills, enrollment/registration and documents, online review and updating of health and demographic information, e-mail reminders, secure messaging to providers, online news from the practice, online consultation and online surveys.

Others offer virtual office visit, symptom assessment, online bill payment, "Ask a Doctor" function and laboratory result report retrieval.

These examples demonstrate currently available functionality. Future functions that Web portals may provide patients include: Medical Home functions to help families to self-manage and co-manage health maintenance (immunizations and growth) and chronic disease (blood glucose measures in diabetes and peak flow measurements in asthma) information. There is evidence that this type of information access can improve patient safety and thereby reduce health care costs (through decreased hospital and emergency department visits) (Fig. 24.3).[25-29]

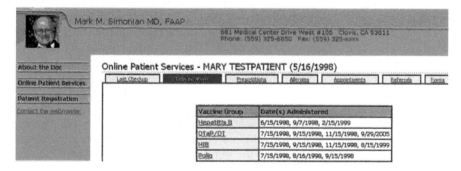

Fig. 24.3 Example of a pediatric office Web portal (Vendor: Connexin. Practice of Mark M. Simonian, MD)

24.4   Case Study (Hypothetical)

Billy D. is a 15 year old who lives with his parents and two younger sisters. His mother and father both work in sales and have challenges bringing their children to the pediatrician's office for scheduled visits. Recently, Billy's parents have noted a drop in his grades and a loss of interest in other activities.

They consult Dr. S. via secure e-mail (through her online practice portal). They have used this in the past and have found it to be a very convenient and confidential adjunct to their long relationship with Dr. S. Dr. S. reviews their message on her daily "e-mail rounds" and considers a differential diagnosis that she shares with the parents via return secure e-mail. In her reply, she explains her concerns, providing additional information by linking to resources from her practice portal: pamphlets from the American Academy of Pediatrics and materials she has written. She asks the parents to complete a validated online questionnaire to screen for behavior problems, depression and substance abuse. They complete the questionnaire that afternoon and the portal Web service alerts Dr. S. by pager when their answers have been submitted. On reviewing their responses, Dr. S. narrows her differential diagnosis of depression and substance abuse, and contacts Billy's mother via phone to discuss the results, requesting that the parents bring Billy in for a face-to-face visit that evening. When Billy comes in, Dr. S. assesses that he is not suicidal and discusses the possibility of a drug screen (consulting the AAP guideline), to which Billy consents. The results of the drug screen are made available to Billy and his parents the following day through their online personal health record (also available through the practice portal) with a follow up visit scheduled. That morning, Dr. S. receives a secure e-mail from Billy, in which he would like to know how to get condoms. Dr. S. replies that Billy should self-schedule a visit that day to pick up condoms and education on their proper use and the risks of pregnancy, sexually transmitted diseases and HIV.

Billy's youngest sister, Sally, was discovered to have insulin-dependent diabetes a year previously and is currently on an insulin pump as part of a clinical trial. Their endocrinologist sends summaries of his consultations to Dr. S's electronic health record as well as to the study coordinator via secure messaging attachments. The parents carry copies of these electronic summaries from their personal health record for Sally on a "smart" card whenever they travel.

During Sally's initial diabetic management on the pump, she had a severe low blood sugar while on a family trip out of town. She was rushed to a local emergency department from which the emergency physician accessed her medical and drug information from her "smart" card through a standard reader and was able to get trend information from her insulin pump. Sally was admitted to the hospital's pediatric observation unit where the pediatric hospitalist, Dr. R., using information from the Medical Home Web service of her PHR (as authorized by her parents), contacted her endocrinologist for guidance on managing and adjusting her insulin pump. The endocrinologist, viewing the trend information from a secure message from Dr. R., was able to specify a modification that made a full inpatient admission unnecessary. Dr. R.'s detailed summary of Sally's care, including data from the observation unit EMR and from the online consultation with the endocrinologist were recorded in Sally's "smart" card and her online PHR. Dr. S., notified by the Medical Home Web service alert of Sally's emergency visit, was able to touch base with Dr. R. and Sally's parents via teleconference between the office and the observation unit prior to discharge.

24.5   Conclusion

A combination of advances in information technology, a maturing of electronic medical records and an evolving business model for patient access to health information is making scenarios such as described in the case study closer to reality than ever before.

Author Disclosure Statement   Mark M. Simonian is a past Board Member of Medem representing the professional societies and served on the Pediatric Advisory Group from the American Academy of Pediatrics to Medem – 1999–2006.

References

1. Hertz A. Section drafting policy on reimbursement for phone care. *AAP News.* 2005;26(6):34.
2. Melzer SM, Poole SR. Reimbursement for telephone care. *Pediatrics.* 2002;109(2):290–293.
3. Kirkland JL, Copeland KC. Telephone charges and payments in a diabetes clinic. *Pediatrics.* 1998;101(4):E2.
4. American Academy of Pediatrics Section on Telehealth Care. Payment for Telehealth Care. American Academy of Pediatrics Website; 2006. Available at: http://www.aap.org/sections/telecare/reimbursement.htm. Accessed December 4, 2008.
5. Liebhaber A, Grossman JM. Physicians Slow to Adopt Patient E-mail Data Bulletin No. 32. Center to Study Health System Change; 2006. Available at: http://www.hschange.com/CONTENT/875/. Accessed December 4, 2008.
6. Katz SJ, Moyer CA. The emerging role of online communication between patients and their providers. *J Gen Intern Med.* 2004;19(9):978–983.
7. American Academy of Pediatrics, Division of Health Policy Research. Periodic Survey of Fellows 51: Use of Computers and Other Technology, Executive Summary. American Academy of Pediatrics; 2003. Available at: http://www.aap.org/research/periodicsurvey/ps51exs.htm. Accessed December 4, 2008.
8. Bauchner H, Adams W, Burstin H. 'You've got mail': issues in communicating with patients and their families by e-mail. *Pediatrics.* 2002;109:954–956.
9. Weingart SN, Rind D, Tofias Z, Sands DZ. Who uses the patient internet portal? The PatientSite experience. *J Am Med Inform Assoc.* 2006;13(1):91–95.
10. Kane B, Sands DZ. Guidelines for the clinical use of electronic mail with patients. The AMIA Internet Working Group, Task Force on Guidelines for the Use of Clinic-Patient Electronic Mail. *J Am Med Inform Assoc.* 1998;5(1):104–111.
11. Gerstle RS, American Academy of Pediatrics Task Force on Medical Informatics. E-mail communication between pediatricians and their patients. *Pediatrics.* 2004;114(1):317–321.

12. Zhou YY, Garrido T, Chin HL, Wiesenthal AM, Liang LL. Patient access to an electronic health record with secure messaging: impact on primary care utilization. *Am J Manage Care.* 2007;13(7):418–424.
13. American Healthcare Information Community (AHIC). Chronic Care Workgroup. Department of Health and Human Services Website; 2008, last update. Available at: http://www.hhs.gov/healthit/ahic/chroniccare/. Accessed December 4, 2008.
14. Medem. Medem Website; 2008. Available at: http://www.medem.com/am/am.cfm. Accessed December 4, 2008.
15. American Academy of Pediatrics. Patient Education Online. Commercially available from the American Academy of Pediatrics; 2008. Available at: https://www.nfaap.org/netforum/eweb/DynamicPage.aspx?webcode=aapbks_productdetail&key=53c87c6f-6dee-4a01-aebb-e1a5b9a8e60f#. Accessed December 21, 2008.
16. National Library of Medicine. MedlinePlus; 2008. Available at: http://medlineplus.gov/. Accessed December 4, 2008.
17. Centers for Disease Control and Prevention. CDC Website; 2008. Available at: http://www.cdc.gov. Accessed December 4, 2008.
18. Food and Drug Administration. FDA Website; 2008. Available at: http://www.fda.gov/. Accessed December 4, 2008.
19. Merck and Co. The Merck Manual Online; 2008. Available at: http://www.merck.com/mmpe/index.html. Accessed December 4, 2008.
20. Medem. Disease Management and Adherence Programs. Available at: http://www.medem.com/node/1098. Accessed December 21, 2008.
21. Medem. Secure Messaging and Online Consultation; 2008. Available at: http://www.medem.com/node/1088. Accessed December 21, 2008.
22. Lewis D. Computer-based approaches to patient education: a review of the literature. *J Am Med Inform Assoc.* 1999;6(4):272–282.
23. Dickerson S, Reinhart AM, Feeley TH, et al. Patient Internet use for health information at three urban primary care clinics. *J Am Med Inform Assoc.* 2004;11(6):499–504.
24. Treweek SP, Glenton C, Oxman AD, Penrose A. Computer-generated patient education materials: do they affect professional practice? A systematic review. *J Am Med Inform Assoc.* 2002;9(4):346–358.
25. Shea S, Starren J, Weinstock RS, et al. Columbia university's informatics for diabetes education and telemedicine (IDEATel) project: rationale and design. *J Am Med Inform Assoc.* 2002;9(1):49–62.
26. Earnest MA, Ross SE, Wittevrongel L, Moore LA, Lin CT. Use of a patient-accessible electronic medical record in a practice for congestive heart failure: patient and physician experiences. *J Am Med Inform Assoc.* 2004;11(5):410–417.
27. Kaplan B, Brennan PF. Consumer informatics supporting patients as co-producers of quality. *J Am Med Inform Assoc.* 2001;8(4):309–316.
28. De Clercq PA, Hasman A, Wolffenbuttel BH. A consumer health record for supporting the patient-centered management of chronic diseases. *Med Inform Internet Med.* 2003;28(2):117–127.
29. Hejlesen OK, Plougmann S, Ege BM, Larsen OV, Bek T, Cavan D. Using the internet in patient-centred diabetes care for communication, education, and decision support. *Stud Health Technol Inform.* 2001;84(Pt 2):1464–1468.

Part V
Informatics and Pediatric
Inpatient Practice

Chapter 25
Overview of Pediatric Inpatient Medication Delivery

George R. Kim and Robert E. Miller

Objectives

- To provide a framework for thinking about medication processes, focusing on medication use and error prevention
- To outline general and pediatric-specific vulnerabilities in medication delivery
- To discuss pediatric-specific issues that technology can address

25.1 Introduction

The term "medication process" includes all aspects of the management of pharmaceuticals used in the care of patients: drug manufacture (creating, packaging, and assuring the quality and safety of medications for human use), pharmaceutical procurement (acquiring, storing, and managing medications for patient care), medication reconciliation (identifying, verifying, and realigning a patient's current drug regimen with the intended care plan when a change in medical care (admission, discharge, transfer) occurs) and medication use. Medication use is the process of prescribing, ordering, compounding, dispensing, and administering drugs, monitoring (and documenting) their effects on patients. It is the last aspect of which this section is an overview, and which is the focus of subsequent sections.

The complexity of each of the above-mentioned processes, within their respective complex environments (chemical manufacturing plants, pharmacies, hospitals, and clinics) makes medication processes inherently error-prone. Of these processes, the largest negative impact on patient health comes from errors in mediation use. Illegible handwriting, numerous human hand-offs of instructions, complex patient data, critical drug dose information and ever-changing formularies of drugs with varying degrees of potency and toxicity all contribute to the vulnerabilities and errors in medication use, and to the challenges of efficiently and safely managing them. Not surprising, adverse drug events (ADEs) result in more than 770,000 injuries and deaths each year in the US and cost up to $5.6 million per hospital.[1]

C.U. Lehmann et al. (eds.), *Pediatric Informatics: Computer Applications in Child Health,* Health Informatics,
© Springer Science + Business Media, LLC 2011

25.2 The Inpatient Medication Delivery Process

Despite its complexity and variations in different settings, the medication use process can be decomposed into several steps that provide a model for analyzing vulnerabilities and for proposing technical approaches to reducing errors (Fig. 25.1):

Prescribing/Ordering (Chapter 26): "Prescribing" is the generation of a formal order (the prescription) by an "authorized prescriber" (a physician, nurse practitioner or physician assistant) for a medication to be given to a patient. A prescription includes identification of: the patient, the ordered drug, the dose, the timing of doses and the route (for pediatrics, this also includes specification of the form of the drug – liquid, suspension, etc.). The formal prescription (order) is sent to the pharmacist either through an intermediary (a unit clerk), a paper form (prescription pad) or computer interface (computerized provider order entry, CPOE).

Prescribing involves shared knowledge of the patient's condition, the current therapy, and pharmacologic information about available drugs. Discussion, correction, and modification may be needed due to constraints (preparation issues, contraindications, drug availability, administrative restrictions) before the order is carried out. The prescribing step is complete when the prescriber and the pharmacist have agreed upon the order to be completed.

Compounding/Dispensing (Chapter 27): "Compounding" has a specific legal definition[2] referring to the physical steps performed by pharmacy staff to prepare a pharmaceutical product for administration to a patient. The safest strategy is to use prepared doses and concentrations of medications, but certain preparations (such as parenteral nutrition and suspensions of drugs in tablet form) are needed when the medical needs of an individual patient that cannot be met by the use of approved commercial drug products. Compounding activities are nonstandard and are prone to errors.

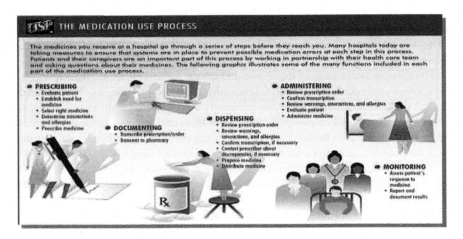

Fig. 25.1 An overview of inpatient medication delivery[3]

"Dispensing" is the provision of drugs with the prescribed instructions (to either a patient or an intermediary) for administration. In institutional ambulatory settings, the pharmacy is increasingly required to manage free samples provided by drug sales representatives. In inpatient settings, dispensing includes proper checking, packaging, and labeling of doses and instructions, time delivery, proper storage until administration, and auditing of handoffs from pharmacy staff to nursing. The compounding/dispensing step is complete when a patient's nurse accepts the medication dose and its instructions for that patient from the pharmacy.

Administering/Monitoring (Chapter 28): "Administering" a drug dose is the last step in delivering a prescribed medication regimen to a patient. It includes understanding of dosing instructions by the patient or an intermediary (in inpatient settings, this may be the nurse). It also includes any final preparation or manipulation of the drug dose (such as mixing with an intravenous carrier) and assurance of delivery (direct observation of oral therapy, intravenous line checking). The administering step is complete when all necessary steps are completed and the dose administration has been documented in a medication administration record.

"Monitoring" is an intrinsic safety function (and the most important part) of medication use. In the ambulatory setting, adverse drug events are based on patient reports and clinical findings. In inpatient settings, nurses and primary care providers document drug effects (favorable and adverse) in the patient record. Adjunct reporting systems track adverse events and reactions for research, and for quality and safety improvement.

Documenting: "Documenting" a drug dose is the creation of a formal record of each of the steps involved in medication use for archiving and for retrieval for clinical and administrative use. This function is an automatic function in HIT applications.

The medication use model emphasizes cognitive and physical activities of the various roles, including communication and record-keeping functions. Improvement of the safety and reliability of the medication use process, and the reduction of process errors, involve analysis of where the model can fail—with what probabilities and with what impacts. One approach to "failure modes analysis" asks the "five wrongs": how frequently and with what impacts do the "wrong drug" or the "wrong dose" via the "wrong route of administration" to the "wrong patient" have? Failure mode and effects analysis is discussed in Chapter 29.

25.3 Automation and Computerization to Improve Safety

Past and current experience in health care (and other industries) suggests that complex and error-prone patient care activities such as the medication process can be reengineered to reduce errors and increase safety through the use of automation and computerization to standardize and streamline work. In prescribing/ordering, computerized provider order entry (CPOE) and clinical decision support (CDS) have been shown to reduce prescribing errors in complex processes such as neonatal parenteral nutrition and continuous infusions (Chapter 26); in compounding/

dispensing, pharmacy information systems (PharmIS, Chapter 27) can reduce errors in intravenous solution admixtures and in administering drugs. Additionally, a number of technologies, including bar-coding, radio-frequency identification (and computer-interfaced supply cabinets), "smart" infusion pumps (Chapter 28) have been explored to improve delivery and safety of medication use.

25.4   Pediatric Specific Issues in Medication Use

The combination of the increased vulnerability of children and infants to medication errors and the specific data needs of pediatric care (Chapters 3–8) suggest that pediatric medication use may benefit from the application of information technology. Special areas of current interest include:

Pediatric drug dosing: Current systems designed for multispecialty use do not uniformly or adequately handle universal weight-dose calculations that are common and vital in pediatrics, including drug dictionaries that reflect age-based dosages and contraindications, clinical decision support rules that handle age and weight-based alerts and reminders and integrate the use of growth charts.

Workflow and human computer interface issues: Pediatric-specific medication workflows include: automatic point-of-ordering weight-based drug dose calculation (with special consideration of the management of low volume doses), incorporation of child growth and development data into documentation and decision support, and just-in-time availability of orders and drugs in emergent situations to optimize care.

Pediatric specialty domains: Children at higher risk for the impact of errors (such as neonates, children with special health care needs (who may be on many medications, with many consultants, and children with cancer) may have more complex care (intensive care, continuous infusions, chemotherapy) that require even more specialized consideration.

Connection to primary care: Pediatrics is a primary care specialty with an emphasis on the medical home concept (especially for children with special health care needs), for which information technology is needed that empowers continuity in terms of medication use and other aspects of pediatric care.

References

1. Agency for Healthcare Research and Quality. Reducing and Preventing Adverse Drug Events to Decrease Hospital Costs. Research in Action, Issue 1. AHRQ Publication Number 01-0020, Rockville, MD; 2001. Available at: http://www.ahrq.gov/qual/aderia/aderia.htm. Accessed December 21, 2008.
2. Nordenberg T. Pharmacy Compounding: Customizing Prescription Drugs. FDA Consumer Magazine; 2000. Available at: http://www.fda.gov/Fdac/features/2000/400_compound.html. Accessed December 21, 2008.
3. United States Pharmacopeia. The Medication Use Process; 2004. Available at: http://www.usp.org/pdf/EN/patientSafety/medicationUseProcess.pdf. Accessed December 21, 2008.

Chapter 26
Prescribing/Ordering: Computerized Order Entry and Decision Support

Christoph U. Lehmann and George R. Kim

Objectives

- To define computerized provider order entry (CPOE) and clinical decision support (CDS)
- To outline their function in pediatric medication use safety
- To guide questions pediatric clinicians should ask during CPOE selection
- To discuss briefly pediatric issues and challenges in CPOE implementation

26.1   Introduction

Institutional adoption of computerized provider order entry (CPOE) and clinical decision support (CDS) has been advocated by the Institute of Medicine (IOM) and others to reduce and prevent medication prescribing errors as part of a global approach to safety (Table 26.1)[1] that includes: fostering an open, nonpunitive, and goal-directed culture and environment for learning and teaching safety improvement, understanding, and anticipating human behaviors and limitations, training and working as a team, and creating robust systems for anticipating and handling the unexpected.

26.2   Definitions

Computerized Provider Order Entry (CPOE, also called POE, Computerized Physician Order Entry or Care Provider Order Entry) is the component of a clinical information system that allows prescribers to enter clinical orders directly into a computer for electronic processing and transmission to appropriate departments and/or individuals for completion. Ambulatory CPOE (ACPOE) may connect

C.U. Lehmann et al. (eds.), *Pediatric Informatics: Computer Applications in Child Health,* Health Informatics,
© Springer Science + Business Media, LLC 2011

Table 26.1 Modified principles from the IOM "*to err is human*" report[1]

Safety principles	Methods to achieve
1. Culture of Safety (p166)	Safety as a corporate priority
	Safety as everyone's responsibility
	Safety efforts are assigned and overseen
	Financial resources for analysis and redesign
	Identification and Dealing with unsafe practitioners
2. Anticipate Human Limitations (p170)	Safe job design
	Avoidance of the need to rely on memory or vigilance
	Use of constraints and forcing functions
	Simplification and standardization
3. Team Work (p173)	Training as a team
	Inclusion of the patient in the planning for safety and care
4. Anticipate the Unexpected (p174)	Proactive approach: identify problems before they become accidents
	Inclusion of recovery plans in the design
	Improving access to timely, accurate information
5. Learning Environment (p178)	Use of simulations
	Encouragement to report errors and hazards
	Non-punitive environment
	Elimination of barriers to communication
	Feedback and learning from errors

intra-clinic activities (Chapter 19), and when it connects ambulatory prescribers to remote pharmacies, it is also called e-Prescribing.[2]

Clinical Decision Support (CDS) is **any** knowledge-based tool that integrates patient data into clinical workflow to improve care quality (and safety), patient satisfaction and outcomes. CDS may:

- Provide users access to patient-specific data and/or medical knowledge
- Guide users' actions or choices in diagnosis and/or therapy
- Deliver timely knowledge-based prompts (such as alerts and reminders) to users and
- Collect and process data about clinical care processes, outcomes, and performance to help users to understand and improve practice[3]

CPOE may be classified according to the clinical environment in which it operates and the degree to which CDS is incorporated. Ambulatory CPOE (see Chapter 19) may vary from "Basic Rx" (printing basic prescriptions without patient data or decision support) to "Advanced Rx-Dx" (full electronic data interchange between physicians' offices and pharmacies with patient-specific decision support).[4] In inpatient settings, almost all CPOE systems include some form of CDS.

26.3   CPOE/CDS Functions

In inpatient settings, CPOE and associated CDS provide prescribing support to a clinician (physician, nurse practitioner, nurse, physician assistant) who is authorized to order medications, laboratory and radiology tests, and treatments, for patients:

- The authorized clinician establishes a therapeutic relationship with a patient and collects data (history, physical examination, laboratory test results) to determine a diagnosis or problem list for the patient.
- Based on the diagnosis or problem list inferred from the collected data, the clinician determines the need for further testing or specific therapies for the patient, according to medical evidence, practice guidelines and clinical constraints (formulary availability, drug interactions).
- The clinician formulates, orders, and documents tests and therapies (using CPOE) that are transmitted to ancillary departments or the pharmacist and nurse for completion. CDS guides the clinician by guiding choices and data entry, by providing knowledge-based prompts and access to information about drugs and the patient.
- In response to test results, alerts, and requests for correction and clarification, the clinician adjusts orders and their documentation as required.

CPOE (depending on the degree of sophistication and CDS) supports and improves the reliability of the prescribing/ordering step by:

- Reducing illegibility and transcription errors by eliminating handwriting
- Standardizing identifiers, names, and codes of clinical entities: drugs, tests, and patients by using data dictionaries and
- Linking patient-specific data and information to the ordering process
- Providing evidence-based order sets
- Automating calculations
- Providing alerts and reminders
- Screening for populations at risk[5]

26.4   Pediatric-Specific Technical Features of CPOE/CDS

Different populations of children have different vulnerabilities and safety needs (Chapters 3–8). Within pediatric care environments, features that should be taken into consideration when designing or choosing CPOE/CDS systems include:

- Universal weight-based dosing
  - Automatic drug dose calculations and rounding
  - Drug dictionaries with up-to-date pediatric-specific dose information
  - Dosing alerts, reminders, and warnings that are age, weight, and drug specific
  - Override ("break the glass") options for specific cases and prescribers (very high or low weight children, impaired drug absorption or clearance, differential tolerances in pain management)

- Special patient identification support features
  - Correct patient identification during ordering
  - Consistent and safe management for disambiguating siblings in multiple births
  - Reconciliation of name changes for infants and children
- Pediatric-specific pharmacy and administration infrastructure (see Chapters 27, 28)
  - Up-to-date pediatric drug information in a CPOE-usable form
  - An experienced, knowledgeable pediatric pharmacist and pharmacy staff
  - Adequate training and support for dispensing equipment appropriate to pediatric care needs (total parenteral nutrition, continuous infusions, chemotherapy)
  - Adequate nursing education and support for administration equipment appropriate to pediatric care needs (smart pumps, appropriate drug forms for pediatric use)
- Pediatric-specific physiologic, developmental, and pharmacologic data and knowledge
  - Growth chart data, with adjustments for prematurity and special conditions (preferably incorporated into CDS)
  - On-demand/just-in-time medical knowledge and patient-specific data (electronic record/digital library/formulary access)
  - Enforcement of timely medication reconciliation
- Increased dosing and decision support in specific risk situations
  - Redundant calculation and rounding support for patients with very low weights
  - Calculation support for standard concentration infusions
  - Smart pumps to deliver very small volumes accurately

26.5   Assessing a CPOE/CDS System for Pediatric Use

Adoption of CPOE/CDS for a pediatric inpatient environment is a team effort that requires a structured and inclusive approach by institutional leadership and clinical users (prescribers, pharmacists, nurses) within the environment:

26.5.1   Pre-Adoption (What Needs to Be Improved and Why?)

1. What types of medication errors occur within a given unit? For which medication?
2. What are the rates of such errors in prescribing, dispensing, and administering drug doses? If not known, what are realistic estimates (or how could they be measured)?

3. What are the effects of these errors on patient outcomes? How have patients been harmed by them? How many sentinel events have arisen from medication errors? What has been done to reduce medication errors?

26.5.2   Planning (What Improvements Will CPOE/CDS Provide and How?)

1. What are the goals of improvement through the use of CPOE/CDS?
2. What features does the proposed CPOE/CDS system (need to) provide to achieve those goals?
3. What training and technical support will be needed for staff?
4. What pediatric-specific features are needed to achieve the goals?
5. If the system is being purchased:
   (a) Does it have these features?
   (b) If so, how has the system performed in similar settings?
   (c) If not, can the features be specified or built? How much added work and time will be required?
6. If the system is being built:
   (a) How will the features be implemented?
   (b) How much work and time will it take?

26.5.3   Benchmarking (How Will the Effect of CPOE/CDS be Measured?)

1. What is the evaluation plan for the system?
   (a) During deployment (roll-out)?
   (b) During ongoing use (maintenance)?
2. What indicators will measure progress and success?
   (a) How will data be collected?
   (b) How will collected data be analyzed?
3. How will results be used for decision-making about the system?

26.5.4   Collateral Effects (What Are the Impacts of CPOE/CDS?)

1. How has the system changed the medication delivery process?
   (a) Do measured indicators support this?
   (b) How has it changed relationships among prescribers, nurses, pharmacists, and patients? Have there been shifts in power or workload?[6]
2. What are downtime (emergent or planned) and recovery procedures?

26.6 Pediatric-Related Organizational Issues

Pediatric care occurs in different institutional environments with varying levels of pediatric expertise (prescribers, nursing, pharmacists). CPOE/CDS must be tailored to fit the needs of the prescribers and the clinical workflow in specific environments in which it operates. Organizational and cultural considerations in pediatric CPOE/CDS adoption include:

- **The need for pediatric leadership and expertise**: Pediatric care may be only one of many competing priorities for a healthcare institution. Medical, surgical, and psychiatric care of children in mixed settings (as may be present in community hospitals) may increase the risks and impacts of medication errors. Pediatricians must act as child advocates in this arena to raise attention of hospital leadership to pediatric patient safety. Pediatricians must also represent the needs of children in development of CPOE/CDS (and other HIT).
- **The need to prioritize pediatric safety**: CPOE/CDS adoption is *part* of a holistic approach to reduce and prevent medication errors, which includes:
  ○ Establishing a child-centric patient safety culture
  ○ Developing communication and shared staff awareness of pediatric care
  ○ Creating an active learning environment that educates staff about pediatric needs and vulnerabilities and that facilitates error reporting[7]
- **The global understanding that pediatric safety and HIT adoption are continuous and iterative**: Adoption of CPOE/CDS (or of any health information technology) requires continuous monitoring and reevaluation of the care process, in which it is embedded. Introduction changes work relationships and may increase stress among staff. Ongoing measurement of system and staff performance, of cultural climate, of errors and of outcomes is needed to assure accurate and safe medication delivery to all pediatric patients.

26.7 Conclusion

The adoption of inpatient CPOE (as with any technology) creates changes within an error prone and complex process (prescribing and ordering of inpatient medications). Pediatricians face technical and organizational challenges in reaping the benefits of error reduction and increased safety for their patients, but they also bring their ability to advocate for the needs of children. Adoption of CPOE goes beyond the selection of a product and involves ongoing consideration of present and future needs of children and the professionals who care for them.

26.8 Case Studies

26.8.1 Study 1: Incorporating Inline Calculators into Commercial CPOE/CDS[8,9]

At the Johns Hopkins Children's Center (JHCC), a commercial CPOE/CDS product was adopted as part of an institution-wide implementation of the product at a multidisciplinary tertiary care center of which JHCC is a part. In turn, JHCC is a multidisciplinary pediatric tertiary care center, including services for pediatric and neonatal critical care, pediatric oncology and numerous surgical services. Deployment of the commercial product was conceived in stages, beginning with general pediatric floors followed by the neonatal intensive care unit and the pediatric critical care unit.

Fitting the CPOE/CDS product to the different sectors of the JHCC required a prolonged concerted effort that required development of:

- Pediatric-specific drug dictionary with over 13,000 manually checked rules for pediatric dosing
- Disease-specific evidence-based order sets, reviewed by clinical faculty from each division in JHCC

Prior to the introduction of the commercial system, clinical calculators had been developed to facilitate the ordering and writing of total parenteral nutrition (TPN) and continuous intravenous infusions. These tools had been developed and made available on public workstations throughout the JHCC and had been in use.

As these functions were not present in the commercial system, a project was undertaken to incorporate the calculators into the functionality of the commercial system. Through cooperation of programmers of the clinical calculators and the CPOE system, a procedure where orders for TPN or infusions were translated into messages to the respective calculators, which returned necessary values to the CPOE system. The benefits of this bidirectional communication between applications which: allowed continued use of the calculators (which had been demonstrated to decrease prescribing errors dramatically) and avoided the need and cost for development and testing of new CDS functionality (by reusing proven technology).

26.8.2 Study 2: CPOE in Pediatric Intensive Care (See Chapter 7)

The publication of two studies on the implementation of the same commercial CPOE system into pediatric critical care units at two different academic medical centers[10,11] demonstrated the importance of anticipating clinical workflow needs, considering implementation and deployment including policy changes. The question of the association of CPOE implementation with increased mortality generated much discussion within the pediatric and informatics literature.[12] Subsequent studies[13,14] support that CPOE does not increase mortality in pediatric critical care.

26.8.3   Study 3: CDS in Pediatric Oncology

Pediatric oncology presents challenges that increase the likelihood of medication errors[15] that result in patient harm (in an already vulnerable population). Issues that contribute to the complexity of the problems in caring for this particularly vulnerable class of patients include:

- Drug dosage calculation challenges (dependent on age, weight, and body surface area)
- Inclusion of many patients in clinical trials (including issues of scheduling, tracking, and billing)
- Complex protocols that combine time-critical surgery, chemotherapy (that may be delivered to different body cavities: intra-thecal, etc.) and radiation treatments of varying intensities[16]
- The need for continuity of care that transcends inpatient/outpatient patient care environment distinctions[17]
- Interruptions, adjustments and delays to individual treatment schedules due to intercurrent illnesses, some as complications of therapy
- The narrow therapeutic profile and high potential for acute and cumulative toxicities of the agents used
- Risks of preventable long-term effects of therapy that may create needs for modifications of treatment protocols and individual schedules

Because of these complexities, global approaches have been used to examine the risks at different steps of ordering chemotherapy[18] and oncology laboratory testing[19] and of the global prescribing-pharmacy processing-administration process.[20] The design, application, and evaluation of clinical decision and workflow support for all phases of pediatric oncology remains an important area of inquiry and development.

References

1. Institute of Medicine. *To Err Is Human: Building a Safer Health System*. Washington, DC: National Academy Press; 1999.
2. Osheroff JA, Pifer EA, Teich JM, et al. *Improving Outcomes with Clinical Decision Support: An Implementer's Guide*. Chicago IL: Healthcare Information and Management Systems Society; 2005.
3. Perrault LE, Metzger JB. A pragmatic framework for understanding clinical decision support. *J Healthc Inf Manag*. 1999;13:2–21.
4. Center for Information Technology Leadership. The Value of Computerized Provider Order Entry in Ambulatory Settings; 2006. Available at: http://www.citl.org/research/ACPOE.asp. Accessed December 21, 2008.

5. Lehmann CU, Kim GR. Computerized order entry and patient safety. *Pediatr Clin N Am.* 2006;53:1169–1184.
6. Ash JS, Sittig DF, Poon EG, Guappone K, Campbell E, Dykstra RH. The extent and importance of unintended consequences related to computerized provider order entry. *J Am Med Inform Assoc.* 2007;14(4):415–423.
7. Pronovost PJ, Berenholtz SM, Goeschel CA, et al. Creating high reliability in health care organizations. *Health Serv Res.* 2006;41(4 Pt 2):1599–1617.
8. Lehmann CU, Conner KG, Cox JM. Preventing provider errors: online total parenteral nutrition calculator. *Pediatrics.* 2004;113(4):748–753.
9. Lehmann CU, Kim GR, Gujral R, Veltri MA, Clark JS, Miller MR. Decreasing errors in pediatric continuous intravenous infusions. *Pediatr Crit Care Med.* 2006;7(3):225–230.
10. Han YY, Carcillo JA, Venkataraman ST, et al. Unexpected increased mortality after implementation of a commercially sold computerized physician order entry system. *Pediatrics.* 2005;116(6):1506–1512.
11. Del Beccaro MA, Jeffries HE, Eisenberg MA, Harry ED. Computerized provider order entry implementation: no association with increased mortality rates in an intensive care unit. *Pediatrics.* 2006;118(1):290–295.
12. Ammenwerth E, Talmon J, Ash JS, et al. Impact of CPOE on mortality rates–contradictory findings, important messages. *Methods Inf Med.* 2006;45(6):586–593.
13. Keene A, Ashton L, Shure D, Napoleone D, Katyal C, Bellin E. Mortality before and after initiation of a computerized physician order entry system in a critically ill pediatric population. *Pediatr Crit Care Med.* 2007;8(3):268–271.
14. Vardi A, Efrati O, Levin I, et al. Prevention of potential errors in resuscitation medications orders by means of a computerised physician order entry in paediatric critical care. *Resuscitation.* 2007;73(3):400–406.
15. van Tilburg CM, Leistikow IP, Rademaker CM, Bierings MB, van Dijk AT. Health care failure mode and effect analysis: a useful proactive risk analysis in a pediatric oncology ward. *Qual Saf Health Care.* 2006;15(1):58–63.
16. Werba BE, Hobbie W, Kazak AE, Ittenbach RF, Reilly AF, Meadows AT. Classifying the intensity of pediatric cancer treatment protocols: the intensity of treatment rating scale 2.0 (ITR-2). *Pediatr Blood Cancer.* 2007;48(7):673–677.
17. Scavuzzo J, Gamba N. Bridging the gap: the virtual chemotherapy unit. *J Pediatr Oncol Nurs.* 2004;21(1):27–32.
18. Kim GR, Chen AR, Arceci RJ, et al. Error reduction in pediatric chemotherapy: computerized order entry and failure modes and effects analysis. *Arch Pediatr Adolesc Med.* 2006;160(5):495–498.
19. Hayden RT, Patterson DJ, Jay DW, et al. Computer-assisted bar-coding system significantly reduces clinical laboratory specimen identification errors in a pediatric oncology hospital. *J Pediatr.* 2008;152(2):219–224.
20. Rinke ML, Shore AD, Morlock L, Hicks RW, Miller MR. Characteristics of pediatric chemotherapy medication errors in a national error reporting database. *Cancer.* 110(1):186–195.

Chapter 27
Dispensing: Pharmacy Information Systems

Sandra H. Mitchell, Michael A. Veltri and George R. Kim

Objectives

- To provide an overview of the roles of pharmacists and pharmacy information systems (PharmIS) in medication management and delivery
- To outline the structure and functionalities of PharmIS
- To distinguish the needs of pediatric medication processes

27.1 Introduction

Medication delivery and administration, especially in inpatient settings, are complex and error prone processes. The multiple dimensions and levels of detail to which specific drugs must be specified, the numbers of handoffs and transformations (calculation and conversion) of patient and drug specific data that must occur, and the manipulations (compounding, dilution, and dose preparation), make medication delivery highly vulnerable to variation and errors of commission and omission.

In pediatrics, these complexities (and the potential for error and harm) are further magnified by the special needs of children: universal weight-based or body surface area-based dosing, the need for alternative drug forms and routes of administration, differential pharmacokinetics in developing physiologic systems and the long-term and cumulative effects of drugs. To improve pediatric medication safety, automation, and information technology (IT) are used to standardize and streamline the drug and associated data processes.

27.2 Roles of Pharmacists and Pharmacy Information Systems (PharmIS)

Pharmacists and pharmacy information systems (PharmIS) are central to two separate but intimately related medication processes: medication management and medication delivery.

C.U. Lehmann et al. (eds.), *Pediatric Informatics: Computer Applications in Child Health,* Health Informatics,
© Springer Science+Business Media, LLC 2011

27.2.1   Medication Management

Medication management (specified by the Joint Commission[1]), consisting of medication selection and procurement (formulary processes) and storage, is primarily the responsibility of the pharmacist and pharmacy staff.

27.2.1.1   Medication Selection and Procurement

The Joint Commission states that medications available for dispensing or administration are selected, listed, and procured based on criteria, which at minimum, must include: indications for use, effectiveness, risks, and costs. The role of pharmacists is to establish criteria and to design, direct, and implement institutional medication selection processes as part of an interdisciplinary team and to manage medication procurement. The institutional list of available medications that results from the selection process is the basis of the clinical formulary and the core of pharmacy IT support.

27.2.1.2   Medication Storage

Medication storage involves comprehensive management of formulary and non-formulary items, patient medications, refrigerated items, controlled substances and expired/damaged/contaminated medications. Medication storage includes controlling the availability of standardized and limited concentrations of drugs (such as intravenous admixtures).

27.2.2   Medication Delivery

Medication delivery, a set of sequential and interrelated steps, is a shared responsibility among providers (clinician, pharmacist, nurse) (see Chapter 25). Pharmacists are responsible for interpreting and translating instructions from a prescriber (prescription) into specific doses of medications, which are subsequently dispensed for administration to a specific patient.

27.2.2.1   Ordering and Prescribing
(Including Transcription/Communication)

In the ordering/prescribing step, a clinician specifies, on the basis of clinical information, a regimen of drugs to be given to a patient. The prescriber transcribes/communicates this regimen to the pharmacist as a formal, standardized message, a prescription, for preparation/dispensing.

To prevent errors in this step, pharmacists need access to clear and unambiguous information about the prescription, the patient for whom it is intended, and the indication for which the drug has been prescribed. The prescription must be complete, and must include sufficient detail, clarity, and legibility, with unambiguous use of numbers, units, and abbreviations. Pharmacists must have ready access to patient-specific data to track/audit prescriptions and to check dosages, presence of potential drug interactions, allergies, or contraindications. Pharmacists also need timely access to prescribers to clarify prescriptions as necessary.

Electronic support for accurate communication of medication orders includes the use of computerized order entry systems (covered in Chapter 26), standard conventions and electronic formats (such as HL7) for writing and encoding prescriptions and unique identifiers for prescribers and patients. The Joint Commission has not yet incorporated this concept into their Medication Management model.

27.2.2.2 Order Checking/Verification, Preparation, and Dispensing

Order checking/verification of a prescription involves identification and correction of errors and ambiguities in the transcribed order and/or determining the adequacy of an available substitution when a desired drug or drug form is not readily available. Pharmacists' familiarity with the clinical domain (such as pediatrics), the clinical condition of the patient and practical considerations (such as alternative drug forms when oral administration is impractical) is essential.

Preparation and dispensing of a drug dose is a pharmacist's assurance that the correct drug for the correct patient and indication is provided at the correct dose and form, for administration at the correct time and schedule, with the correct directions, and checked for any contraindications. Pharmacist information needs include: patient-specific data including age, weight, height, current medications, allergies and diagnoses and physiologic parameters that determine drug absorption and clearance (such as liver and renal functional test results), general medical knowledge of the pharmacology, toxicology, and drug interactions of prescribed drugs and practical knowledge about pharmacy availability, substitutions, contraindications, and interactions.

Information technology resources that support this step include: electronic health records, drug-specific information libraries for prescribers, nurses and patients, formulary and inventory management systems (including controlled access cabinets, barcoding, and radio-frequency identification) and disease-specific order sets. The role of pharmacists is central in creating and maintaining systems that provide information support about drugs and proactively provide decision support to prevent errors in the ordering/prescribing and administration steps of the medication delivery process.

27.2.2.3 Administration and Monitoring

Administration is the direct delivery or application of a drug to a patient, and in inpatient settings is frequently performed by a nurse. Nursing actions within the context of medication delivery include: receipt of drugs from pharmacy, retrieval of locally stored drug doses intended for patients, checking, and matching of drug doses to patients according to schedule, checking for contraindications, administering the medication properly, recording administered doses, and monitoring the patient. Nursing information needs include: general disease and drug-specific knowledge and patient-specific data regarding medications and other care (Chapter 28).

27.3   Pharmacy Information Systems (PharmIS)

Pharmacy information systems (PharmIS)[2–4] are computerized systems that support the management and dispensing of drugs, including inventory, reporting, and cost tracking. In many cases, they are comprised of a central database (data on drugs in the formulary), interfaces (views) that provide access to information (such as inventory reports) and clinical decision support (CDS). PharmIS may act as a standalone system (accessible to pharmacy staff only) and/or may be connected to computerized provider order entry (CPOE), electronic medical records (EMR) and/ or electronic medication administration records (eMARs) as part of an integrated health information technology (HIT) system.

27.3.1   Central Database

The central database manages current and detailed information about drugs used within an institution. Functions of the central database should include the ability to:

- Store and make available pharmacologic knowledge about formulary drugs, including drug interactions and patient information sheets in a form accessible to users (according to language and literacy levels)
- Import and update drug information from commercially available data dictionaries
- Link patient-specific drug information, including current diagnoses, medications, allergies, and contraindications and nonformulary drugs
- Track cumulative dosages of identified drugs (such as chemotherapy)

Newer functionalities include abilities to:

- Interoperate with other data systems, such as ePrescribing networks and pharmacy benefits management systems
- Provide paperless package inserts

Pediatric specific functionality should include:

- Weight and body-surface area based dosing information and calculation support
- Age-based pharmacologic data

27.3.2   Interfaces

Interfaces connect the central database to other information systems and to users (including patients). Selection of pharmacy information systems may be based in part on the interfaces that are provided or that are possible (that may be negotiated with a vendor). Interfaces may provide:

- Physical access to pharmacy information for users
  - Computer workstations (online access to drug libraries, handbooks)
  - Telephone (direct consultation with an on-site pharmacist in the case of standalone databases)
  - Mobile devices (handheld/wireless)
- Print media (handbooks, brochures)
- Functional tools to help users locate information
  - Search engines
  - Calculators for doses, body surface area
  - Reference charts to normal values
- Integration with clinical information and workflows
  - Electronic medical records
  - Computerized provider order entry
  - Electronic medication administration records
- Interoperability with external information systems
  - Financial information systems
  - Benefits information systems
  - Commercially available data dictionaries

Specific configurations for interfaces between a PharmIS and CPOE include: complete integration of the two systems, a bidirectional interface, a unidirectional interface or not using an interface. Each has advantages and disadvantages and these should be considered carefully when deciding on a system.[2]

27.3.3   Clinical Decision Support

Clinical decision support (CDS) provides "clinicians, patients or individuals with knowledge and person-specific or population information, intelligently filtered or presented at appropriate times, to foster better health processes, better individual patient care."[5] Functionalities of PharmIS CDS include:

- Checking doses based on allowed dose ranges
- Detecting known allergy and drug interactions
- Identifying and flagging duplicate orders/therapies
- Providing patient and drug-specific warnings
- Intercepting drug incompatibilities (intravenous admixtures)

27.3.3.1 Checking Doses Based on Allowed Dose Ranges

Robust dose-checking functionality should be considered a mandatory safety feature for any PharmIS, especially if it is intended for use at a health-system caring for pediatric patients. Common dosing errors include decimal errors (10-, 100-, or 1,000-fold errors) and other miscalculations. More sophisticated dose checking may include considerations of renal and hepatic function according to known serum drug levels or cumulative (lifetime) doses of specific medications (such as in cancer chemotherapy). Currently most advanced functionalities are not widely available in machine-usable forms.

Most PharmIS require the final ordered dose to be entered, either manually or via a CPOE system, into its database to support operations (labeling, billing, etc.) and for dose range checking. The mathematical calculations (i.e. dose per kilogram or Body Surface Area (BSA) single and/or total daily dose) require access to the appropriate data (such as weight, height, and age).

An ideal pediatric PharmIS should allow configuration for dose range calculations (such as for BSA, which requires both weight and height) to use published algorithms or to individualize algorithms for a specific institution (such as when consensus is lacking[6] particularly in pediatrics). Appropriate dose check values for any specific medication may also vary by administration route, and therefore, the ability to vary these, either in user built data or through a configurable CDS system, is desirable.

Some dose checking features may be configured directly within the PharmIS application itself and performed according to institution-defined limits, or by a separate CDS system running in tandem with the PharmIS. The former will offer more flexibility as it is dependent on users defining and configuring the rules. The advantage of this customizability should not be underestimated. Alert fatigue,[7] a phenomenon where users of a system begin to ignore alerts after the validity or importance of previously viewed the alert warnings are felt to be minimal, can leave even the most well-intentioned users vulnerable to missing significant alerts. The drawback of institutional adjustment of alerts is the amount of labor and clinical expertise that are required to develop and maintain optimum rates of alert response.

Interfacing of the PharmIS with a third party CDS system allows updating of the CDS by subscription to a service. Such a service provides periodic (monthly, quarterly, or semiannually) updates, based on peer-review and evidence. Although maintaining the data in such a system is as simple as applying the provided update disk, these systems do not typically offer local editing of content that may contribute to alert "noise."

In PharmIS that allow configurable dose checking rules, all personnel involved must be familiar with the clinical and technical aspects of the configuration tool and developed rules must be tested extensively before deployment. Systems vary in design details and critical functionality may or may not be available. For pediatrics, significant dose variations may exist for many drugs according to patient age or weight. Such a situation might lead to conflicting rules such as allowable high dose limits for one patient group that would be overdoses in another group (and would be missed). Rules and data across the clinical systems within an institution (such as CPOE and PharmIS) should be as consistent as possible. Differences in tolerances for errors or flexibility may lead to conflicting alerts (such as a situation where a CPOE system that does not display a dosage warning to a prescriber, but for which the linked PharmIS provides a dosage error to the pharmacist.

Example of dose range check:

Drug "X" has the following dose limits

Pediatric limits:

Per Dose: 25–50 mg/kg

Per Day: 50–100 mg/kg [daily dose usually divided twice per day (every 12 h)]

Adult limits:

Per Dose: 1,000–2,000 mg

Per Day: 2,000–4,000 mg [daily dose usually divided twice per day (every 12 h)]

In a 12 kg pediatric patient – if the prescriber orders 300 mg per dose every 12 h, the 300 mg value is the one needed by most PharmIS, as it reflect the final dose to be compounded, labeled, dispensed, and administered. For Dose Screening, however, the 300 mg value must be divided by the weight in order to check it against the above parameters (i.e. 300 mg per dose/12 kg = 25 mg/kg/dose; 25 mg/kg/dose × 2 doses per day = 50 mg/kg/day). It should also be checked against maximum adult doses to assure that, in an example of a larger adolescent pediatric patient, the correct mg/kg dose is not in excess of the adult maximum doses.

27.3.3.2   Detecting Known Allergy and Drug Interactions

Another essential PharmIS CDS function is allergy checking/screening,[8] which requires linkage to an accurate and current patient allergy profile (which must be maintained and available to the PharmIS). Although drug allergy checks should be comprehensive and include chemically related drugs with known cross-reactive potential (such as is known penicillin with piperacillin or cefotaxime), this is challenging because of the lack of an available evidence-based standard coding scheme of cross-reactivity potentials and an effective method to distinguish (or notate a distinction) between true allergy (such as anaphylaxis) and individual intolerance (such as nausea to narcotics) to a medication. Most systems do not differentiate these two phenomena, and it is unknown if doing so would improve safety in this area.

As with automated dose checking, allergy screening rules may be provided by an interfaced third party CDS system or may be configured locally. Allergy checking functionality is currently available on many PharmIS. The same advantages and challenges regarding their set-up, customizability, and maintenance discussed for dose checking apply to allergy and interaction screening.

Drug-interaction checking[9] should also be considered core CDS functionality. This clinical check is frequently performed through a separate and tandem CDS system. As with other clinical alerting systems, noise, and alert fatigue are concerns, although most third party system databases are typically conservative and inclusive (i.e. theoretical, potential, and low-risk interactions are included in warnings), with limited ability to filter these.

In this case, filtering may be available through the PharmIS, which may be used to filter warnings from the third party CDS data bases secondarily through natural language or logical processing (such as suppression of "interaction significance: minor" and "level of documentation: theoretical," etc.). Knowledge and control of the PharmIS filtering interfaces and of which drug interaction combinations are being filtered is essential. In addition to the technical challenges this approach poses are issues of sharing proprietary knowledge of the CDS third-party vendors.

Drug interaction functionality is present in most systems. An important configuration consideration is the type of medication orders or circumstances that are included in interaction checking. For example, a drug that has been discontinued for a patient, but which has a prolonged half-life, may need to be considered regarding possible interactions when new drugs are prescribed. This may include drugs which are given once in a sustained-release form or in patients (such as those with renal or hepatic failure) with impaired excretion of a previously administered drug (which may not be listed as active).

27.3.3.3   Identifying and Flagging Duplicate Orders/Therapies

A PharmIS should automatically screen patient medication profiles for duplicate therapies. This issue may occur in geriatric and home health populations,[10] but may occur in any patient. One difficulty in screening for duplication lies in how it is defined. "Duplicate orders" may refer to an exact medication match (one drug at one dose for a given schedule), while duplicate therapies may be considered different drugs that have the same indication or be of the same classes (such as furosemide and chlorothiazide (for diuresis) or ibuprofen and naproxen (for pain)). Differentiation of true alerts from clinically acceptable and appropriate "duplications" (such as tapering doses of a drug or multiple routes of administration for nursing discretion) may be challenging. Current experience of many is that the noise of these types of alerts often far exceeds perceived benefit. Solutions may include local configuration of PharmIS alerts (instead of utilizing a third-party CDS product) or suppression of specific duplicate alerts (that are known to be "noisy").

27.3.3.4   Providing Patient and Drug-Specific Warnings

Other patient and drug-specific warnings that have been provided in PharmIS CDS include drug-laboratory test, drug-pregnancy, drug-lactation, and age-specific interactions or warnings. The usefulness of some of these messages varies, as they may not be context sensitive. For example, a warning that a specific drug may cause a false-positive urine toxicology screen is significant only if one is ordered, otherwise it is noise. Some PharmIS CDS systems may screen warnings appropriately (such as displaying drug-pregnancy and/or lactation warnings only for female patients of childbearing age), but in many cases, such warnings are of significance to the primary clinician (when they are not noise) and would be better included in a CPOE or eMAR system.

27.3.3.5 Intercepting Drug Incompatibilities (Intravenous Admixtures)

Incompatibilities of drugs in intravenous (IV) admixtures are undesired but sometimes chemically predictable phenomena that reduce or negate medication potency (through precipitation, inactivation, neutralization, absorption, etc.) of an active component of the mixture. Some incompatibilities depend on relative admixture component concentrations and other factors (temperature, exposure to light, etc.).

An IV component compatibility screening tool within a PharmIS CDS system has tremendous usefulness. The ability to check an entire IV profile on-demand and to provide incompatibility warnings prior to admixture would have great utility. Currently, systems are hindered by the fact that the necessary calculations that determine compatibility problems do not occur until the order for the admixture has been entered. One workaround would be to provide this calculation in CPOE, but currently, IV compatibility integration into PharmIS CDS is only in its infancy.

27.4 Special Workflows

Certain medication delivery workflows pose greater risk to patients (either higher likelihood or impact of error), which create the need for special precautions to reduce errors. Cancer chemotherapy requires complex protocols that may be interrupted due to the current health status of the patient and drugs of high toxicity. PharmIS may provide alternative scheduling and lifetime medication dose tracking for drugs of cumulative toxicity.[11,12] Continuous infusions are frequently used in critical care and require calculation support as well as the required use of standard concentrations.[13]

27.5 Conclusion

Within pediatric medication delivery processes, the most valuable component of any pediatric pharmacy process is a qualified and experienced pediatric pharmacist and pharmacy staff who actively participate in clinical care of inpatients (such daily work rounds).[14,15] As much of medication management and checking/dispensing is invisible to the rest of the clinical staff, this expertise provides an additional layer of error catching and safety in medication ordering. In a recent study,[16] pediatric clinical pharmacists were effective in intercepting prescribing errors, but did not capture potentially harmful medication administration errors.

In addition to the presence of trained pediatric pharmacists, the role of PharmIS in error catching as part of an integrated medication delivery system that includes connection to CPOE and electronic medication administration records is central. The continuing evolution of PharmIS and PharmIS CDS as well as participation of clinical pharmacists in development of CPOE, eMAR, and other tools within the medication delivery cycle will be important in reducing errors and improving quality of the pediatric medication use system.

27.6   Case Study: Elimination of the "Rule of Six" in Pediatric Continuous Infusions[17]

At a 180 bed tertiary pediatric academic center, a redesign project to reduce continuous infusion medication errors and to transition safely to Joint Commission mandated standardized infusion concentrations (SC)[13] was undertaken. After an initial assessment of baseline infusion order error rates, a Web-based calculator[18] was developed in 2003 to reduce errors, using the "Rule of Six" resulting in a significant and sustainable decrease in prescribing errors. The Joint Commission requirement for transition of all infusions to standard concentrations[19] led to: (a) specification of standard concentrations for 51 infusion drugs, (b) redesign of the infusion calculator with an interface to the hospital census and additional decision support to facilitate use of SC, (c) construction of pre-built choices into the associated PharmIS for SC (thus eliminating pharmacist calculations) and (d) incorporation of syringe "smart" pumps for infusions. This facilitated transition to standard concentrations for infusions with a further reduction in error rates.

The success of the system and its subsequent incorporation into a commercial CPOE system was the result of its multidisciplinary approach which included the expertise of pediatric clinical pharmacists. This expertise, which included knowledge about medication stability, usual and extreme doses, appropriate flow/infusion rates, concentration limits (in peripheral vs. central infusions), and commercially available dosage forms was essential for developing drug-specific SCs for pediatric infusions.

References

1. Rich, Darryl S. New JCAHO medication management standards for 2004. *Am J Health-Syst Pharm.* 2004;61:1349–1359.
2. Chaffee BW, Bonasso J. Strategies for pharmacy integration and pharmacy information system interfaces, Part 1: history and pharmacy integration options. *Am J Health Syst Pharm.* 2004;61(5):502–506.

3. Chaffee BW, Bonasso J. Strategies for pharmacy integration and pharmacy information system interfaces, Part 2: scope of work and technical aspects of interfaces. *Am J Health Syst Pharm.* 2004;61(5):506–514.

4. Chaffee BW, Townsend KA, Benner T, de Leon RF. Pharmacy database for tracking drug costs and utilization. *Am J Health Syst Pharm.* 2000;57(7):669–676.

5. Osheroff JA, Teich JM, Middleton BF, Steen, EB, Wright A, Detmer DE. A Roadmap for National Action on Clinical Decision Support. American Medical Informatics Association; 2006. Available at: http://www.amia.org/inside/initiatives/cds/. Accessed December 21, 2008.

6. Liem RI, Higman MA, Chen AR, Arceci RJ. Misinterpretation of a Calvert-derived formula leading to carboplatin overdose in two children. *J Pediatr Hematol Oncol.* 2003;25(10):818–821.

7. van der Sijs H, Aarts J, Vulto A, Berg M. Overriding of drug safety alerts in computerized physician order entry. *J Am Med Inform Assoc.* 2005;13(2):138–147. Available at: http://www.jamia.org/cgi/content/abstract/13/2/138. Accessed December 21, 2008.

8. Kuperman GJ, Gandhi TK, Bates DW. Effective drug-allergy checking: methodological and operational issues. *J Biomed Inform.* 2003;36(1–2):70–79.

9. Pham PA. Drug-drug interaction programs in clinical practice. *Clin Pharmacol Ther.* 2008;83(3):396–398.

10. Alkema GE, Wilber KH, Simmons WJ, Enguidanos SM, Frey D. Prevalence of potential medication problems among dually eligible older adults in Medicaid waiver services. *Ann Pharmacother.* 2007;41(12):1971–1978.

11. Koren G, Schechter T. Cancer chemotherapy in young children: challenges and solutions. *Pediatr Blood Cancer.* 2007;49(7 Suppl):1091–1092.

12. Green DM, Grigoriev YA, Nan B, et al. Congestive heart failure after treatment for Wilms' tumor: a report from the National Wilms' Tumor Study group. *J Clin Oncol.* 2001;19(7):1926–1934.

13. Hennessy SC. Developing standard concentrations in the neonatal intensive care unit. *Am J Health Syst Pharm.* 2007;64(1):28–30.

14. Leape LL, Cullen DJ, Clapp MD, et al. Pharmacist participation on physician rounds and adverse drug events in the intensive care unit. *JAMA.* 1999;282(3):267–270.

15. Kucukarslan SN, Peters M, Mlynarek M, Nafziger DA. Pharmacists on rounding teams reduce preventable adverse drug events in hospital general medicine units. *Arch Intern Med.* 2003;163(17):2014–2018.

16. Wang JK, Herzog NS, Kaushal R, Park C, Mochizuki C, Weingarten SR. Prevention of pediatric medication errors by hospital pharmacists and the potential benefit of computerized physician order entry. *Pediatrics.* 2007;119(1):e77–e85.

17. Veltri MA, Ascenzi J, Clark JS, et al. Successful Elimination of the "Rule of Six" in an Academic Children's Hospital Through a Medication-Use-System Redesign and Standardization of Continuous Infusions. American Society of Health-Systems Pharmacists 2006 Mid Year Meeting [Poster]; 2006. Available at: http://www.ashpadvantage.com/bestpractices/2006_papers/veltri.htm. Accessed December 21, 2008.

18. Lehmann CU, Kim GR, Gujral R, Veltri MA, Clark JS, Miller MR. Decreasing errors in pediatric continuous intravenous infusions. *Pediatr Crit Care Med.* 2006;7(3):225–230.

19. Joint Commission. Transition to standardized drug concentrations by the end of 2008. *Jt Comm Perspect.* 2005;25(4):3–5.

Chapter 28
Medication Administration and Information Technology

Catherine Garger, Carol Matlin, George R. Kim and Robert E. Miller

Objectives

- To present a framework for thinking about medication administration and errors
- To discuss healthcare information technology interventions in the context of the model
- To focus on pediatric-specific issues

28.1 Introduction

Medication administration is the final step in the medication delivery cycle before a prescribed drug reaches a patient. In ambulatory settings, the patient, or in the case of children, the parent or guardian is responsible for accepting prescribed medications from the pharmacist and following directions regarding direct administration of drug doses. In inpatient settings, it is principally the bedside nurse who administers prescribed medications. A study of inpatient settings suggests that interventions by pediatric clinical pharmacists, while effective for intercepting prescribing errors, may be ineffective in intercepting harmful administration errors.[1]

28.2 The Steps of Medication Administration

The steps of the inpatient administration process assure the "5 Rights" of medication safety (Right patient, Right medication, Right dose, Right time, Right route) in delivering a drug dose to a patient. These steps include:

1. *Medication reconciliation*: the development and maintenance of shared knowledge of a patient's prescribed medications by the entire health team and what is actually being given. Development of this shared knowledge begins when a patient is admitted to an inpatient unit and current drug regimen is checked, corrected, and recorded as part of the care process. The principal prescriber should have this information in the patient record where it is available to nursing and other

C.U. Lehmann et al. (eds.), *Pediatric Informatics: Computer Applications in Child Health,* Health Informatics,
© Springer Science + Business Media, LLC 2011

team members. Shared awareness is maintained, reviewed, and updated by staff on patient rounds, at nursing shift changes and other handoffs. Knowledge of the drug regimen is summarized and communicated when the patient is discharged to home or transferred from the unit.

2. *Medication storage and retrieval*: the handling of medications prior to delivery and administration to the patient is usually a shared function between pharmacy and nursing. For formulary drugs, pharmacy personnel deliver labeled drug doses to the care unit. For controlled drugs, the nurse formally acknowledges receipt of the doses. In most cases, doses are placed in secure storage until actual delivery to the patient. Storage facilities may provide environmental control (such as temperature). Emergency drugs may be stored for rapid access by nursing during resuscitation. Special items (such as chemotherapy and biological materials (live vaccines, breast milk)) may need to be stored, prepared, and tracked separately.

3. *Dose preparation and verification*: the reconstitution of a drug dose into its final form before delivery or application to the patient may be performed by pharmacy or on the unit. The nurse identifies and checks patient, drug, dose, and form, other constituents (oral or intravenous carrier fluids) and the route by which the drug dose are to be given.

4. *Dose delivery/application (and verification)*: the action of giving a drug dose directly to a patient according to prescription/order and assuring that the dose has been delivered/applied to the patient (according to the 5 Rights), usually performed by nursing, but the patient and/or family may be involved (such as in patient-controlled analgesia). In the case of children on oral medications, it may involve direct observation that swallowing has occurred. For inhaled medications, the respiratory therapist may hold the responsibility for dose preparation and administration, or it may be shared with nursing.

5. *Monitoring*: observation and response as needed for a patient's reaction to a drug dose, usually performed on a regular basis by nursing in conjunction with prescribers and other care providers.

6. *Documentation*: systematic tracking and recording of a patient's planned drug dosing schedule (including biological products and investigational drugs), drug doses administered (or omitted) and other clinical observations, performed principally by nursing. For prescribers, the order sheet/prescription form/ order entry system tracks ordering of medications. For nursing, the medication administration record (MAR) is the principal documentation and tracking tool.

28.3   Medication Administration Risks

Studies suggest that approximately 20% of all adverse patient events are related to medications. In a study of medication errors in an inpatient acute care setting, approximately 40% of errors were deemed to be due to problems during the medication ordering process; 10% were associated with the order-transcription and verification steps, 10% with pharmacy dispensing and the remaining 40% with the medication administration process. Specific conditions or issues increase the risk of harm to patients in medication administration by increasing the probability or impact of errors.

28.3.1   General Risks

- *ISMP high-risk drugs*[2] have higher administration complexities or toxicities.
- *Investigational drugs* pose added risks to patients due to their experimental nature and undocumented interactions with disease states and other drugs.
- *Sound (or look)-alike medications* increase the risk for "wrong drug."
- *Central venous catheters* pose a risk for preventable blood stream infections.
- *Continuous infusions* (including total parenteral nutrition) make drugs and their effects (including toxicities) immediately available on delivery.

28.3.2   Pediatric and Neonatal Specific Risks

- *Alternative routes of administration* for the same drug may result in wrong-form/ wrong-dose/wrong route errors. Rectal and intramuscular routes (which may be dosed differently) are frequently used when intravenous and oral routes are unavailable.
- *Smaller margins for errors* due to smaller absolute dose volumes may result in acute errors of high impact (decimal place errors or cumulative errors over time, such as for chemotherapeutic drugs).
- *Prescriber unfamiliarity with pediatric dosing* by clinicians who care for children infrequently (such as general surgeons and/or non-pediatric residents on rotation on pediatric services) requires higher vigilance in catching errors prior to administration.
- *Alternative (liquid) forms of medications* require carrier fluids that may interact with other drugs.
- *Multiple births*, especially in neonatal intensive care, increase the risk for "wrong patient" errors.
- *Variability in redundant patient identification* by infants and young children when caretakers are unavailable (such as in intensive care) may increase the risk for "wrong patient" errors.
- *Breast milk*, a bodily fluid that is infant nutrition and that may serve as a medium for infectious agents, is prone to administration errors. Reported NICU breast milk management errors have included "wrong route"[3,10] and "wrong patient"[4] errors (with concerns of infection). In addition, prolonged storage of breast milk has been associated with decreases in bactericidal and antioxidant capacity.[5,6]
- *Continuous infusions using standard infusions in very low weight neonates* have posed challenges.

28.4   Information Technology in Medication Administration

The medication administration step represents a "last chance" to intercept an error. Interventions to reduce errors include those in the prescribing/ordering and transcribing/dispensing steps plus:

28.4.1   Bar-Coding

Bar-coding technology involves labeling of an object (medication package, patient identification bracelet) with a machine-readable printed tag and identification with an optical scanner at the point of administration. For individual medication doses, the bar code contains the National Drug Code (NDC), which includes the drug company labeling the package for sale, the name of the drug and its dose. For inpatients, the patient identification bracelet bar code contains the hospital patient number,[7] and scanning allows and enforces matching of patient medical record number to drug dose.

In pediatrics (and in other domains), medications from the manufacturer may be supplied in multidose packs that must be separated and recoded (with the possibility of mislabeling). Use of bar-coding has been associated with interception of "wrong drug" and "wrong dose" errors, as well as "wrong time" and drug storage errors, and doses for which no order was given. Reported errors and failure points associated with the use of bar-coding include: mislabeling of drug dose, missing bar codes, inability to scan bar codes, manual overrides or workarounds (such as scanning a patient identification from the patient chart instead of the patient's identification bracelet), failure to scan bar codes, wrong patient and system unavailability.

In neonatal intensive care units, infants are at risk for medication errors,[8] including "wrong route" errors[9,10] and patient misidentification, particularly in the case of multiple births[11] and with similar medical record numbers, similar sounding surnames. Wristbands that are missing or that contain incorrect or incomplete information may be a frequent occurrence.[12] For errors in breast milk administration, a comprehensive approach has been proposed.[13]

28.4.2   Radio-Frequency Identification (RFID)

RFID appliances or "tags" consist of an embedded integrated circuit that can process and store information from a radio-frequency signal and an antenna that receives and transmits the signal.[14] Current RFID (approved for patient use) consists of passive devices that require an external radio transmitter to operate, while active (self-powered) devices have yet to be approved. Identifying information (including personal health information) can be stored on RFID device (or "tag") and accessed by exposure to a specific radio-frequency (RF) at a sufficiently close range. Its advantage over bar-coding is that it does not require "line of sight" to operate.

RFID has been used as a clinical inventory tracking tool[15] and was approved by the US Food and Drug Administration in 2004 for use as an implantable device for patient identification. Debates on the benefits and risks for patient information being used for nonmedical issues, as well as provider responsibilities in obtaining informed consent have arisen.[16,17] RFID is envisioned as a replacement for bar-coding with current barriers being cost and privacy concerns.

In pediatrics, RFID has been used to relax children in radiology suites by giving them control over the environment (lighting, sound)[18,19] to reduce the need for sedation and in newborn nurseries (as part of a comprehensive plan[20] that uses the infant and mother's wrist bands) to prevent infant abductions and matching infant-mother pairs (using proximity alerts).[21]

28.4.3 "Smart" Infusion Pumps

"Smart" infusion pumps are devices with internal programmable computer control systems that provide complex and precise control over intravenous infusions, which presents unique opportunities and challenges with respect to patient safety and workflow. Smart pumps are now the preferred method for intravenous therapy administration in the acute care setting, particularly for pediatric and critically ill patients, and have largely supplanted gravity-fed drip infusions. It is estimated that as of 2006, 37% of US hospitals used smart infusion pumps.[22]

Advantages of smart pumps include: administration of low flow rates that cannot be achieved with drip infusions, precise timing of intermittent injections and bolus injections, control over patient administered intravenous medications (such as patient controlled analgesia, PCA) and management of administration schedules that use circadian rhythms or other complex protocols. Depending on pump design, control over *continuous infusions* results from frequent small "pulsed" (bolus) deliveries ranging from nanoliters to microliters, while control over *intermittent infusions* alternates high and low infusion rates to deliver therapy and to keep the venous catheter open respectively. For on-demand medications such as *patient (or parent)-controlled analgesia* (PCA), smart pump computers manage the basal rates and dose maximums (lock-outs) to reduce pain while avoiding toxicity.

In the acute care setting, two ranges of pumps are used: *large-volume pumps* use peristaltic pumps to control intravenous fluid delivery, while *small-volume* pumps use controlled syringes to deliver medications into an intravenous system. Both ranges use embedded microprocessors to control the fluid delivery rate and other capabilities of the pump. In home settings, *implanted pumps* (such as for insulin therapy) manage bolus and basal doses and provide alarms and integration to monitors (such as glucometers) and home computers.

Smart pumps can be integrated into a hospital medication delivery system and can be programmed and updated from a central server via a local or wireless network with customized drug libraries. Additionally, some pumps support bar coded medication labels, which can further reduce errors by automating patient and medication identification. Other interfaces from smart pumps are possible, to computerized order entry systems or to pager-driven alert systems, but to date few institutions have implemented these.

Errors (some resulting in morbidity and mortality) that have been associated with the use of smart pumps include: dosing errors due to pump hardware problems,[23,24] misconnections of intravenous lines,[25] inaccurate programming of the pump/incorrect dosing,[26] electrical short-circuit[27] and alert overrides.[28] In pediatrics, smart pumps have been helpful in conjunction with other technologies to reduce errors in administration of continuous infusions using standard concentrations,[29] but there is need for further research.[30]

28.4.4 Electronic Medication Administration Records (eMARs)

In inpatient and residential care settings, the medication administration record (MAR) is the principal coordination and documentation tool for nursing and others (principally respiratory therapists) involved in the direct delivery of drug doses to patients. In some cases, documentation of a drug dose (such as an intravenous "push" dose of a specified drug for resuscitation) given by another provider may be documented by a nurse on behalf of the provider.

Paper versions of the MAR are patient-specific records that provide a temporal listing of scheduled and given drug doses. The paper MAR is manually populated by the nurse according to prescribed drug orders (from CPOE or paper orders), and completed (scheduled or emergent) doses are signed-off by the nurse (or respiratory therapist). The portion of the MAR in current use is kept with the active nursing record (which includes nursing assessments and problem lists), while completed orders are archived with the remainder of the patient chart. The MAR also provides communications to other members of the care team regarding informal (handwritten notes) but important details of the medication schedule.

Electronic versions of the MAR (eMARs) provide similar functions as paper versions, with added functionalities of drug dose information linkage from computerized provider order entry (CPOE) and pharmacy information systems (PharmIS), drug dose schedule alerts, auto-adjustment of future scheduled doses based on schedule changes and control over data entry rights (restrictions to nurses and respiratory therapists). Without modifications, eMARs may not afford unstructured entry of ad hoc notes that allow informal communication of important details among providers.

Standalone eMARs surprisingly do not change the cognitive workflow of nurses,[31] who must still go through the outlined steps to assure the "five rights." The principal exception may be increased time in checking or verifying medication doses (which may require computerized sign-off by a colleague).[32] Nursing satisfaction with the fit of the technology into workflow and its acceptance are essential, and perceptions of ineffective technology may induce overrides and workarounds ("first order problem-solving"[33]) that defeat the purpose of the technology.

Linkages of eMARs to bar-coding provide functionalities of positive identification of patient wristbands to drug doses, double-checking of dose times and interception of errors.[34] The incorporation of these into an inpatient closed-loop (end-to-end integrated medication cycle) system has been shown to reduce prescribing and administration errors, increase patient identity confirmation prior to administration and increase time required for task completion.[35]

Successful adoption, deployment, and use of eMARs depends on many human and organizational factors, including nursing leadership (particularly at the level of the clinical care unit) that is aligned with institutional leadership that promotes HIT as a path to patient safety and the presence of clinical nurse champions,[36] sufficient nursing education and technical support. Understanding nursing resistance to adoption[37] may give directions to efforts to improve it. Structured educational programs must provide nurses with (a) an overview of the incorporation of HIT (such as eMARs) into medication administration and how it will change their work, (b) hands-on training with tools that uses scenarios that match the particular user's work tasks and (c) an opportunity to demonstrate competence via simulation.

Monitoring and evaluation of problems occurring at deployment[38] and in operation[39] may provide data for further refinements to the system. Problems, when reported, may arise from: lack of staff knowledge about the patients, medications, equipment (including system capabilities) or procedures; failure to follow correct procedures or lack of standard protocols; failures of communications or transcription; or systems issues.

Particular administration problems may persist: where dual medication administration records (paper and electronic) exist, requiring duplicate entry and the opportunity for errors[34]; during patient transfers between institutions[40] care units (where duplication or omission of doses may occur)[41] and in domains where care is complex (such as pediatric cancer chemotherapy).[42]

28.5 Conclusion

Medication administration is a step in the medication delivery cycle that is vulnerable to errors. Health information technologies may help to mitigate some of the vulnerabilities, but it is still a largely human controlled process, even with closed-loop applications. Even with reductions in prescribing errors, there remains much work to be done in reducing medication administration errors.

28.6   Case Studies

28.6.1   The VA Bar Code Medication Administration System

The US Department of Veterans Affairs (VA) Bar Code Medication Administration
(BCMA) system is an integral part of the Veterans Health Information Systems
and Technology Architecture (VistA),[43] the VA's comprehensive electronic record
system, used by all VA inpatient facilities, outpatient clinics, nursing homes, and
long-term care facilities across the US.

VistA's Computerized Patient Record System's (CPRS) graphical user interface
(GUI) supports provider order entry (CPOE), including real-time communication
of clinical reminders, access to problem-allergy-medication lists, laboratory, radiology, and pathology data. It also provides access to clinical notes, consultations,
discharge summaries; and other functions (Fig. 28.1).

The VA developed a bar code medication administration system (BCMA) in
1995. In the BCMA, patients wear bar-coded wristbands and unit-dose medications
are bar-coded in the pharmacy before delivery to a patient's medication drawer.
The BCMA shares data with the CPRS through the VistA database, using wireless laptop computers mounted on wheeled medication carts. During medication
rounds, nurses scan patients' wristbands with a bar code reader connected to the
laptop to access up-to-date medication order data in BCMA (entered into CPRS by
physicians and verified by pharmacists in the VistA database). When a nurse scans

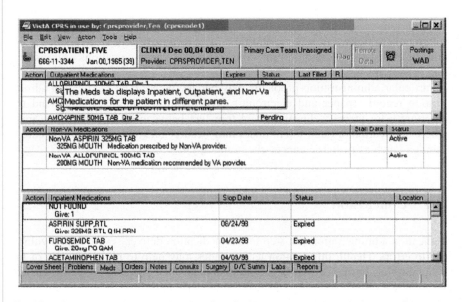

Fig. 28.1 CPRS screen listing medications for a fictitious patient. Tabs at the bottom of the screen
show other CPRS functions

a dose, it is automatically documented as administered when the dose bar code number matches the order number for the drug/dose/form/time, as displayed on the primary BCMA screen. If there is a mismatch on any parameter, an alert box is presented. The BCMA also automatically updates the electronic medication administration record (eMAR) with the time of administration and operator identification when the medications are scanned as "administered" (Fig. 28.2).

Logistic problems encountered during widespread deployment of the BCMA throughout the VA system included equipment procurement, bar code print quality, pharmacy coverage and lack of standardization of medication administration policies and practices (across VA hospitals). Ethnographic observation and analysis of medication administration practices pre- and post-BCMA deployment provided insight into unanticipated negative effects:

- Unexpected automated functions (such as removal of missed doses from the BCMA display)
- Degraded coordination between nurses and physicians
- Bypassing scanning (manual data entry) to increase efficiency
- Increased anxiety regarding and prioritization of audited activities
- Decreased capacity for complex sequences (such as steroid tapers)
- Variable flexibility in handling system failures[44]

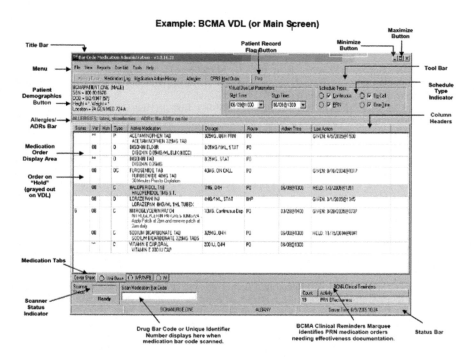

Fig. 28.2 Bar code medication administration (BCMA) user interface

The next generation of BCMA, using a "breakthrough" collaborative process, incorporated IV medications and STAT verbal orders prior to pharmacy verification[45] and solved a number of problems encountered in the first generation.

28.6.2   RFID vs Bar Coding and Pragmatics

The superiority of one technology over the other is a matter of practicality. Bar coding requires "line of sight" and two hands to operate when a handheld scanner is used, but is cheaper than RFID tags. Once adopted, changing strategies can be costly (retagging all medications with RFID), so a parsimonious combined approach may be useful. In one Pennsylvania hospital, RFID was used to tag IV fluid bags (which were difficult to scan with bar coding due to the irregular surface on which bar codes were placed).[46]

The use of RFID devices has been extended to prevent infant abductions from hospitals. As a security-sensitive area of the hospital, maternal-infant areas must (per Joint Commission) have a multidisciplinary plan to prevent misidentification of infants ("baby-switching") and/or abductions.[47] Incidental reports of abduction prevention[48] attributing success to RFID devices do not emphasize all the components needed for an abduction-proof system.[49]

References

1. Wang JK, Herzog NS, Kaushal R, Park C, Mochizuki C, Weingarten SR. Prevention of pediatric medication errors by hospital pharmacists and the potential benefit of computerized physician order entry. *Pediatrics*. 2007;119(1):e77–e85.
2. Institute for Safe Medical Practices (ISMP). ISMP's List of High-Alert Medications; 2007. Available at: http://www.ismp.org/Tools/highalertmedications.pdf. Accessed December 21, 2008.
3. Vanitha V, Narasimhan KL. Intravenous breast milk administration–a rare accident. *Indian Pediatr*. 2006;43(9):827.
4. Warner B, Sapsford A. Misappropriated human milk: fantasy, fear, and fact regarding infectious risk. *Newborn Infant Nurs Rev*. 2004;4(1):56–61.
5. Martínez-Costa C, Silvestre MD, López MC, Plaza A, Miranda M, Guijarro R. Effects of refrigeration on the bactericidal activity of human milk: a preliminary study. *J Pediatr Gastroenterol Nutr*. 2007;45(2):275–277.
6. Hanna N, Ahmed K, Anwar M, Petrova A, Hiatt M, Hegyi T. Effect of storage on breast milk antioxidant activity. *Arch Dis Child Fetal Neonatal Ed*. 2004;89(6):F518–F520.
7. Cochran GL, Jones KJ, Brockman J, Skinner A, Hicks RW. Errors prevented by and associated with bar-code medication administration systems. *Jt Comm J Qual Patient Saf*. 2007;33(5):293–301, 245.
8. Snijders C, van Lingen RA, Molendijk A, Fetter WP. Incidents and errors in neonatal intensive care: a review of the literature. *Arch Dis Child Fetal Neonatal Ed*. 2007;92(5):F391–F398.
9. Bridge L. Reducing the risk of wrong route errors. *Paediatr Nurs*. 2007;19(6):33–35.
10. Ryan CA, Mohammad I, Murphy B. Normal neurologic and developmental outcome after an accidental intravenous infusion of expressed breast milk in a neonate. *Pediatrics*. 2006;117(1):236–238.
11. Gray JE, Suresh G, Ursprung R, et al. Patient misidentification in the neonatal intensive care unit: quantification of risk. *Pediatrics*. 2006;117(1):e43–e47.

12. Howanitz PJ, Renner SW, Walsh MK. Continuous wristband monitoring over 2 years decreases identification errors: a College of American Pathologists Q-Tracks Study. *Arch Pathol Lab Med.* 2002;126(7):809–815.
13. Drenckpohl D, Bowers L, Cooper H. Use of the six sigma methodology to reduce incidence of breast milk administration errors in the NICU. *Neonatal Netw.* 2007;26(3):161–166.
14. Wikipedia. Radio-Frequency Identification; 2007. Available at: http://en.wikipedia.org/wiki/Radio-frequency_identification. Accessed December 21, 2008.
15. Grey M. Tracking with RFID. Brigham and Women's is keeping tabs on expensive equipment and valuable devices with the help of an indoor positioning system. *Healthc Inform.* 2007;24(11):25–27.
16. Levine M, Adida B, Mandl K, Kohane I, Halamka J. What are the benefits and risks of fitting patients with radiofrequency identification devices. *PLoS Med.* 2007;4(11):e322.
17. Sade RM, American Medical Association Council on Ethical and Judicial Affairs. Radio Frequency ID Devices in Humans. American Medical Association; 2007. Available at: http://www.ama-assn.org/ama1/pub/upload/mm/369/ceja_5a07.pdf. Accessed December 21, 2008.
18. Anastos JP. The ambient experience in pediatric radiology. *J Radiol Nurs.* 2007; 26(2):50–55.
19. Campbell BC, Anastos J. Can CT scans be 'fun'? Innovative CT suite gives children greater control over the environment to ease their fears. *Healthc Exec.* 2006;21(1):36–37.
20. The Joint Commission. Root causes: practical approaches for preventing infant abductions. *Jt Comm Persp Patient Saf.* 2003;3(10):7–8.
21. Miller RS. Preventing infant abduction in the hospital. *Nursing.* 2007;37(10):20, 22.
22. Vanderveen T. Smart Pumps: Advanced Capabilities and Continuous Quality Improvement. Patient Safety and Quality Healthcare; 2007. Available at: http://www.psqh.com/janfeb07/smartpumps.html. Accessed December 21, 2008.
23. Syed S, Paul JE, Hueftlein M, Kampf M, McLean RF. Morphine overdose from error propagation on an acute pain service. *Can J Anaesth.* 2006;53(6):586–590.
24. Steffen M, von Hintzenstern U, Obermayer A. Critical infusion incident caused by incorrect use of a patient-controlled analgesia pump. *Anaesthesiol Reanim.* 2002;27(4):107–110.
25. Elannaz A, Chaumeron A, Viel E, Ripart J. Morphine overdose due to cumulative errors leading to ACP pump dysfunction. *Ann Fr Anesth Reanim.* 2004;23(11):1073–1075.
26. Vicente KJ, Kada-Bekhaled K, Hillel G, Cassano A, Orser BA. Programming errors contribute to death from patient-controlled analgesia: case report and estimate of probability. *Can J Anaesth.* 2003;50(4):328–332.
27. Doyle DJ, Vicente KJ. Electrical short circuit as a possible cause of death in patients on PCA machines: report on an opiate overdose and a possible preventive remedy. *Anesthesiology.* 2001;94(5):940.
28. Rothschild JM, Keohane CA, Cook EF, et al. A controlled trial of smart infusion pumps to improve medication safety in critically ill patients. *Crit Care Med.* 2005;33(3):533–540.
29. Larsen GY, Parker HB, Cash J, O'Connell M, Grant MC. Standard drug concentrations and smart-pump technology reduce continuous-medication-infusion errors in pediatric patients. *Pediatrics.* 2005 July;116(1):e21–e25.
30. Conroy S, Sweis D, Planner C, Yeung V, Collier J, Haines L, Wong IC. Interventions to reduce dosing errors in children: a systematic review of the literature. *Drug Saf.* 2007;30(12):1111–1125.
31. Eisenhauer LA, Hurley AC, Dolan N. Nurses' reported thinking during medication administration. *J Nurs Scholarsh.* 2007;39(1):82–87.
32. Hurley AC, Bane A, Fotakis S, et al. Nurses' satisfaction with medication administration point-of-care technology. *J Nurs Adm.* 2007;37(7–8):343–349.
33. Vogelsmeier AA, Halbesleben JR, Scott-Cawiezell JR. Technology implementation and workarounds in the nursing home. *J Am Med Inform Assoc.* 2008;15(1):114–119.
34. Larrabee S, Brown MM. Recognizing the institutional benefits of bar-code point-of-care technology. *Jt Comm J Qual Saf.* 2003;29(7):345–353.
35. Franklin BD, O'Grady K, Donyai P, Jacklin A, Barber N. The impact of a closed-loop electronic prescribing and administration system on prescribing errors, administration errors and staff time: a before-and-after study. *Qual Saf Health Care.* 2007;16(4):279–284.

36. Wideman MV, Whittler ME, Anderson TM. Barcode Medication Administration: Lessons Learned from an Intensive Care Unit Implementation. Advances in Patient Safety: From Research to Implementation. Vol 3, AHRQ Publication Nos. 050021 (1–4). Agency for Healthcare Research and Quality, Rockville, MD; 2005: 437–451. Available at: http://www.ahcpr.gov/downloads/pub/advances/vol3/Wideman.pdf. Accessed December 21, 2008.
37. Kirkley D, Stein M. Nurses and clinical technology: sources of resistance and strategies for acceptance. *Nurs Econ.* 2004;22(4):195, 216–222.
38. Kim GR, Miller MR, Ardolino MA, Smith JE, Lee DC, Lehmann CU. Capture and classification of problems during CPOE deployment in an academic pediatric center. *AMIA Annu Symp Proc.* 2007:414–417.
39. Wakefield BJ, Uden-Holman T, Wakefield DS. Development and Validation of the Medication Administration Error Reporting Survey. Advances in Patient Safety: From Research to Implementation. Volumes 4, AHRQ Publication Nos. 050021 (1–4). Agency for Healthcare Research and Quality, Rockville, MD; 2005. Available at: http://www.ncbi.nlm.nih.gov/books/bv.fcgi?rid=aps.section.8223. Accessed December 21, 2008.
40. Keatings M, Martin M, McCallum A, Lewis J. Medical errors: understanding the parent's perspective. *Pediatr Clin North Am.* 2006;53(6):1079–1089.
41. Bayley KB, Savitz LA, Rodriguez G, Gillanders W, Stoner S. Barriers Associated with Medication Information Handoffs. Advances in Patient Safety: From Research to Implementation. Volumes 3, AHRQ Publication Nos. 050021 (1–4). February 2005. Agency for Healthcare Research and Quality, Rockville, MD; 2005. Available at: http://www.ncbi.nlm.nih.gov/books/bv.fcgi?rid=aps.section.4074. Accessed December 21, 2008.
42. Rinke ML, Shore AD, Morlock L, Hicks RW, Miller MR. Characteristics of pediatric chemotherapy medication errors in a national error reporting database. *Cancer.* 2007;110(1):186–195.
43. United States Department of Veteran Affairs. Veterans Health Information Systems and Technology Architecture (VistA) Monograph; 2006. Available at: http://www.va.gov/vista_monograph/. Accessed December 21, 2008.
44. Patterson ES, Cool RI, Render ML. Improving patient safety by identifying side effects from introducing bar coding in medication administration. *J Am Med Inform Assoc.* 2002;9:540–553.
45. Mills PD, Neily J, Mims E, Burkhardt ME, Bagian J. Improving the bar-coded medication administration system at the Department of Veterans Affairs. *Am J Health Syst Pharm.* 2006;63(15):1442–1447.
46. Young D. Pittsburgh hospital combines RFID, bar codes to improve safety. *Am J Health Syst Pharm.* 2006;63(24):2431, 2435.
47. Shogan MG. Emergency management plan for newborn abduction. *J Obstet Gynecol Neonatal Nurs.* 2002;31(3):340–346.
48. Sullivan L. RFID System Prevented A Possible Infant Abduction. Information Week; 2005. Available at: http://www.informationweek.com/story/showArticle.jhtml?articleID=166400496. Accessed December 21, 2008.
49. Cesario SK. Selecting an infant security system. *AWHONN Lifelines.* 2003;7(3):236–242.

Chapter 29
Understanding and Preventing Errors

Michael Apkon

Objectives

- To provide a framework for understanding and studying errors and risk
- To discuss root cause analysis and Failure Modes and Effects Analysis in terms of the framework
- To outline and illustrate the place of informatics in error-proofing processes

29.1   Introduction

Medical care requires the coordinated action of many actors to provide fail-safe care across time, space, and specialty. Patients are subjected to dangerous procedures and potentially toxic medications where the margins of safety are thin. The processes we use to decide which procedures and medications are appropriate as well as those used to perform or deliver them effectively rely on people to perform flawlessly regardless of the environmental and system factors that hinder performance. The results are inevitable: error and failure are inescapable properties of the healthcare system. Lucien Leape[1] reminds us that we must "accept the notion that error is an inevitable accompaniment of the human condition, even among conscientious professionals with high standards." However, each error or failure also provides an opportunity to learn how complex systems function and to develop strategies that will reduce the likelihood and risk of failure. Whereas failure is inevitable, learning is optional.

29.2   Failures, Errors, Accidents, and Risk Reduction

A number of terms can be used to describe breakdowns of the processes of care, only some of which put patients or staff at risk. Failure refers to a condition where a desired outcome is not achieved. Whereas failure represents a property of the overall system, errors refer to a deviation from the most appropriate action or sets

C.U. Lehmann et al. (eds.), *Pediatric Informatics: Computer Applications in Child Health,* Health Informatics,
© Springer Science+Business Media, LLC 2011

Fig. 29.1 Hazards and harm

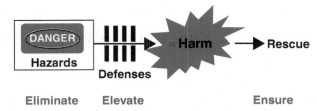

of actions by individuals. Although errors may well contribute to system failures, not all failures are caused by errors.

The risks of errors being committed or other failures occurring are examples of dangers or hazards in the environment that can contribute to harm or other undesirable effects. James Reason is an organizational safety expert who has developed a useful and widely used model relating these hazards to harm.[2] In Reason's model (Fig. 29.1), hazards are an inevitable property of our systems. Organizations typically provide multiple layers of defenses that prevent, detect, or intercept potential failures and provide a means of protecting the system from causing harm. However, we must recognize that these defenses are incomplete. For example, defenses might not be developed for certain hazards or they might not operate under every possible condition. When hazards are not intercepted, there is the potential to cause harm or loss and result in, what Reason terms, an accident.

This model of accident causation suggests three broad strategies for system improvement: (1) eliminating hazards; (2) elevating defenses; and, (3) ensuring rescue should an accident occur. Improvement requires not only an awareness that errors, failures, and accidents occur, but also an understanding of how they occur and a mechanism to evaluate and prioritize potential countermeasures.

These strategies can be incorporated into information systems to prevent failures of those systems. Additionally, information systems can be used as mechanisms to implement each of these strategies in reducing failures for other systems.

29.3   Root Cause Analysis

Preventing recurrent failure requires identifying the underlying cause or causes. The ability to look back on a sequence of events and discern the factors that led away from the desired outcome seems straightforward in the light of knowing how things turned out. However, investigators are biased by knowing the outcomes, an effect known as hindsight bias.[3] Hindsight bias causes investigators to see the sequence of events as occurring under conditions where trajectories could be predicted. Investigators also are prone to working back from the point of failure and identifying the closest contributor without regard to any number of contributing factors and conditions. Root Cause Analysis (RCA) refers to a structured approach to investigation in order to avoid these and other biases in defining the contributors to failure. The purpose of RCA is to determine: what happened; why it happened; and what countermeasures could be developed to prevent recurrence.

In defining the event to be analyzed (i.e. what happened), it is important to capture in chronologic order the sequence of events as well as the prevailing conditions. It is also important to develop a picture of the event that does not include assigning blame or causation which could bias the RCA process.

At the surface, RCAs are intended to dig beyond the most readily imaginable cause. In its simplest form, RCAs ask "why." Taichi Ohno, the person credited with developing Toyota Motor Company's revolutionary approaches to quality management,[4] proposed asking "why" five times ("5 whys") in order to uncover the causes beneath the cause. The questions can continue until either the results are beyond control, trivial, or unknowable.

As an example of applying the *5 Why* approach, consider the hypothetical case of a child exposed to a 50-fold excess rate of morphine infusion with resultant hypoventilation and hypoxemia. Why did this occur? At first consideration, it might have appeared to occur because the patient's nurse loaded a Patient-controlled-analgesia pump with a 50-fold higher concentration of narcotic but did not adjust the infusion rate used to infuse the drug cassette that had just completed infusing. Such an occurrence could be viewed as an error. However, we might ask, why did the drug infusion proceed without interception by the standard operating procedure requiring double checking process? We could find that double checking did not occur. Why? Because there might be a culture tolerating deviations from the procedure and it has been common to omit double checks. Alternatively, a second nurse might not have been available and there might have been considerable pressure to complete the task quickly to alleviate the patient's discomfort. We might also ask why the nurse selected the wrong drug cassette from the automatic dispensing device that supplied the medication on the patient care unit. We could find that she had been forced to make a selection of two solutions when the machine should have only offered the correct cassette. Why might the two solutions have been offered? They could have been offered because the patient's order had expired and no drug order had been dispatched to the dispensing device requiring the nurse to override the normal checks and balances in the system. Why might the order have been allowed to expire? It could have expired because no systems existed to alert the physician, nurse, or pharmacist that expiration was imminent. This would be consistent with the existing practice of reordering only after an infusing medication cassette became empty.

In examining the example above, one can see that, were we to be satisfied with the explanation that the dosing failure resulted from "nurse error," we might be satisfied to censure or retrain the offender. Had we stopped there, we might have done nothing to alter the underlying factors that created the conditions under which the nurse could err. Having delved further, we can identify a number of strategies that could reduce the likelihood of future failure such as; increasing accountability for double checking, procedures to prevent order expiration and stock-outs in the dispensing devices that force workarounds, and automatic systems to intercept dosing errors.

The Five-Why tool is consistent with what Gano has termed the "Cause and Effect Principle"[5] which says that causes and effects are one and the same: the cause of one effect is typically the effect of another cause earlier in a chain of causation.

Each effect is the consequence of at least one cause and one condition that allows or predisposes the effect to occur. In the example above, the nurse selection the wrong drug cassette was a causative action leading to the ultimate effect of administering the wrong drug concentration whereas the fact that the patient's order had expired and the fact that the dispensing device had two different drug concentrations were both contributing conditions that allowed an incorrect selection to be made. These cause/condition and effect relations form an infinite chain that can be examined as far back as one wants. However, once the causes and conditions become trivial or beyond control, there is little value of pursuing further. The Five-Why's work backwards along that chain.

Whereas the Five-Why approach to conducting an RCA is relatively unstructured, a number of other approaches rely on more structured approaches to ensure that specific areas of risk are interrogated to define contributors to failure. One example of a structured approach is the use of cause and effect diagrams that enumerate contributors to failure from a set of prespecified domains. These diagrams are called Ishikawa diagrams after one of quality management's founding fathers, Kaoru Ishikawa. They are also called "fishbone" diagrams because of their resemblance to a fish's skeleton. Key domains are shown as lines off the arrow leading to the specific problem. Potential causes are shown as branches of these key domain lines and the contributors to these causes are shown as braches from these branches. Key domains for consideration often follow the mnemonic, "5M's and a P" for: measurements, machines, materials, methods, mother-nature (the environment) and people. The application of this tool to the example above might identify the contributors (List 29.1, Fig. 29.2).

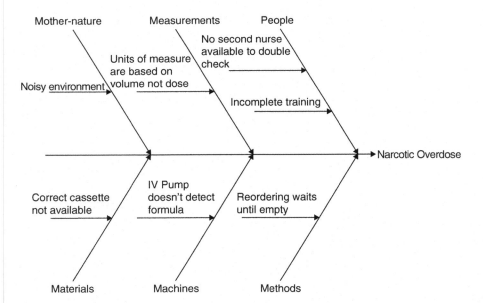

Fig. 29.2 Cause-effect diagram

List 29.1 Cause and effect

- Machines
  - ○ IV pumps cannot detect the strength of the formulation they are infusing
- Materials
  - ○ The correct cassette of morphine was not available
- Methods
  - ○ Reordering of medication does not occur until the next dose is required
- Measurements
  - ○ The unit of measurement for the IV pump is based on volume infused rather than the dose administered
- Mother-nature (environment)
  - ○ Noise contributed to distraction at the time the nurse was checking
- People
  - ○ Nurse was incompletely trained
  - ○ No second nurse was available to cross-check the IV pump settings

Other structured approached to RCA rely on formal sets of questions intended to examine specific possible causes. The National Center for Patient Safety of the Veteran's Affairs Administration has developed a set of Triage Cards[TM6] that provide a series of questions to explore causes and conditions related to: training; communication; staff fatigue; environmental factors; rules and policies; and, failures of barriers or controls. These questions serve as an alternative to the Five-Why approach and ensure a broad scope for investigation. The questions follow a logical thread where affirmative answers prompt a deeper level of questioning.

The relationships between causes, conditions, and effects can be displayed graphically in order to clarify the relationships. Logical relationships can be developed and tested for consistency in explaining the chain and the ultimate effect to be investigated.[5,7] This helps ensure a comprehensive analysis and may help identify causes or conditions which may be altered to prevent recurrence.

29.4 Failure Mode and Effects Analysis

Root Cause Analysis can be helpful in identifying holes in defenses and risk points only after a failure or near miss has occurred. Moreover, each RCA presents one view of failure and no specific way of aggregating or integrating experiences over time. Nor does RCA provide an approach to prospective risk identification and reduction. Failure Mode and Effects Analysis (FMEA) provides an approach to understanding the riskiest components of processes in order to prioritize the development of countermeasures. FMEA can be used prospectively to identify risk points, can be used as a way to integrate information across RCAs, and can be used to compare the relative riskiness of alternative process designs.

FMEA is a tool developed by reliability experts and used in a number of industries to systematically evaluate complex processes with respect to the types of failures experienced, the consequences of those failures, and the likelihoods of specific failure types occurring.[8–10] FMEA considers risk to be a consequence of not only the likelihood of failure occurring, but also the severity of the consequence of failure and the ease with which failures are detected prior to the consequences occurring. Failures that occur more frequently, cause more significant harm, or which can not be detected before harm occurs are considered higher risk than other failure types.

FMEA is a multistep process described in List 29.2.

List 29.2 Failure mode and effects analysis

- Characterize the elements or steps of the process
- Identify modes of failures
- For each process element, score each of the following (10 point scales are common)
  ○ Severity (S) of failure, if not detected prior to causing harm
  ○ Likelihood of occurrence (O) for each failure
  ○ Likelihood that failures will escape detection (D) before causing harm
- For each calculate a risk-priority-number (RPN) to assess riskiness
  ○ $RPN = S \times O \times D$
- Prioritize countermeasures to improve those process elements with the highest RPN

FMEA is generally conducted by a multidisciplinary team so that a range of perspectives are applied to the analysis. FMEA begins by identifying the steps in a process and then identifying all of the ways that each component of a process might fail. For each failure mode, the consequences of failure are identified and then the severity, likelihood of occurrence for each failure, and the likelihood of detection in time for corrective action are evaluated. Typically, the severity, likelihood, and detectability are characterized according to a 5 or 10 point scale. Data to character-ize the severity and likelihoods of occurrence and detection may come from direct measurement, the literature, or expert opinion. The results of root cause analyses provide important information that helps characterize each of these parameters.

FMEA has been applied to a diverse set of healthcare processes such as medication administration,[8,11–13] blood product administration,[14] case management,[15] diagnostic testing,[16] as well as medical device use and maintenance.[17–19] FMEA is also applied in planning new processes where it can be used to forecast risk so that safer processes can be selected at the time of design. For example, one hospital applied FMEA to the process for electronic ordering of chemotherapy in advance of moving from handwritten orders.[20] This led to specific decisions about the imple-mentation of ordering and documentation systems that were believed to create a safer system. Similarly, another hospital used FMEA to plan the introduction of "smart" IV pumps that incorporated dose-error prevention software.[21] This process led to a better ability to anticipate and plan for failures as well as to design care processes that minimized risk.

29.5 Error Proofing

Both RCA and FMEA help identify risk points and contributors to failure. Although both approaches imply that countermeasures or corrective actions will be taken to prevent recurrence and lower the risk of failure overall, neither approach offers tools to guide the improvement process. In looking at failures in complex systems involving the action of individuals, human error is a special case that requires particular consideration. Even when multiple contributors outside the realm of error contribute to failure, human error is often a proximate cause of the failure.

By recognizing certain patterns or types of error, it is possible to identify specific strategies to reduce the risk of error or the consequences of errors. These strategies can be incorporated into the design of systems including the design of information systems. Takeshi Nakajo[22] recognized that tasks require sets of specific functions. When those functions are not applied correctly, tasks are not completed correctly and an error occurs. Error prevention strategies work to minimize the likelihood of occurrence. Although not all errors cause consequences, some do result in abnormalities that can be identified. In some cases, those abnormalities reflect harm of some sort. In other cases, there may be a warning between the occurrence of that abnormality and harm. Even when errors occur, strategies that minimize their effects can also protect patients from harm. This schema is illustrated in Fig. 29.3.

The functions that are called upon for task completion include: memory, perception, attention, judgment, and motion (or action). In the narcotic overdose example above, the task of refilling the medication cassette in the infusion pump might have required each of these. The nurse might have been required to remember the correct drug formulation and dose if it were not available at the point of drug dispensing. She would have needed to perceive or recognize that the medication she chose was of a different concentration than intended. She exercised judgment in choosing an alternative strategy in overriding safety checks on the drug dispensing system when the correct formulation was unavailable. Actions were required to check the

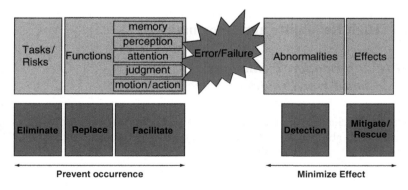

Fig. 29.3 Error proofing strategies

medication vial and compare it with the medication order. Throughout the task, attention was required to ensure that the standard operating procedure was followed correctly.

The likelihood of error or failure would be reduced if tasks could be eliminated. One could consider the overall task of replacing the medication cassette. Were the cassettes to hold a larger volume, the task of replacement would not be required as frequently which would reduce the likelihood of harm over the course of therapy. One could also consider the component tasks of the replacement process. If the task of choosing, whether to wait for the patient's medication drawer to be refilled or to override the dispensing machine and choose an alternative mechanism for dispensing, were eliminated, there would not be an opportunity for error.

The likelihood of error would also be reduced if certain functions could be replaced. For example, the function of memory could be replaced by information systems that make the correct dose retrievable at the dispensing machine. Alternatively, functions could be facilitated so that they would be less error prone. Electronic calculators are examples of mechanisms to facilitate the action of performing mathematical operations to reduce the likelihood of mistakes.

Even when errors occur, harm can be prevented by detecting abnormalities early. In the example of the patient receiving a narcotic infusion, monitoring blood oxygenation or exhaled carbon dioxide could detect respiratory depression as a consequence of an overdose before any permanent harm occurs. When abnormalities are detected and even when they are not, there may be opportunities to mitigate harm or rescue. In continuing the overdose scenario, respiratory depression could be reversed using pharmacologic antidotes or a patient may be resuscitated with mechanical ventilation and supported until the medications are metabolized.

Innovative solutions that reduce error may arise from any number of creative processes. Seeking solutions that eliminate tasks, replace or facilitate function, detect abnormalities, or enable rescue provide a useful framework and helps generate a broad range of countermeasures for consideration.

29.6   High Reliability and Informatics

29.6.1   Information Technology and Error-Proofing Strategies

Information technology can be incorporated into each of the error-proofing strategies described above. For example, computerized physician order entry (CPOE) solutions could be used to eliminate tasks, replace or facilitate actions, improve detection of abnormalities and help ensure rescue.

Consider the ordering of methotrexate, a potent cancer chemotherapeutic agent that is administered in doses based on body surface area which is calculated based on a patient's height and weight. It is common to monitor serum methotrexate levels to prevent toxicity. It is also common to administer folinic acid (Leucovorin) which is an antidote to methotrexate and rescues healthy cells from methotrexate's toxic effects at the conclusion of therapy. We can examine how CPOE could be used to develop an error-prevention strategy to prevent methotrexate toxicity.

CPOE applications could eliminate the task of cumbersome calculations for body surface area by recalling height and weight data stored as a component of other tasks. The application could also calculate appropriate methotrexate doses thereby eliminating the task of that manual calculation. CPOE could also replace the action of handwriting with the action of typing or selection from pick-lists. This would be expected to have the result of improving legibility and preventing certain handwriting interpretation errors. A multitude of functions could also be facilitated electronically. For example, memory could be facilitate through the use of order sets that combine orders for leucovorin and methotrexate level monitoring along with the methotrexate order itself. Perception of potentially worrisome laboratory values that might influence the medication ordering could be facilitated through the use of alerts. Judgment could be facilitated by making drug information, patient-specific information such as history or laboratory values, or disease management protocols available at the point of ordering. The detection of abnormalities such as a high methotrexate level could be improved by forcing or automating the ordering of drug level monitoring at the time of medication ordering. Rescue could be better assured if information systems also monitored the results of drug level monitoring and provided alerts to appropriate caregivers that the patient is in danger and requires immediate changes in therapy. Failures to rescue could be reduced further were that information system to require a timely response to the alert and escalate the notification to the next caregiver in line should no response be received.

Evidence supports the potential benefits of informatics solutions in reducing error. For example, computerized physician order entry systems can reduce medication prescribing errors.[23–26] In addition, computerized decision support systems can improve performance and diagnosis.[27–29] It is important to recognize, however, that whereas it is possible to conceive, design, and build informatics solutions intended to reduce error and improve performance, implementation does not guarantee impact. Systems can fail to have their intended impact for any number of reasons including users ignoring or rejecting computerized advice,[30] having difficulty using the systems,[31] or challenges in integrating the tools into caregiver's workflow.[32] One strategy for optimizing the impact of informatics solutions is to design and implement considering the failure modes of the information systems themselves.

29.6.2 Failure Modes in Informatics Solutions

Although information systems may confer substantial benefits in reducing error, they often substitute different tasks and functions than would be required in completing a process without them. Accordingly, because of human factors, their use will be subject to other kinds of errors. For example, ordering a medication from pick-lists of groups of medications requires caregivers to perceive the differences among medications. This can result in errors where similarly sounding or similarly spelled medications could be chosen instead of the correct medication. Scanlon describes an error of that type where phenobarbital was ordered instead of phenytoin.[33]

Computerized ordering may also require greater reliance on memory when data is presented on sequential screens whereas handwriting orders may be able to be completed with the relevant data spread out before the caregiver. Koppel and colleagues studied failure modes for the use of computerized ordering and identified two broad categories of error sources: "information errors" which related to fragmented data access and poor integration across systems; and, "human–machine interface flaws" that were produced when the electronic workflow did not correspond to work organization.[34] The errors Koppel describes can also be examined using the human factors framework in Fig. 29.3. Memory figures prominently as the design of systems may require the user remember which patient medications are being ordered for as one moves deeper into the ordering process when patient selection occurs early. Similarly, users may be relied on to recall the patient's medication lists as they order new medications and may not be able to review the list while ordering because of design limitations. Users may also erroneously rely on CPOE systems rather than memory for dosing information, making assumptions that choices displayed in ordering systems reflect acceptable doses when in fact they may reflect units of distribution from the pharmacy. One can find examples of errors in using each of the functions described in the human factors framework (Table 29.1).

This suggests that error-proofing strategies may be useful in the design and implementation of information systems. The fact that information systems may not meet their objective in reducing error combined with the potential for introducing new error modes, argues for the rigorous evaluation and testing of systems prior to broader implementation.

Table 29.1 Human factor errors in CPOE	Function used	Example of error
	Memory	Failure to recall which patient was selected as the user moves through ordering screens[34]
	Perception	Choosing the wrong medication from pick lists[33, 34]
	Attention	Failure to attend to all components of a task such as discontinuing orders when medication orders can not simply be changes[35]
	Judgment	Accepting orders that are part of order sets even when they may be contraindicated[35]
	Motion or action	Keyboard entry errors[35]

29.7   Case Study: RCA, FMEA, and Error Proofing in Continuous Infusions

Drug infusions are commonly used in Intensive Care Units to deliver sedative and vasoactive medications. These infusions require that a mass of medication be added to a volume of diluent and then infused at a rate that is then typically titrated to effect. Voluntary reporting of near miss and adverse events revealed instances where drug infusions were formulated incorrectly, infused at incorrect rates, or prepared at concentrations that required either unmanageably low or excessively high infusion rates. These experiences caused a multidisciplinary team to examine and redesign the process used to prepare and infuse medications. The details of this work have been published elsewhere.[8] Key elements of this project are described here to illustrate the processes of RCA, FMEA, and error proofing.

The team evaluated errors experienced within our ICU as well as errors reported in the literature. Two major error modes were identified: incorrect drug doses delivered; and, inappropriate rates of fluid administration but correct drug doses. Although the proximate contributor to incorrect dosing may often be a miscalculation, there are multiple contributors that underlie this first error mode, many of which are identified in List 29.3.

List 29.3 Contributors to incorrect dosing of drug infusions

- Machines
  - Existing IV pumps require titration in increments of 1 ml/h
  - Computerized physician order entry incapable of necessary calculations
- Materials
  - Medication and diluent solutions come in preestablished mass/volumes – requires recombination in correct proportions to arrive at correct infusion solution
- Methods
  - No standard method in use – prescribers free to choose among several (e.g. "rule of sixes") or use their own approach
  - All methods in use are cumbersome, requiring multiple calculations and multiple independent variables
  - Doses typically expressed in different units (e.g. mcg/kg/min) than infusions (ml/h)
- Measurements
  - Medications commonly delivered already in solution – requires multiple conversions to add correct mass of medication to correct volume of diluent
- Mother-nature (environment)
  - Bedside formulation subject to many environmental distractions that can interrupt attention or workflow
- People
  - People have different abilities to calculate correctly without assistance
  - People have been taught different methods
  - Often perceived to have insufficient staff for timely double-check

Although it is tempting to define countermeasures effective against each of these contributors, the team recognized that different failures occurred with different likelihoods. Moreover some failures are potentially detectable as in calculation errors that are found on double-check whereas other failures are undetectable as in placing an incorrect mass of medication into the diluent solution. It was also important to recognize that the two failure modes were not equivalent in severity: it was thought to be more dangerous to infuse the medication at the wrong dose compared to the correct dose at too high a fluid administration rate.

Recognizing that a redesigned infusion process would need to be compared against the existing process, the team conducted a FMEA to characterize the riskiness of the original and improved infusion processes. The FMEA takes into account differences in likelihood of failure, ease of detection, and the severity of the consequences of failure. The FMEA identified three risky elements of the original infusion process: calculating the required formulation; preparing the formulation by combining drug and diluent; and programming the infusion pump, particularly at the time of dose changes. It is important to note that although mistakes in preparing the infusion solution are likely less common than calculation errors, preparation errors are considered riskier in this analysis because they are not detectable after they are committed whereas calculation errors can be detected by double-checking.

A number of improvements were identified to reduce the risk of these processes. It is useful to consider these improvements in the framework of the error-proofing strategies described above. The task of formulation was eliminated entirely for some infusions by purchasing premanufactured solutions. This required a change from formulations being defined at the point of care to being standardized with fixed concentrations of medications. Formulations were also eliminated by increasing the "hang-time" of the solutions thereby reducing the number of solutions formulated over a course of therapy.

The functions of "action" required to formulate solution in the more error-prone environment of the bedside was replaced by formulation in a central pharmacy by dedicated staff specifically trained to the task. The functions of judgment as to the correct rates of fluid administration were replaced as part of standardizing concentrations because the standards were designed to allow appropriate fluid administration rates. The functions of "action" required to calculate the solution formulations were enhanced by a set of readily accessible internet-based calculators which drew from the standard concentration library.

Detection of errors was also enhanced by having the calculators print out a spreadsheet intended to be placed at the bedside which presented a set of dose/infusion-rate combinations. This is intended in part to enhance the ability to identify errors in pump programming. In addition, standardization itself makes detection of anomalous prescriptions easier.

Together, these improvements reduced the riskiness of the infusion delivery process considerably. The ability to prospectively model the impact of these improvements was helpful in communicating the need for radical changes in practice including the need to standardize and give up individual autonomy in deciding how to formulate infusions.

29.8   Conclusion

Healthcare delivery is a complex process requiring the coordinated action of many actors, movement of information across time and space, and decision making in the face of frequent uncertainty. Given this complexity, it is not surprising that errors and failures occur. At the same time, we are compelled to do better. Improving the safety and effectiveness of care requires us to understand the processes used to deliver care and the ways that they fail to achieve their desired objectives. Disciplined approaches to root cause analysis facilitate developing a deeper understanding and avoiding the hindsight bias that otherwise may truncate the investigation prematurely. When processes are at risk for repeated failure, failure mode and effects analysis can help one to understand the contributors to risk across multiple failure points. FMEA helps focus the development of countermeasures where they may have the greatest impact.

Just as structuring the analysis of failures using RCA and FMEA can optimize learning, disciplined error-proofing techniques can optimize solution finding and accelerate the trajectory of improvement. Eliminating hazards, elevating defenses, and ensuring rescue are general strategies that work together to prevent harm in error-prone systems.

The import and impact of the problems we seek to solve together with a lack of familiarity with the tools described above can intimidate some individuals and teams from embarking on a structured improvement journey. This, coupled with the desire for quick action can lead to identifying and apparently rectifying the most easily identifiable "cause" although this approach is less likely to result in reducing the likelihood or impact of future failure. It is a mistake to assume that the tools described here are applicable only for certain types of failures, are applied only by interdisciplinary teams, or must take extended periods of time. Rather, these tools are intended to guide thinking across a wide range of error situations and are helpful to individuals or teams. Perhaps the best way to gain familiarity with this way of thinking is to simply jump in.

References

1. Leape LL. Error in medicine. *JAMA*. 1994;272:1851–1857.
2. Reason J. *Managing the Risks of Organizational Accidents*. Burlington, VT: Ashgate; 1997.
3. Fischhoff B. Hindsight not equal to foresight: the effect of outcome knowledge on judgment under uncertainty. *J Exp Psychol Hum Percept Perform*. 1975;1(3):288–299.
4. Womack JP, Jones JT, Roos D, Sammons-Carpenter D. *The Machine That Changed the World*. New York: Harper Collins; 1990.
5. Gano DL. *Apollo Root Cause Analysis*. Yakima, Washington, DC: Apollonian; 1992.
6. Veterans Affairs, National Center for Patient Safety. NCPS Triage Cards™ for Root Cause Analysis; 2001. Available at: http://www.va.gov/ncps/CogAids/Triage/index.html. Accessed December 21, 2008.

7. Baigan JP. NCPS Root Cause Analysis Tools. Veterans Affairs, National Center for Patient Safety; 2008. Availabe at: http://www.patientsafety.gov/CogAids/RCA/index.html. Accessed December 21, 2008.
8. Apkon M, Leonard J, Probst L, DeLizio L, Vitale R. Design of a safer approach to intravenous drug infusions: failure mode effects analysis. *Qual Saf Health Care.* 2004;13:265–271.
9. Grissinger M, Rich D. JCAHO: meeting the standards for patient safety. Joint Commission on Accreditation of Healthcare Organizations. *J Am Pharm Assoc (Wash).* 2002;42:S54–S55.
10. DeRosier J, Stalhandske E, Bagian JP, Nudell T. Using health care failure mode and effect analysis: the VA national center for patient safety's prospective risk analysis system. *Jt Comm J Qual Improv.* 2002;28:209, 248–267.
11. Adachi W, Lodolce AE. Use of failure mode and effects analysis in improving the safety of i.v. drug administration. *Am J Health Syst Pharm.* 2005;62:917–920.
12. Robinson DL, Heigham M, Clark J. Using failure mode and effects analysis for safe administration of chemotherapy to hospitalized children with cancer. *Jt Comm J Qual Patient Saf.* 2006;32:161–166.
13. Kunac DL, Reith DM. Identification of priorities for medication safety in neonatal intensive care. *Drug Saf.* 2005;28:251–261.
14. Burgmeier J. Failure mode and effect analysis: an application in reducing risk in blood transfusion. *Jt Comm J Qual Improv.* 2002;28:331–339.
15. [No authors listed]. FMEA (failure mode analysis): a new QI tool to help improve case management processes. *Hosp Case Manag.* 2003 Mar;11(3):33–36.
16. Nichols JH, Bartholomew C, Brunton M, et al. Reducing medical errors through barcoding at the point of care. *Clin Leadersh Manag Rev.* 2004;18:328–334.
17. Ridgway M. Analyzing planned maintenance (PM) inspection data by failure mode and effect analysis methodology. *Biomed Instrum Technol.* 2003;37:167–179.
18. Wehrli-Veit M, Riley JB, Austin JW. A failure mode effect analysis on extracorporeal circuits for cardiopulmonary bypass. *J Extra Corpor Technol.* 2004; 36:351–357.
19. Willis G. Failure modes and effects analysis in clinical engineering. *J Clin Eng.* 1992;17:59–63.
20. Kozakiewicz JM, Benis LJ, Fisher SM, Marseglia JB. Safe chemotherapy administration: using failure mode and effects analysis in computerized prescriber order entry. *Am J Health Syst Pharm.* 2005;62:1813–1816.
21. Wetterneck TB, Skibinski KA, Roberts TL, et al. Using failure mode and effects analysis to plan implementation of smart i.v. pump technology. *Am J Health Syst Pharm.* 2006;63:1528–1538.
22. Nakajo T. A method of identifying latent human errors in work systems. *Qual Reliab Eng Int.* 1993;9:111–119.
23. Kaushal R, Shojania KG, Bates DW. Effects of computerized physician order entry and clinical decision support systems on medication safety: a systematic review. *Arch Intern Med.* 2003;163:1409–1416.
24. Potts AL, Barr FE, Gregory DF, Wright L, Patel NR. Computerized physician order entry and medication errors in a pediatric critical care unit. *Pediatrics.* 2004;113:59–63.
25. Shulman R, Singer M, Goldstone J, Bellingan G. Medication errors: a prospective cohort study of hand-written and computerised physician order entry in the intensive care unit. *Crit Care.* 2005;9:R516–R521.
26. Huertas Fernandez MJ, Baena-Canada JM, Martinez Bautista MJ, Arriola Arellano E, Garcia Palacios MV. Impact of computerised chemotherapy prescriptions on the prevention of medication errors. *Clin Transl Oncol.* 2006;8:821–825.
27. Garg AX, Adhikari NK, McDonald H, et al. Effects of computerized clinical decision support systems on practitioner performance and patient outcomes: a systematic review. *JAMA.* 2005;293:1223–1238.
28. Berner ES, Maisiak RS, Cobbs CG, Taunton OD. Effects of a decision support system on physicians' diagnostic performance. *J Am Med Inform Assoc.* 1999;6:420–427.
29. Steele AW, Eisert S, Witter J, et al. The effect of automated alerts on provider ordering behavior in an outpatient setting. *PLoS Med.* 1995;2:e255.

30. Killelea BK, Kaushal R, Cooper M, Kuperman GJ. To what extent do pediatricians accept computer-based dosing suggestions? *Pediatrics.* 2007;119:e69–e75.
31. Johnson CW. Why did that happen? Exploring the proliferation of barely usable software in healthcare systems. *Qual Saf Health Care.* 2006;15 Suppl 1:i76–i81.
32. Apkon M, Mattera JA, Lin Z, et al. A randomized outpatient trial of a decision-support information technology tool. *Arch Intern Med.* 2005;165:2388–2394.
33. Scanlon M. Computer physician order entry and the real world: we're only humans. *Jt Comm J Qual Saf.* 2004;30:342–346.
34. Koppel R, Metlay JP, Cohen A, et al. Role of computerized physician order entry systems in facilitating medication errors. *JAMA.* 2005;293:1197–1203.
35. Walsh KE, Adams WG, Bauchner H, et al. Medication errors related to computerized order entry for children. *Pediatrics.* 2006;118:1872–1879.

Chapter 30
Error Reporting Systems

David C. Stockwell and Anthony D. Slonim

Objectives

- Provide a framework for quality and safety improvement
- Outline traditional and electronic error collection methods and tools, their strengths and weaknesses
- Describe an example of the use of trigger tools in pediatrics

30.1 Introduction

The ability to detect errors in medicine is an important starting point for programmatic interventions aimed at improving patient safety. While information technology has the ability to improve many aspects of healthcare, the optimization of error reporting can ultimately improve error reduction because of the focus it brings to system defects.

30.2 Quality, Safety, and Errors

The healthcare industry has become increasingly focused on outcomes. The Institute of Medicine (IOM) reports on healthcare quality were intended to improve the healthcare services delivered to individuals and populations,[1-3] and discussions on quality, safety and errors are more prominent as a result.

30.2.1 Quality

Quality of care is defined in terms of health outcomes for individuals and populations. Thus, institutional improvements in care delivery should result in measurable improvements in outcomes. For adult medicine, core quality measures are well

C.U. Lehmann et al. (eds.), *Pediatric Informatics: Computer Applications in Child Health,* Health Informatics,
© Springer Science+Business Media, LLC 2011

defined. The Joint Commission requires accredited hospitals to collect and submit performance data on care for three of the following conditions: acute myocardial infarction, heart failure, pregnancy and related conditions, community acquired pneumonia. These measures are publicly reported by the Department of Health and Human Service (DHHS) and are linked to reimbursement.[4] For pediatrics, quality measures have only recently become available for inpatient asthma care but little else. Despite this limitation, pediatric institutions have been proactive in identifying, defining and sharing quality measures publicly.[5]

30.2.2 Safety

Safety is the first step in achieving healthcare quality. Safe care minimizes risks and optimizes benefits. Medical care involves medications, procedures and treatments that offer benefits but also have inherent risks that can result in patient harm.

The first step in increasing safety is to improve communication about risks and potential side effects of interventions. Thus, communication with the *patients and their families* is a central focus of safety initiatives. Improving communication within the *medical team* is important in addressing safety, and not surprisingly, the IOM promotes "effective team functioning,"[1,2] as many safety problems are due to the lack of communication and coordination between members of the healthcare team. Improving communication within the provider team can improve outcomes,[6] and successful team dynamics are essential to achieve the goal of delivering safe healthcare.

30.2.3 Errors

An error is a problem in the process of care.[7] Processes are sequences of operations or events that produce outcomes. Examples of healthcare processes include: insertion and removal of central venous catheters, preparation, administration and documentation of vaccine delivery and medication ordering, dispensing and administration.

Etiologies of errors are multi-factorial. The complexities of processes create opportunities for error at any step. Human knowledge deficits in performing a task can be difficult to identify and correct. Errors of omission, such as failure to utilize DVT prophylaxis in ICU care when indicated (many pediatric patients do not require this but post-menarchal females should receive it unless contraindicated),[8] may also occur. A recent study that involved patients in adult ICUs and on the wards suggested that patients in the United States receive, on average, only half of the recommended care that they should receive.[9]

30.3   Medical Error Classification Systems

A number of classification schemes have been proposed to more fully describe medical errors, which occur when care becomes unsafe. The IOM used a system that classified medical errors as diagnostic errors, treatment errors, preventative errors and "others error." (1) A recent review of the topic added procedural errors and nosocomial infections.[10] Table 30.1 provides examples of these medical error categories in pediatrics.

30.4   Existing Error Identification and Detection Methods

Medical error identification is an (under-appreciated) opportunity for improving care. To take advantage of these opportunities, institutional leadership should promote practices and attitudes that encourage error identification and reporting (Table 30.2).

After errors (such as sentinel events) are detected, investigation and system/process redesign can help to prevent their recurrence. Currently no ideal infrastructure for error identification exists, and traditional data collection on medical errors within institutions consists of:

Table 30.1   A classification schema for medical errors in pediatrics[10]

Category	Examples
Diagnostic Errors	Tachypnea attributed to upper respiratory infection when pneumonia exists
	Failure to recognize meningitis as a cause of headache
	Failure to identify cyanosis in a child with congenital heart disease
	Gastroenteritis diagnosed when appendicitis is the etiology of abdominal pain
Treatment Errors	Any violation of "Five Rights" of medication administration:
	Right Patient, Right Drug, Right Route, Right Dose, Right Time
	Incorrect patient given abdominal CT
	Administering enteral feeds into a central venous line
Nosocomial Infections	Hospital acquired RSV infection
	Catheter related blood stream infection
	Infection related to placement of external ventricular drain
Procedural Errors	Inappropriate interpretation of chest X-Rray leading to incorrect placement of thoracostomy tube
	Hemothorax following central line insertion
	Placement of tympanostomy tube in opposite ear
Prophylactic Errors	Failure to treat ongoing hyperglycemia
	Failure to provide preoperative antibiotics in child with structural heart disease
	Failure to provide adequate antibiotic prophylaxis for Pneumocystis jiroveci in immune suppressed patients

Table 30.2 Critical steps in increasing error reporting

- Institute timely investigation, actions and communication after errors are identified
- Focus on improving systems rather than blaming individuals
- Encourage identification and documentation of errors without punitive repercussions
- Establish anonymous, accessible and redundant (paper and electronic) error/incident reporting systems
- Benchmark system performance ("Days without an accident") and report to staff

30.4.1   Root Cause Analysis (See Chapter 29)

30.4.2   Chart Review

The oldest form of error/adverse event detection is random audits of the medical record. This method arose out of retrospective research projects designed to identify medical errors. This process is time consuming, has low yield, relies upon a small sample size, is expensive and has considerable interobserver variability.[11] However, this method is more sensitive in identifying individual errors. This method is not typically utilized outside of the research setting due to its high cost and large amount of labor required to identify errors.[11]

30.4.3   Incident Reporting

Incident reporting involves completing a standard report about an adverse event after it has occurred. This report is then routed for review to assess quality and safety process breakdowns leading to error. Incident reports are the most commonly available data upon which patient safety improvements are made. These reports are typically monitored by the hospital's risk management department.

From performance improvement and research perspectives, incident reports are inadequate because of their inherent biases. First, incident reports represent only the "tip of the iceberg" in terms of the events that are reported.[12] It is estimated that this method identifies approximately 5% of all hospital errors.[11] Second, there are biases associated with what is reported and more importantly, what is not reported. Finally, like many aspects of any safe healthcare environment, incident reporting also depends on a positive cultural norm that encourages reporting.[13] Practitioners are less likely to report if they believe the filing will lead to blame to either them or a colleague for the adverse outcome.[13] Further, safety programs and interventions that are implemented based on these rare events may actually perturb the system of care further and lead to adverse events in other areas. Nonetheless, incident reports provide fundamental information on what the front line staff believes are important issues. Practitioners and staff who take the time to complete incident reports need support and regular feedback on the types and frequencies of reported errors and need a system in place for correcting the identified errors.[13]

30.4.4   Direct Observation

Direct observation of steps has been implemented to identify errors in the
medication administration process.[14] This involves a dedicated staff member (usually a pharmacist or nurse) monitoring the occurrence of medication errors at each
step of the process from prescribing to dispensing. This approach improves the
identification of medication errors when compared to voluntary incident reporting.
However, while potentially an improvement in the quantity of reported errors, this
method has its limitations as well: the high cost of a dedicated staff member for the
task and reporting bias based upon the explicit "job" of the reporters.[15]

30.4.5   Mortality and Morbidity Conferences

Mortality and Morbidity (M&M) conferences are a traditional approach for identifying and addressing adverse events that result in significant harm or patient death.
While M&M conferences provide an opportunity to detect system and practitioner
level deficiencies and add value to the detection of diagnostic medical errors, their
format is inconsistent. Some departments engage in rigorous examination of errors
while others perform superficial reviews. The effectiveness and utility of M&M
conferences in improvement is unproven,[16] and frequently no documentation of
conclusions or actions arising from these conferences is available, so the ability
to track effectiveness or to detect trends is lost.[16] Furthermore, with this approach,
there is a historical tendency to focus on the performance of a particular practitioner
rather than on the system of care. Both approaches are necessary if errors are to
be reduced.

M&M conferences are retrospective and reactive when error identification and
reduction activities need to be systematic and proactive. Strategies to preserve
the M&M's utility in medical care include: using a template that addresses the
contributions of the system and practitioner in the adverse event, multidisciplinary
(nursing, respiratory therapy, etc.) participation, inclusion of morbidity (in addition
to mortality), and using data about adverse events with appropriate benchmarks
when available to help guide practice. Finally, providing a systematic structure for
improving the identified flawed processes and communication of these findings and
solutions are important to maintaining a culture of safety.

30.4.6   Limitations of These Tools

Traditional assessment techniques like M&M conferences, incident reports and
chart review will often fall short in producing meaningful results in terms of identifying errors. Errors are often missed due to the reliance of staff to initiate the investigation. This is often approached cautiously depending on the culture of the
institution. Fear of retribution and institutional inertia in "fixing problems" can be

a powerful disincentive to completion of incident reports or objective participation in an M&M conference. Also these techniques often vary in their identification of near misses or absorbed events.

Since it is difficult to even encourage error reporting it is therefore almost impossible to track the number of reports and identify trends. Dependence on incident report rates as a measure of safety (error rates) is erroneous since the denominator of errors is not known. Campaigns to empower staff to report without retribution may help to increase reporting rates. Workplace cultural issues, such as poor staff morale, perceptions about retribution or leadership inactivity can dramatically decrease rates.[17] and severely limit staff identification of errors.

Another difficulty with these tools is that while the investigation into the source of the error, the communication of findings to staff and the translation of actionable recommendations may be poor or inappropriate. Thus, new procedures, forms and guidelines the critical phase of explaining the learned lessons to physicians, nurses and other staff often does not occur.[17-19]

Focus on only the most serious events may miss numerous opportunities (near-misses, no harm errors or low severity errors) for correcting dangerous situations. Since all of these methods (except for direct observation) are reactive, recall may not be precise and may introduce inaccuracies, detection methods may not consider prevented errors (*near misses*) and errors that occurred but from which no harm resulted (*absorbed events*).[17]

Each of these methods is used locally and therefore does not benefit from the broad range of experiences in a multi-institutional setting to guide error reduction and safety optimizations.[1,20-22] Few collaborative efforts focus on the multi-institutional approach to improving care and formally sharing their strategies. Currently, patient safety efforts are viewed negatively as inadequacies in care and as potential opportunities for litigation rather than an opportunity to share information that can improve safety in the industry.[1,2] Hence, patient safety interventions need to provide a broader view that takes into account the efforts of multiple institutions' ideas and strategies.[1,20-22]

30.5   Electronic Solutions

Information technology solutions address some of the limitations of existing error detection methods. In the airline industry, after recognizing that one of the barriers to improving safety was poor communication, leadership created a reporting system whereby members of the industry could learn from previously made mistakes and avoid repeating similar situations.[23] It was acknowledged that having centralized reporting would allow all airlines to benefit from the mistakes of others. This simple method is credited with greatly improving the safety of the airline industry. In healthcare, individual providers or institutions may learn from past mistakes but other providers and institutions are forced to make similar errors rather than to learn from the collective knowledge of the industry. Several factors conspire to limit this approach. Admission of mistakes in medicine is not part of the cultural norm. Concern over liability and public disclosure and how that may affect recruitment of patients minimize the open disclosure.

30.5.1 Electronic Incident Reporting

Some institutions have developed internal electronic anonymous reporting systems. Having one institutional model may help to increase participation and reduce confusion and frustration with the submission process. The reporter completing the online form also benefits from true anonymity. Finally, if the process is well designed and submission of these forms is not overly laborious then near-miss and adverse event collection may increase.[24]

Limitations of electronic incident reporting parallel those of their paper equivalents. Electronic reporting may increase the number of submitted reports, but the reporting bias associated with a large fraction of errors and near misses that are not gathered is a major problem. Also while the reporting may be improved the real benefits of incident reports are not the reports themselves but as a way to identify the problems within the healthcare environment and act on them. Inaction after the report is submitted will stifle improvement. Finally lack of coordinated reporting does not allow for learning from other hospitals that have benefited from learning from their own mistakes and then making their experiences public.

Recently several Web-accessible, anonymous error reporting programs designed for hospitals and health systems to systematically collect, analyze, and report medication errors have been created. Academic systems have developed confidential, voluntary error reporting systems at the organizational level. Patient Safety Net was developed by the University HealthSystem Consortium, a coalition of 87 academic medical centers. The Patient Safety Net is a software program and database, accessible via the Internet, for "Safety Report" entry by health care workers and clinicians.[25] Large healthcare systems can streamline the approach to incident reporting, identify trends within their own institutions and ensure action on the identified errors.

The United States Pharmacopeia is the official public standards-setting authority for all prescription and over-the-counter medicines, dietary supplements, and other healthcare products manufactured and sold in the United States. United States Pharmacopeia sets standards for the quality of these products and works with healthcare providers to help them reach the standards. They have created a subscription based national, Internet-accessible database that hospitals and health care systems use to track and trend adverse drug reactions and medication errors. Hospitals and health care systems participate in this system called MEDMARX voluntarily and subscribe to it on an annual basis. MEDMARX is a quality improvement tool, which facilitates productive and efficient documentation, reporting, analysis, tracking, trending, and prevention of adverse drug events. Individual hospitals can compare their own data to the database and allow for benchmarking.

It allows subscribing facilities to learn valuable lessons from the experiences of other users.[26]

Federal agencies have developed systems for broad oversight of medication errors. The Food & Drug Administration has developed and is improving a system of voluntary reporting of adverse events associated with the use of Agency-approved products. The Agency's MedWatch program receives about 25,000 adverse event and medical product problem reports annually, mostly from health care professionals and consumers. The MedWatch data are entered into Food & Drug Administration's Adverse Events Reporting System, which also receive 270,000 manufacturers' reports. The manufacturers' reports, which must be filed periodically, are based on information provided by physicians and other health care providers.[27]

Another important Food & Drug Administration program is the Vaccine Adverse Events Reporting System. It received more than 14,000 reports of adverse reactions in FY 2002, most of which were volunteered by health care providers, patients and their parents.[28]

To ensure the safety of the blood supply, the Food & Drug Administration's Center for Biologics Evaluation and Research requires all blood banks to promptly report fatalities connected with blood transfusions and donations. The Center for Biologics Evaluation and Research regulates the collection of blood and blood components used for transfusion or for the manufacture of pharmaceuticals derived from blood and blood components, such as clotting factors. It also establishes standards for the products themselves. In addition, the Center operates a web-based voluntary reporting system for rapid identification of supply shortages affecting blood, blood components and reagents.[29]

Also in blood administration, collaboration with University of Texas Southwestern and Columbia University by way of a National Institutes of Health funded project called the Medical Event Reporting System for Transfusion Medicine (MERS-TM). The MERS-TM tracks transfusion errors through a no-fault, standardized reporting system.[30]

30.5.2 Administrative Coding

Administrative data such as diagnosis and procedure codes have been utilized to screen for complications that occur during the course of hospitalization.[31] The coding data represents one of the few sources of clinically relevant data.[11] The codes provide direct and indirect evidence of the clinical state of the patient, comorbid conditions and the progress of the patient during the hospitalization or clinic visit.

However, since these administrative codes are typically generated for reimbursement and legal documentation their accuracy and appropriateness for clinical studies may be unreliable. There are errors within the coding itself, it is not in real-time and therefore cannot be addressed during a hospitalization or clinic visit. And unfortunately adverse event codes are rarely used in practice.[32]

30.5.3 Automatic Triggers

A new method for identifying errors is via "automatic triggers." Triggers are computerized data that *may be associated with* an error or adverse event (such as an order for naloxone as a signal that an overdose of morphine has occurred). Unlike most other error identification programs discussed, this type of error detection can occur in real-time (such as monitors within CPOE systems). Thus, triggers have the potential to prevent worsening clinical situations while a patient is still hospitalized. A computerized surveillance system monitors for the occurrence of any trigger, as defined by the hospital or outpatient clinic.[33,34] Typically the triggers are from lab values (e.g. hypoglycemia, hyperkalemia) medication records (e.g. reversal agents like naloxone), microbiology laboratory triggers (e.g. new positive blood culture), radiology triggers (e.g. use of the word "fall" in the study's justification) or administrative data (e.g. readmission within 24 h).[11]

With electronic clinical information, these types of triggers can be an excellent way to augment a robust adverse event detection program. Triggers can augment chart reviews (both paper and electronic), allowing more effective and time-efficient pickup of errors than random or unscreened reviews.[35] Other advantages of triggers include a consistent methodology for identifying adverse events over time. This consistency can produce more reliable results after interventions are made to address the adverse events. Therefore the progress of an institution or clinic can be tracked and trended.

The use of natural language processing (NLP) to detect adverse events is evolving. The goal of NLP is to convert electronic narrative documents into a coded form suitable for computer based analysis. The coding is based on pattern matching. Therefore documents such as discharge summaries, clinical notes and daily progress notes can be searched for the occurrence of adverse events.[36]

Triggers have been used to develop a successful (nonelectronic) error identification program in neonatology that identifies errors at higher rates than existing methods. Researchers found a positive predictive value of each identified trigger to be 38%. Since neonatal intensive care units are complex environments, the possibility for error is quite high (Chapter 4). In a published study, the trigger-based program captured several previously unidentified instances of nosocomial infection, catheter infiltrates, abnormal cranial imaging and unplanned extubations. Although this program used manual chart review, the methodology can be adapted to an automated electronic form.[37] This approach has been extended to other areas of inpatient pediatrics.[43]

Outpatient use of triggers is also possible. As the use of electronic medical records increases in outpatient pediatric practices the ability to utilize triggers grows. Outpatient triggers have been utilized in an outpatient geriatric setting[38] and in other primary care clinics.[39]

Barriers to computer based screening to identify errors and adverse events are the low positive predictive value of their results. Therefore it is important to verify the accuracy of the system. Both internal and external validations are important.[11]

30.6 Conclusion

Incident reporting is the most commonly used method of collecting data on errors. Its inherent selection biases prevent it from providing accurate measures of safety, nevertheless, what it identifies can help guide improvement efforts. Electronic solutions provide greater access to separate facilities with the possibility for learning from other institutions.[42] To succeed in collecting data on errors, institutions must:

- Create an environment conducive to reporting: The term "just culture" has evolved out of error reporting literature and describes a work environment in which frontline personnel feel comfortable in reporting and disclosing errors.
- Promote professional accountability in reporting: A just culture recognizes that individuals should not be held accountable for system failings over which they have no control, but it does not tolerate conscious disregard of clear risks to patients or gross misconduct.[40]
- Promote and communicate system accountability: It is important to document results, share stories, and disseminate results.[18] Error detection is useless unless action is taken.[41] A just culture combined with effective communication and strategies for decreasing the likelihood of errors engages staff in identifying them and improving the processes of care.

No individual solution is adequate. The use of complementary methods of identifying errors increases reporting and provides better understanding of the processes of care and greater opportunities for improving the delivery of care.

30.7 Case Study: An Adverse Event Trigger in Hyperkalemia

During the course of treatment for a severe RSV infection and subsequent respiratory failure, a 4 month old was given high doses of loop diuretics to improve respiratory function and to hasten weaning from mechanical ventilation. As is common with loop diuretics, this patient's potassium level steadily decreased. In order to avoid severe hypokalemia, enteral potassium supplements were initiated.

Following successful extubation, the child required fewer diuretics, but still required them to improve respiratory function. Two days later the child was transferred to the respiratory ward. As her respiratory function improved the diuretics were discontinued. Via the use of an electronic adverse event trigger, it was recognized on the third day on the ward that the child had increasing potassium levels. This notified the adverse event coordinator to investigate the issue. Shortly after arrival to the ward the coordinator noticed that the potassium supplements were still being administered and the likely source of hyperkalemia. After advising the team that this may have been an oversight, the potassium supplements were discontinued before any adverse events secondary to hyperkalemia occurred.

References

1. Institute of Medicine Committee on Quality of Health Care in America. *To Err is Human Building a Safer Health System*. Washington, DC: National Academy Press; 2000.
2. Institute of Medicine Committee on Quality of Health Care in America. *Crossing the Quality Chasm: A New Health System for the 21st Century*. Washington, DC: National Academy Press; 2001.
3. Lohr KN, ed. *Medicare: A Strategy for Quality Assurance*. Washington, DC: National Academy Press; 1990.
4. US Department of Health and Human Serrvices. Hospital Compare; 2008. Available at: http://www.hospitalcompare.hhs.gov/. Accessed December 21, 2008.
5. Cincinnati Children's Hospital Medical Center. How Cincinniati Children's Measures Up; 2008. Available at: http://www.cincinnatichildrens.org/about/measures/. Accessed December 21, 2008.
6. Stockwell DC, Slonim AD, Pollack MM. Physician team management affects goal achievement in the intensive care unit. *Pediatr Crit Care Med*. 2007;8(6):540–545.
7. Skiba M. Strategies for identifying and minimizing medication errors in health care settings. *Health Care Manag*. 2006;25:70–77.
8. Pronovost PJ, Thompson DA, Holzmueller CG, et al. Defining and measuring patient safety. *Crit Care Clin*. 2005;21(1):1–19, vii.
9. McGlynn EA, Asch SM, Adams J, et al. The quality of health care delivered to adults in the United States. *N Engl J Med*. 2003;348(26):2635–2645.
10. Slonim AD, Pollack MM. Integrating the Institute of Medicine's six quality aims into pediatric critical care: relevance and applications. *Pediatric Crit Care Med*. 2005;6:264–269.
11. Bates DW, Evans RS, Murff H, et al. Detecting adverse events using information technology. *J Am Med Inform Assoc*. 2003;10(2):115–128.
12. Cullen DJ, Bates DW, Small SD, Cooper JB, Nemeskal AR, Leape LL. The incident reporting system does not detect adverse drug event: a problem for quality improvement. *Jt Comm J Qual Improv*. 1995;21:541–548.
13. Taylor JA, Brownstein D, Christakis DA, et al. Use of incident reports by physicians and nurses to document medical errors in pediatric patients. *Pediatrics*. 2004;114:729–735.
14. Buckley MS, Erstad BL, Kopp BJ, et al. Direct observation approach for detehcing medication errors and adverse drug events in a pediatric intensive care unit. *Pediatr Crit Care Med*. 2007;8(2):145–152.
15. Stockwell DC, Slonim AD. Detecting medication errors: a job for six sigma. *Pediatr Crit Care Med*. 2007;8(2):190–192.
16. Friedman JN, Pinard MS, Laxer RM. The morbidity and mortality conference in university-affiliated pediatric departments in Canada. *J Pediatr*. 2005;146:1–2.
17. Pronovost PJ, Miller MR, Wachter RM. Tracking progress in patient safety: an elusive target. *JAMA*. 2006;296:696–699.
18. Pronovost PJ, Wu AW, Sexton JB. Acute decompensation after removing a central line: practical approaches to increasing safety in the intensive care unit. *Ann Intern Med*. 2004;140:1025–1033.
19. Wears RL, Janiak B, Moorhead JC, et al. Human error in medicine: promise and pitfalls, part 2. *Ann Emerg Med*. 2000;36:142–144.
20. Joint Commission. *Medical Errors, Sentinel Events, and Accreditation*. A report to the Association of Anesthesia Program Directors.
21. Leape LL, Bates DW, Cullen DJ, et al. Systems analysis of adverse drug events. *JAMA*. 1995;274:35–43.
22. Roos NP, Black CD, Roos LL, et al. A population-based approach to monitoring adverse outcomes of medical care. *Med Care*. 1995;33:127–138.
23. Vicente K. *The Human Factor: Revolutionizing the Way People Live with Technology*. New York: Routledge.

24. Miller MR, Clark JS, Lehmann CU. Computer based medication error reporting: insights and implications. *Qual Saf Health Care.* 2006;15(3):208–213.

25. University Health System Consortium. Patient Safety Net (PSN), Learn More; 2008. Available at: http://www.uhc.edu/11851.htm. Accessed December 21, 2008.

26. US Pharmacopeia. MEDMARX National Database Website; 2008. Available at: https://www. medmarx.com/. Accessed December 21, 2008.

27. US Food and Drug Administration. MedWatch Website; 2008. Available at: http://www.fda. gov/medwatch/. Accessed December 21, 2008.

28. US Department of Health and Human Services (DHHS). VAERS - The Vaccine Adverse Event Reporting System Website; 2008. Available at: http://vaers.hhs.gov/. Accessed December 21, 2008.

29. US Food and Drug Administration. Center for Biologics Evaluation and Research (CBER) Website: Blood; 2008. Available at: http://www.fda.gov/cber/blood.htm. Accessed December 21, 2008.

30. Medical Event Reporting System - Transfusion Medicine (MERS-TM); 2008. Available at: http://www.mers-tm.org. Accessed December 21, 2008.

31. Slonim AD, LaFleur BJ, Ahmed W, et al. Hospital-reported medical errors in children. *Pediatrics.* 2003;111(3):617–621.

32. Honigman B, Lee J, Rothschild J, et al. Using computerized data to identify adverse drug events in outpatients. *J Am Med Inform Assoc.* 2001;8(3):254–266.

33. Rozich JD, Haraden CR, Resar RK. Adverse drug event trigger tool: a practical methodology for measuring medication related harm. *Qual Saf Health Care.* 2003;12:194–200.

34. Resar RK, Rozich JD, Simmonds T, et al. A trigger tool to identify adverse events in the intensive care unit. *Jt Comm J Qual Patient Saf.* 2006;32(10):585–590.

35. Jha A, Kuperman G, Teich J, et al. Identifying adverse drug events: development of a computer-based monitor and comparison with chart review and stimulated voluntary report. *JAMIA.* 1998;5(3):305–314.

36. Melton GB, Hripcsak G. Automated detection of adverse events using natural language processing of discharge summaries. *J Am Med Inform Assoc.* 2005;12(4):448–457.

37. Sharek PJ, Horbar JD, Mason W, et al. Adverse events in the neonatal intensive care unit: development, testing, and findings of an NICU-focused trigger tool to identify harm in North American NICUs. *Pediatrics.* 2006;118: 4:1332–1340.

38. Field TS, Gurwitz JH, Harrold LR, et al. Strategies for detecting adverse drug events among older persons in the ambulatory setting. *J Am Med Inform Assoc.* 2004;11(6):492–498.

39. Singh H, Thomas EJ, Khan MM, et al. Identifying diagnostic errors in primary care using an electronic screening algorithm. *Archives of Internal Medicine.* 2007;167(3):302–308.

40. Marx D. *Patient Safety and the 'Just Culture': A Primer for Health Care Executives.* New York: Columbia University; 2001. Available at: http://www.mers-tm.org/support/Marx_Primer.pdf. Accessed December 21, 2008.

41. Wachter RM. The end of the beginning: patient safety five years after 'to err is human'. Health Aff (Millwood); 2004: Suppl W4–534–45. Available at: http://content.healthaffairs.org/cgi/content/abstract/hlthaff.w4.534. Accessed December 2008.

42. Williams SK, Osborn SS. The development of the National Reporting and Learning System in England and Wales, 2001–2005. *Med J Aust.* 2006;15;184(10 Suppl):S65–S68.

43. Takata GS, Mason W, Taketomo C, Logsdon T, Sharek PJ. Development, testing, and findings of a pediatric-focused trigger tool to identify medication-related harm in US children's hospitals. *Pediatrics.* 2008;121(4):e927–e935.

Part VI
Frontiers in Pediatric Informatics

Chapter 31
Communities of Pediatric Care and Practice

Joseph H. Schneider

Objectives

Upon completion of this chapter, the reader should be able to discuss and formulate questions about the following issues regarding the electronic exchange of clinical information:

- The need for accessible health information in providing quality care and the roles of Health Information Exchanges (HIEs) in providing "anytime, anywhere" health information
- Key issues affecting the formation and success of HIEs
- Key pediatric issues that must be addressed in designing HIEs

31.1 Introduction

The impact of Hurricane Katrina in 2005[1] on health care infrastructures abruptly clarified the need for and value of "anytime, anywhere" access to health information by health care providers during disasters. The development of Health Information Exchanges (HIEs) to meet that need has faced and continues to face technical, business, and adaptive challenges in creating sustainable child health information systems. Key issues in HIE development for child health are the inclusion of pediatric-specific data and guardian-related privacy/security issues. As HIE developers address these issues in designing regional information systems, experts in both child health and informatics must be included in the planning and implementation to achieve successful development, diffusion, and sustainability of HIEs.

31.2 Case Study 1: Hypothetical Scenario

Samuel and his aunt got off the plane in Dallas after the long ride from New Orleans. His mother had died in a car accident in New Orleans a week ago and he was now a 4 month old refugee thanks to Hurricane Katrina. Born prematurely, he had

C.U. Lehmann et al. (eds.), *Pediatric Informatics: Computer Applications in Child Health,* Health Informatics,
© Springer Science+Business Media, LLC 2011

a number of problems that his aunt was only beginning to learn about from his pediatrician. However, they were about 500 miles from home and the pediatrician's office, with Samuel's records, were nine feet under water.

Samuel was having difficulty breathing. His aunt explained that he had run out of his home oxygen this morning. An internist who was helping to triage the planeload of people put Daniel on oxygen, thought he heard wheezing when he listened to Samuel's lungs, and wrote for albuterol. That seemed to make Samuel's breathing easier. They were placed on a bus to the Dallas Convention Center. When Samuel and his aunt arrived at the Convention Center he was finally examined by a pediatrician. His aunt knew, that he had been in the hospital for a month at birth and had some vaccinations. She also knew that he used inhalers and took some medicines but she didn't know why. She also wasn't sure of Samuel's exact birth date.

The pediatrician did the best she could to diagnose Samuel's problems. She hoped that he didn't have any allergies. There was a loud holosystolic heart murmur over the left sternal border. She was able to get him to the children's hospital where a large ventricular septal defect was diagnosed with left to right shunt. The medications he needed were restarted in time and slowly his fluid overload was corrected.

A few days later the pediatrician was able to connect to the Houston Immunization Registry through a friend and she learned that Samuel's pediatrician in Louisiana had participated in LINKS, the Louisiana immunization registry. The Houston registry had an emergency link to LINKS that was made possible because they were developed by the same vendor. With some work, the pediatrician was able to retrieve Samuel's history and avoided having to revaccinate him.

Samuel's medical record wasn't available at the time that he needed critical care. In this regard, he wasn't different than most other children if their medical need occurs away from where their medical record is stored. Even in the age of Electronic Medical Records (EMRs), it is not unusual for medical records to be unavailable in emergencies. Children with Special HealthCare Needs (CSHCN) are often the most affected as their care can be fragmented across multiple specialists. Samuel spent days without critical medications and was under diagnosed at the airport triage by an adult medicine physician unfamiliar with pediatric conditions. He also underwent an expensive cardiac workup that simply confirmed what was already recorded in his birth hospital, which was now closed, and in his pediatrician's office, which was nine feet under water. Luckily Samuel's vaccination history was in a registry, which saved him at least from having to repeat this portion of his medical care.

31.3 Health Information Exchange: Definitions and Goals

It is estimated that in 14% of primary care visits clinical information is missing,[2] enough to affect care adversely in 44% of those visits. For complex patients (such as children with special health care needs (CSHCN)), missing information is three times more likely. In many cases, practitioners will construct records anew, based on patient or parent verbal histories, while requesting photocopied medical records only occasionally. For CSHCNs, the volume and complexity of record processing and transfer is time and resource intensive and error-prone for both the sending and the receiving physician.

To provide quality (safe, timely, effective, efficient, equitable, and patient-centered[3] care through "anytime, anywhere" access to patients' health information regardless of the situation (mobile or transient patients and practitioners, displacements due to disasters or situational changes, etc.), Health Information Exchange (HIE) has been pursued. HIE is defined as the "electronic mobilization or movement of healthcare information across organizations within a region or community…while maintaining the accuracy of the information being exchanged."[4] "HIE" also refers to any initiative or organization that performs this function. An HIE either contains selected health data of its members or provides a means of accessing it. As of 2007, approximately 130 HIEs were in various stages of formation.[5]

Goals for HIEs include:

- *Clinical goals* (e.g., decreasing medical errors arising from insufficient information at the point of care and facilitating disease management including patient-specific education)
- *Public health goals* (e.g., improved bio-surveillance and medical research)
- *Economic goals* (e.g., the elimination of the need to repeat tests)
- *Patient empowerment goals* (e.g., patient access to personal health records and improved health information quality through patient management of their record)

Financial benefits[6] of a standardized national HIE have been estimated at $77.8 billion annually once fully implemented, and this has provided incentive to form HIEs in both private and public sectors. HIEs have traditionally been nongovernmental entities, but with federal, state, and local government support. Constituents and stakeholders of HIEs include physicians, hospitals, payors, employers, laboratories, public health departments, professional associations, pharmacies, and patients with leadership originating from any of these groups.

HIEs and the data contained within them are distinct from Medical Homes[7] and are *complementary* to them. While Medical Homes collect, centralize, and coordinate medical data about individual patients through a primary care physician, HIEs permit pooling, dissemination, and sharing of medical data about many patients from many providers through a sponsoring organization and infrastructure.

31.4 HIE Types: CHINs, Registries, and RHIOs

31.4.1 Community Health Information Networks (CHINs)

In the 1990s, community health information networks (CHINs) promised that sharing patient information would be good for patients and would save money and lives. Most CHINs failed for a variety of reasons,[8] among them technical issues, such as a lack of a widespread Internet infrastructure, lack of financing, disagreements on governance, unresolved privacy/security issues and barriers from hospital and practitioner competition. Many of these issues continue to face current HIEs.

31.4.2   Registries

Despite the mostly false start of CHINs, public health efforts to aggregate patient information have partially succeeded through registries. Examples of registries include:

- Immunization information systems (IIS)[9]
- State newborn metabolic[10] and hearing[11] screening registries
- Lead poisoning databases[12]
- Birth defect and rare disease[13] registries
- Tumor[14] registries

While these often are governmental entities, the net result for the patient can be the same as a nongovernmental HIE if the health data is made available to clinicians. In the case of vaccine registries, an electronic link from the Houston vaccine registry to the LINKS system in Louisiana was credited with saving a large number of children from revaccination following Hurricane Katrina (Boom J., 2005).

An example of a registry that provided effective and timely access to health information is *www.katrinahealth.org*, a Website created by a public–private collaboration following Hurricane Katrina. It pooled medication and other data from pharmacy benefits companies, e-prescribing networks, insurers, Medicaid, and the Veteran's Administration. To use the Website, physicians and pharmacists would obtain security clearance that gave them access to medication histories of refugee patients from areas affected by the hurricane.

The experience with *katrinahealth.org* illustrated some of the positives and negatives that HIEs face.[15] Among the positives were that it did aid care, as 30% of queries were successful in obtaining health information. Among the many negatives was that finding the right patient was difficult as the system required five pieces of matched identifying information to retrieve a record. Children, with frequent name changes and caretakers who often might not even know birthdays, were probably affected more by this.

31.4.3   Regional Health Information Organizations (RHIOs)

In mid 2004, Dr. David Brailer was appointed the first National Health Information Technology Coordinator. During his tenure, he fostered the growth of Regional Health Information Organizations (RHIOs). A RHIO has been defined by the National Alliance for Health Information Technology as both "an organization that oversees and governs the exchange of health-related information among organizations according to nationally recognized standards [and] a health information organization that brings together health care stakeholders within a defined geographic area and governs health information exchange among them for the purpose of improving health and care in that community."[16]

The creation of RHIOs got a major boost with the issuance of the "Goals of the Strategic Framework" by the Office of the National Coordinator for Health Information Technology in July 2004.[17] In 2005, 65% of CIOs from academic medical centers surveyed, indicated that they were participating in or forming a RHIO.[18] In 2006, over 160 RHIOs were counted by the e-Health Initiative.[19] Following David Brailer's resignation in 2006, literature references to RHIOs decreased significantly (by late 2007), with "Health Information Exchange" becoming the more global term for the various types of organizations pursuing this function.

31.5 HIE Functions

A full description of the functions of HIEs is beyond the scope of this chapter, but an excellent summary of these can be found in the Conference Workbook of the *Development of State Level RHIOs Consensus Conference.*[20] Key functions include:

- Creating data standards and policies for data aggregation from remote sources
- Providing a central data repository for aggregated data
- Providing pointers to remote data

Although most HIEs[21] have a master patient index, not all have a central data repository.

Types of access to remote data include:

- ***Transactional***: unfiltered health data (e.g., the weight of a child at each visit and date of care at one clinic)
- ***Analytical***: filtered/processed data provided as value-added reports (e.g., comparison of a child's weight to normal values and plotting them on a growth chart)

Most HIEs provide transactional data in their early stages. The demand for efficient, appropriate, and rapid presentation of health information from multiple locations and systems may increase the prevalence of analytic data. Tools such as clinical dashboards to aggregate, consolidate, and visualize data will be needed to provide added value and to sustain HIEs.

31.6 HIEs Relationships to EMRs and PHRs

Electronic Medical Records (EMRs) and Personal Health Records (PHRs) are two primary sources of patient data that HIEs can tap. Important concepts regarding the linkage of HIEs, EMRs, and PHRs include:

- Data relevance
- Connection and access
- Data reconciliation
- Data sources

31.6.1 Data Relevance

An EMR typically contains much more information than what is needed for sub-sequent care. An example is the timing of individual inpatient medication doses that usually would not be useful in an outpatient follow up visit. As EMR and e-prescribing adoption increases, the amount of information available to HIEs will be overwhelming.[22] Critical information, such as medications on which a patient is discharged from the hospital, is useful if summarized. One of many value-added functions that HIEs can provide is aggregation and transmission of "medication reconciliation" data ("a complete list of a patient's current medications, including herbal supplements and vitamins, reconciled with new medication orders to ensure that no duplications, adverse interactions, incorrect dosages or omissions occur").[23] Both hospitals and providers have struggled with providing complete listing of all the medications that patients are on across all their locations of care.

HIE developers must decide which EMR/PHR data is important for aggrega-tion. Important elements might include advance directives, problem lists, procedure histories, allergies, medications, immunizations, medical supplies, durable medical equipment and laboratory/radiology test results. Other information, such as family and social history, may be important but have less value to the function of the spe-cific HIE. A number of HIEs, e.g., Northern Illinois Physicians for Connectivity, are using the ASTM Continuity of Care Record Standard (CCR). The CCR was developed by clinicians and it contains a core set of health information designed to be transmitted from one care location to another. HL-7 has worked with ASTM to create the Continuity of Care Document, a document compatible with both the CCR and the Clinical Document Architecture of HL-7.

31.6.2 Connection and Access

Once HIE developers have decided what information to collect, the next question is how to obtain it. Some HIEs have data repositories and others do not. Each model has limitations when handling EMRs and PHRs. The assumption of an HIE without a repository is that the HIE-EMR/PHR connection is always available. If any EMR/PHR connection is interrupted, the HIE will have incomplete information. This is of particular concern in disasters, such as Hurricane Katrina, where PHRs are more vulnerable to interruption than physician or hospital-based EMRs.

Alternatively, an HIE using a central repository of data has only the most recently *accessed* data from EMR/PHRs. It may not necessarily be the most *recent* data. Connectivity and availability are still issues, because if the EMR/PHR data is updated locally without connection to the HIE, then the HIE records are incom-plete. If a HIE performs analytic processing of data, then it also needs to store and track the database versions on which specific reports have been based, for auditing, corrections, and medico-legal purposes.

31.6.3 Data Reconciliation

A key consideration in connecting EMR/PHRs to a HIE is data standardization and reconciliation. For example, a parent may not recall or relate an element of medical history at one location, e.g., a history of appendicitis during a dermatology office visit. Even if it was provided, the dermatologist may not consider it important enough to enter into their EMR and so the HIE will have an inconsistency between the dermatologist's record and that of another provider. How is the HIE to determine whether the patient had appendicitis?

For transactional HIE data, presentation of all available information from all visits to all providers without filtering is time-consuming for clinicians to reconcile, and often, this is not done. For analytical HIE data, the need to reconcile discrepancies in both a central repository (if one exists in the HIE) and the source system (EMR/PHR) may be more important because errors and inconsistencies will persist if uncorrected. Data sources that require HIE reconciliation include PHRs[24] (allowing patients to review and directly correct their own records), claims, pharmacy fulfillment and EMRs.

31.6.4 Data Sources

The need to identify data sources relates to reconciliation. Physicians generally trust clinical information (examination, test results) obtained directly from other physicians over that reported by patients. A concern over allowing patient-provided PHR information into EMRs and HIEs is that physicians using the information will want to know the source (physician or patient/parent). This adds burdens on processing, transmission, and presentation, with functionality that is typically not part of an EMR/PHR.

The intersection of PHRs and HIEs seems ideal in terms of improving data quality, but this is not the direction that most HIEs have been planning to take. In a study evaluating HIE proposals in 2004, most planned to have a repository (78%), results delivery (74%), and reminders (71%) but only 6% proposed PHR functionality,[8] although the PHR has been noted to be of importance in the development of the National Health Information Infrastructure and HIEs.[25] Given the historical absence of electronic PHRs and the new complexities that exist once they are electronic, it is not surprising that HIEs have not moved rapidly in this direction, but it is reasonable to expect this trend to develop.

31.7 HIEs and Children's Health

The issues surrounding the formation and continued success of HIEs have been well described,[20] including:

- Understanding opportunities and obstacles including marketplace characteristics
- Generating regional support for participation, particularly among physicians, hospitals, and other key stakeholders and identifying and supporting champions
- Creating the business case for development and obtaining funding
- Establishing a governance structure
- Assessing information technology capabilities and needs; and
- Developing health information standards and policies, particularly with respect to pediatrics.

31.7.1 Understanding the Opportunities and Obstacles Including Marketplace Characteristics

Among the many factors for HIE success is a thorough understanding of marketplace dynamics. Marketplaces differ dramatically in terms of their ability to form and support an HIE and their willingness to include pediatrics.

Questions that should be answered include:

- Are physician groups, hospitals, payors, medical societies, etc. willing to work together?
- Is there a dominant group, hospital, or payor in the area?
- Is the region contiguous with other states and likely to need a multistate HIE?
- Is penetration of EMR use significant enough to allow a clinically useful volume of data to be electronically captured?
- Is there acceptance of the idea of a HIE among the population of the region, particularly with regard to concerns over privacy?

With regard to child health, EMR use by pediatricians may be lagging versus other physicians. If so, children's data would be underrepresented in such a HIE. The presence of more than one children's hospital or more than one medical school in a region can contribute to competitive roadblocks that hold back progress with respect to children's health information. Pediatricians and child heath providers are typically not the dominant medical force in most locations. Aligning with the dominant forces – e.g., groups, hospitals, and payors – without alienating other nondominant participants is critical.

31.7.2 Generating Regional Support for Participation by All Parties, Particularly Physicians, Hospitals, and Other Key Stakeholders

It is critical to identify and cultivate champions knowledgeable about child health and informatics to identify and overcome obstacles. While one might expect that child health would be an easiest focus for coalition, frequently it is forgotten in the initial stages of HIE formation. Failure to consider pediatrics can have severe consequences to how children's health information is represented in the HIE.

In larger markets, children's hospitals or the department of pediatrics of a medical school may be a source of support for pediatrics in an HIE. In areas without a children's hospital or medical school, the hospital medical director of pediatrics may need to take the lead. Alternatively, the state pediatric society may provide assistance.

Champions need support. A significant portion of pediatric payments come from Medicaid, which historically has paid poorly. As a result of this relatively poorer funding source for pediatricians, they may not have the time or resources to "work" all of the connections that need to be made to generate support for the HIE. Planners are well-advised to provide adequate support for their champions, particularly child health advocates including pediatricians.

31.7.3 Creating the Business Case for Development and Obtaining Funding

While initial funding of many HIEs is from grants, it is important that the HIE provides identifiable services that generate a stream of funding. Starting with the basics such as supporting medication reconciliation is a way to gain credibility and funding, as this function in particular has been extremely difficult for hospitals to accomplish successfully. Quantifying savings to users is critical.

One way for a HIE to provide value to child health practitioners is to make state registry information available through the HIE. Frequently individual physicians have had difficultly electronically accessing immunization and birth screening records in a way that is supportive of their workflow. The difficulty and rewards of incorporating these into each HIE vary by region, but the net result in terms of added value is often significant. Of note, pediatricians do not gain financially in any significant way by gaining access to this information and so it is payors, including state Medicaid programs that probably should fund these efforts.

31.7.4 Establishing a Governance Structure

Governance is probably one of the most important tasks in the formation of a HIE. Key tasks include:

- Determining what kind of legal form the HIE will take
- Establishing a mission and vision statement that is inclusive and fair for all parties and
- Determining who will be on the governing structure (e.g., Board of Directors)

Access to child healthcare information through the HIE is probably not affected much by the most common legal forms of HIEs. Perhaps the most important aspect of this component of HIE formation is that pediatricians must be present during the formation of the HIE to avoid having to play catch-up.

A strong mission and vision statement that explains the need to focus on children's healthcare issues is critical. Even a simple phrase such as *"The needs of vulnerable populations, such as children, will be kept paramount"* can be used by child health advocates when difficult decisions need to be made once the HIE is functional.

Finally, obtaining at least one representative of children's health on the governing structure is a necessity. This individual should have a thorough understanding of the special informatics needs of children's health and the workings of physician practices and hospitals in the care of children.

31.7.5 Assessing Information Technology Capabilities and Needs

Information technology capabilities within states and local regions differ widely. As mentioned above, there can also be significant differences between subgroups of physicians within a region.

A key function of a HIE beyond governance can be to provide the means through which all providers, especially those with limited means, can participate electronically in the HIE, using an EMR as part of their normal workflow. This can be done by having HIE developers identify preferred EMR vendors, which reduces the costs to each practice of vendor investigation. It can also be done by providing support for obtaining funding for EMRs, such as providing a way that health plans and hospitals can be better assured that the funding that they can provide to physicians under the relaxed Stark regulations will have payoffs through data sharing. Efforts to support their members also indirectly support HIEs financially, as the quality and value of the data in the HIE increases as physician participation increases. Therefore, efforts by HIEs to support the conversion of physicians to EMRs should be high on the list of tasks to be done.

Nationally, pediatricians have lower EMR adoption rates than other types of physicians.[26, 27] Because pediatricians typically do not provide care for Medicare patients, they are also generally not eligible for EMR implementation support through Quality Improvement Organizations. Financially, because of their increased reliance on Medicaid, they often lack the capital for EMR purchases and implementation. HIE planners need to recognize these technology capability needs and limitations in their planning.

It is also important for planners to note that the EMR products that may be the most appropriate for HIE members who provide care for adults are not necessarily good for pediatric care. This will be covered more in the next section. Lists of preferred EMR vendors prepared by HIEs should include choices that match the needs of pediatricians. The American Academy of Pediatrics (AAP) can be an excellent source for information on "pediatric-friendly" EMRs.[28] The AAP has annually supported Pediatric Documentation Challenges that identify EMRs with excellent pediatric functionality and its members rank pediatric EMR products on the Web.[29]

31.7.6 Developing Health Information Standards and Policies

HIE leadership must consider four dimensions of health information standards:

- *Identification of data standard needs* (Data dictionaries, terminologies, unit reporting conventions): Consistency of data field names, their content and the level of detail that is specified in EMR/PHRs for use in HIEs is essential. For children's health information, items such as tests may have highly specific names and abbreviations and use different normal ranges than corresponding tests for adults. HIEs will need to provide a process to include such standards.
- *Identification standards* (Patient identifiers): Controversies on mandatory national patient identifiers make its implementation unlikely despite support for its use for children.[30] Numerous organizations support the use of a voluntary healthcare identifier and there are numerous approaches to this with proposed standards.[31] The significant risk of misidentification of patients using classical healthcare identifiers (name and date of birth) for children make considerations for its use (either voluntary or involuntary) important.
- *Authentication standards* (Provider and requestor identifiers): Much of this has been simplified by the establishment and implementation of the National Plan and Provider Enumeration System (NPPES).[32]
- *Pediatric standards in EMRs for HIEs*: Pediatric requirements for EMRs have been articulated by the AAP[30]. These need to be considered during HIE formation and expansion. These include special data representation, processing, and administrative needs (see Table 31.1). Unless a HIE is able to display its information through a pediatric-compatible EMR, challenges will exist for both "transactional" and "analytic" HIEs. The challenge to HIEs and pediatrics is that while EMRs have dramatically improved over the last 3 years in their ability to handle these issues, the battle to incorporate these features at the HIE level has just begun.

Table 31.1 Special data needs for pediatric EMRs for HIEs[30]

Special Data Representation Needs

Presenting growth information (i.e., height, weight, head circumference and body mass index from a variety of locations where the child has received care) in specialized growth charts in order to get an accurate picture of the child's development.

Tracking multiple name changes in a way that allows for searching on any one of them. For example, a child could be named "Girl of Mary Smith" at her birth hospital if the hospital uses the mother's maiden name, "Sally Jones" at her pediatrician's office and "Sally Samuels" at a different pediatrician's office once she is adopted and moves across town. In between, Sally may have adopted a special nickname that she would want to have used. Each location of care could have a different name for this child and only the HIE would have all three. Robust algorithms for matching this child's multiple names (short of a voluntary or mandatory health identifier) need to exist at the HIE level to handle these situations.

Reporting age-based normal values, especially those that differ across institutions. For example, sick neonates can easily have a respiratory rate of 100 breaths per minute, but this would be flagged as grossly abnormal by most adult-based systems and many would not even allow a

(continued)

Table 31.1 (continued)

value greater than 99. HIEs need to report appropriate age-based normals in order to be useful, but these are often not available from adult-based EMRs. Where age-based normals do exist, they frequently vary by institution.

Reporting fetal surgery and prenatal maternal factors. EMR vendors are slowly recognizing that these are an important parts of a child's EMR.

Special Data Processing Needs

EMRs with good pediatric functionality have the built-in capability of doing special processing on the following items:

Medications ordering in mg, cc, or tsp and calculated in mg/kg and mg/m².

Immunizations recording with easy to use decision support and registry interfaces

Complex developmental analyses

A problem that HIEs may face is that the pieces of these (particularly immunizations and developmental analyses) may be in different EMRs as children move and change pediatricians. HIEs may find it difficult to do the analysis necessary to provide value in these areas.

Special Administrative Needs

There are many of these issues, but some of the more difficult for EMRs and therefore HIEs include:

Adolescent privacy. With different rules in many states, this area currently is one of the weakest areas of pediatric EMRs. The problem for HIEs is that the rules that EMRs use to protect privacy may be independent of the data in an EMR and therefore are not transmitted to the HIE with the data. The data then becomes unintentionally available.

Guardianship, adoption, foster care and custodial versus financial responsibility. The complexity that exists in pediatrics, where a child may have a guardian who is not financially responsible for the care

Length of data retention time. HIEs that provide data storage are subject to the rules governing pediatric medical records, which vary significantly by jurisdiction.

Medical record production. Clinicians who use HIEs that provide screen-only views need to be concerned that the medical decisions that they are making are supported only by their notes, as the HIE may be unable to demonstrate in a court of law what the clinician actually saw. This would be particularly true for HIEs without a data repository.

31.8 Conclusion

There are many other challenges to HIEs, including:

• The ability of patients to "opt-in" or "opt-out" of the HIE. "Opt-in" refers to the situation where an individual patient must actively sign up for participation. "Opt-out" refers to where the individual is included in the HIE unless they request not to be included. Of the two, better participation is usually achieved with the "opt-out" model.

• The need for HIEs to avoid duplicate entries from multiple input sources. The same medication information, for example, can come from pharmacies, payors, and physicians. A HIE must be able to filter the duplicates if it is to provide efficient information.

• The disposition of medical information in the event of bankruptcy. It is likely that some of the new HIEs will not survive. If these are built using the model where the HIE stores patient data, it is unclear what happens to any data which the HIE contains.

HIEs represent a tremendous opportunity to improve the quality and efficiency of care that is provided to children. However, they face many challenges and the long-term survivability of many is questionable. HIE planners should strongly consider including pediatricians in their development and management. Pediatricians should take an active role in HIEs as failure to do this could lead to systems that are not pediatric-friendly.

31.9 Case Studies

31.9.1 The Indiana Network for Patient Care (INPC)

The INPC is a sustained (30 years +) city-wide clinical informatics network that leverages the success of the Regenstrief Medical Record System (RMRS) throughout Indianapolis and providers in the state of Indiana. Through the efforts of a group of clinical informaticians led by Clement MacDonald MD, the RMRS was able to realize three goals: (a) to make "just-in-time" information available to authorized clinicians, (b) to assist in diagnosis and prevention through support of the record-keeping process and (c) to aggregate clinical information for multiple uses. In 2004, the INPC was operational in all five major hospital systems in Indianapolis as well as all county and state public health departments, 20 primary care sites, 3,000 specialists, 30 school health sites and four homeless organizations (95% of inpatient and non-office based ambulatory care in Indianapolis), serving 390,000 emergency, 165,000 inpatient and 2.5 million ambulatory visits per year. Data input from clinical systems included: laboratory results, inpatient, and outpatient summaries, medication lists, and radiology, operative and pathology reports, tumor and immunization registry data, pharmacy prescription data and other information. The central data store is a series of federated databases located at the Regenstrief Institute. Secure data connections transfer data in the HL7 messaging standard, using domain-specific terminologies (LOINC for laboratory results, CPT-4 for procedures, ICD-9 for diagnoses and National Drug Codes (NDC) and RxNorm for drug names). Records within the federated data store use a central global patient registry. The system supports many applications including a system for child health (Child Health Improvement through Computer Automation (CHICA)) that provides pediatric decision support at the point of care.[33]

31.9.2 An Electronic Health Record-Public Health System Prototype

A prototype for an electronic health record for public health that links (via HL7 messages) from EHRs to multiple public health systems (newborn metabolic screening, newborn hearing screening, immunization, and communicable disease registries) has been described.[34]

References

1. American Academy of Pediatrics. Hurricane Katrina, Children, and Pediatric Heroes: Hands-on Stories by and of Our Colleagues Helping Families During the Most Costly Natural Disaster in US History. *Pediatrics*. 2006;117:S355–S460.
2. Smith PC, Araya-Guerra R, Bublitz C, et al. Missing clinical information during primary care visits. *JAMA*. 2005;293(5):565–571.
3. Institute of Medicine. *Crossing the Quality Chasm: A New Health System for the 21st Century*. Washington, DC: Institute of Medicine, National Academy Press; 2001.
4. AHIMA e-HIM Workgroup on HIM in Health Information Exchange. Health Information Management (HIM) Principles in Health Information Exchange. *J AHIMA*. 2007;78(8) (September 2007): online version for members only. Available at: http://www.ahima.org/hie/index.asp. Accessed December 21, 2008.
5. e-Health Initiative. Fourth (and fifth) Annual Survey of Health Information Exchange at the State, Regional and Community Levels; 2007, 2008. Available at: http://www.ehealthinitia-tive.org/HIESurvey/2007Survey.mspx. Accessed December 21, 2008.
6. Walker J et al. The Value of Health Care Information Exchange and Interoperability. Health Affairs; 2005: Supplement 24: 10–18. Available at: http://content.healthaffairs.org/cgi/content/full/hlthaff.w5.10/DC1. Accessed December 21, 2008.
7. American Academy of Pediatrics Medical Home Initiatives for Children with Special Needs Project Advisory Committee. The medical home. *Pediatrics*. 2002;110(1 Pt 1):184–186.
8. Overhage et al. (2004) Communities' readiness for health information exchange: the national landscape in 2004. *J Am Med Inform Assoc*. 2004;12:107–112.
9. Boom JA, Dragsbaek AC, Nelson CS. The success of an immunization information system in the wake of Hurricane Katrina. *Pediatrics*. 2007;119(6):1213–1217.
10. Kim S, Lloyd-Puryear MA, Tonniges TF. Examination of the communication practices between state newborn screening programs and the medical home. *Pediatrics*. 2003;111(2):e120–e126.
11. Hayes D. State programs for universal newborn hearing screening. *Pediatr Clin North Am*. 1999;46(1):89–94.
12. Papadouka V, Schaeffer P, Metroka A, et al. Integrating the New York citywide immunization registry and the childhood blood lead registry. *J Public Health Manag Pract*. 2004;Suppl:S72–S80.
13. Watson MS, Epstein C, Howell RR, et al. Developing a national collaborative study system for rare genetic diseases. *Genet Med*. 2008;10(5):325–329.
14. Dishop MK, Kuruvilla S. Primary and metastatic lung tumors in the pediatric population: a review and 25-year experience at a large children's hospital. *Arch Pathol Lab Med*. 132(7):1079–1103.
15. Markle Foundation, American Medical Association, Gold Standard, RxHub, SureScripts Lessons from KatrinaHealth; 2006: 15–18. Available at: http://www.markle.org/downloadable_assets/katrinahealth.final.pdf. Accessed December 21, 2008.
16. National Alliance for Health Information Technology (NAHIT). Press release: NAHIT Releases HIT Definitions; 2008. Available at: http://www.nahit.org/pandc/press/pr5_20_2008_1_33_49.asp. Accessed December 21, 2008.
17. US Department of Health and Human Services Office of the National Coordinator for Health Information Technology. Goals of Strategic Framework; 2004. Available at: http://www.hhs.gov/healthit/goals.html. Accessed December 21, 2008.
18. Sprague C. The Role of Academic Medical Centers in Regional Health Information Organizations. Presentation at the Greater Chicago Chapter of the Health Information Management Systems Society (HIMSS), November 10, 2005.
19. e-Health Initiative. Improving the Quality of Healthcare Through Health Information Exchange; 2006. Available at: http://toolkits.ehealthinitiative.org/assets/Documents/eHI-2006HIESurveyReportFinal09.25.06.pdf. Accessed December 21, 2008.

20. State-level HIE. Reports; 2008. Available at: http://www.slhie.org/reports.asp. Accessed December 21, 2008.
21. Halamka J et al. Health care IT collaboration in Massachusetts: the experience of creating regional connectivity. *J Am Med Inform Assoc*. 2005;12:596–601.
22. Basch P. Data Excess and Document Overload: Barriers and Disincentives to an Interconnected / Interoperable Healthcare System" in Connecting for Health: A Public Private Collaborative, edited by The Data Standards Working Group; 2003: 90. Available at: http://www. connectingforhealth.org/resources/dswg_report.pdf. Accessed December 21, 2008.
23. Healthcare Management Council, Inc (HMC). Medication Reconciliation. HMC Wiki: Collaboration for Hospital Performance Improvement; 2008. Available at: http://wiki. hmccentral.com/index.php/Medication_reconciliation. Accessed December 21, 2008.
24. Tang P et al. Personal health records: definitions, benefits, and strategies for overcoming barriers to adoption. *J Am Med Inform Assoc*. 2006;13:121–126.
25. Stead WW et al. Achievable steps toward building a national health information infrastructure in the United States. *J Am Med Inform Assoc*. 2005;12:113–120.
26. Kemper AR, Uren RL, Clark SJ. Adoption of electronic health records in primary care pediatric practices. *Pediatrics*. 2006;118(1):e20–e24.
27. Burt CW, Hing E, Woodwell D, Centers for Disease Control. Electronic Medical Record Use by Office-Based Physicians: United States, 2005; 2008. Available at: http://www.cdc. gov/nchs/products/pubs/pubd/hestats/electronic/electronic.htm. Accessed December 21, 2008.
28. American Academy of Pediatrics Council on Clinical Information Technology (COCIT). COCIT Website. Available at: http://www.aap.org/visit/medinfo.htm. Accessed August 1, 2008.
29. American Academy of Pediatrics Council on Clinical Information Technology. Electronic Medical Record (EMR) Review Project Website. Available at: http://www.aapcocit.org/emr/. Accessed August 1, 2008.
30. Spooner SA. Council on Clinical Information Technology, American Academy of Pediatrics. Special requirements of electronic health record systems in pediatrics. *Pediatrics*. 2007;119(3):631–637.
31. ASTM International. ASTM E1714 - 07 Standard Guide for Properties of a Universal Healthcare Identifier (UHID); 2007. Available at: http://www.astm.org/Standards/E1714.htm. Accessed December 21, 2008.
32. Department of Health and Human Services. National Plan and Provider Enumeration System Website; 2008. Available at: https://nppes.cms.hhs.gov/NPPES/NPIRegistryHome.do. Accessed December 21, 2008.
33. Biondich PG, Grannis SJ. The Indiana network for patient care: an integrated clinical information system informed by over thirty years of experience. *J Public Health Manag Pract*. 2004;Suppl:S81–S86.
34. Orlova AO, Dunnagan M, Finitzo T, et al. Electronic health record - public health (EHR-PH) system prototype for interoperability in 21st century healthcare systems. *AMIA Annu Symp Proc*. 2005:575–579.

Chapter 32
Developing Pediatric Data Standards

S. Trent Rosenbloom and Joy Kuhl

Objectives

- To provide a clinical rationale for clinical data standards
- To give a brief overview of the types of data standards
- To illustrate the use of data standards in implementing a growth chart into an electronic record system

32.1 Introduction and Background

A major goal of Electronic Health Record (EHR) systems is to collect, store, and make available high-quality clinical information to healthcare providers whenever and wherever it is needed.[1] This clinical information can help inform decision making, as well as supply data for research and drive quality assessment. To support clinical decision making, EHR systems typically make available many types of clinical information, including lists of a patient's allergies, medications, or diagnoses, the results from laboratory testing and narrative documents expressing healthcare providers' clinical observations and impressions.[2-5] The methods used by EHR systems to aggregate and display clinical information can impact healthcare providers' workflow and decisions related to patient care.[2,5,6]

For example, a single medical center may use more than one laboratory for testing blood, including a central laboratory and one in the emergency department. In the case that the child with abdominal pain has her blood tested for inflammation in the emergency department, and then has the same test in clinic the next day as follow-up with her physician, the physician would likely expect that the results are aggregated together in the EHR system. If the results from the emergency department are not easily seen alongside the results from the follow-up testing, the physician may not see them and may request additional subsequent testing and withhold any change in therapy while awaiting those results. A physician concerned that the abdominal pain may be due to a serious illness, such as appendicitis, may obtain a CT scan or ultrasound rather than waiting for a third blood test result. If, by contrast, the results are all displayed together in the EHR system,

C.U. Lehmann et al. (eds.), *Pediatric Informatics: Computer Applications in Child Health,* Health Informatics, the physician will be able to make decisions and prescribe the necessary therapies more efficiently.

Standards are principles and rules designed to ensure that methods used and products created reliably and consistently conform to expectations. Software standards in particular exist to align the structure and data contained in disparate computer systems and application programs.[7] Typically, such standards detail the minimum set of functions that the software provides, the methods used to achieve those functions, and the formatting of the data structure. The goal of standards is to ensure that both data and users' experiences are similar from one computer system to another, and that information can flow easily between computer systems.[7-9] Standards for EHR systems and clinical data may include specifications for the terms used to represent medical entities and the relationships between entities and individual patients. For example, medication standards may include details about what words and spellings to be used to represent each medication, ingredient, dosing frequency and dose form, as well as the data structure that links a given medication to the dates that it was started or refilled and to the patient who is taking it.

Standards for clinical data exist with the primary objective of enabling it to be aggregated, shared, and exchanged within and among various EHR systems.[8,9] The ability for data to be shared among computer systems without loss of detail or meaning is termed "interoperability." For data to be maximally interoperable, it must be normalized to a single form and content. This single form and content is a standard.

32.2   Types of Clinical Data Standards

Data standards designed to support aggregation and exchange generally consist of three components, each of which may be defined using a terminology or a guideline: (1) the scope and content of the standard; (2) the syntax and formatting of the content; and (3) the actual semantics and words used to represent the content. We will consider each of these types of standards.

32.2.1   Content, Function, and Quality Standards

One major purpose of software standards for EHR systems is to define the core set of functions, features, and activities that such systems should support. Defining necessary functions, with descriptions of each, ensures that system developers, evaluators, and users all have similar expectations of what EHR systems do (and do not do). A listing of desired functions, features, and activities serves as a standard for content or quality, because it defines the minimum set of content that a piece of software should provide, and against which its quality can be judged.

For example, an EHR system designed to support pediatric practice should perform several basic functions. The American Academy of Pediatrics (AAP) Task Force on Medical Informatics recently published the statement, "Special Requirements for Electronic Medical Record Systems in Pediatrics." The Task Force's report includes a listing of desirable pediatric EHR system attributes, with formal definitions of how they envision the attributes to be implemented.[10] The Task Force categorized the quality standards as relating to data representation, data processing and system design. The specific standards are listed in Table 32.1.

Table 32.1 Standards for data representation in EHR systems[10]

Content	
Growth data	Permit recording, graphic display, special calculations of growth patterns, and comparing a child's growth against population-based percentiles and other normal ranges
Patient identifier	Provide for assignment immediately at the time of birth or prenatal testing, accommodate temporary names, and allow searching for multiple names for a single patient.
Special terminology	Common terms used for pediatric preventive care (e.g., "developmental milestones" and "anticipatory guidance") and exam findings (e.g., "weak cry,", "bulging fontanelle," and "umbilical granuloma")
Age-based normal ranges	Allow the user to easily compare a patient's vital signs and laboratory results with age-based normal ranges
Time of birth	Use the time of birth to calculate the patient's exact age in the first days and weeks of life
Data processing	
Prescribing	Dosing and decision support should be based on the age and weight or body surface area of the child, and should include child-friendly formulations (e.g., elixirs and chewable tablets)
Immunizations	Efficient recording and effective display and printing of immunization data, with reminders and decision support, and ability to change with vaccine guideline updates
Parental documentation	Permit parents to review or append chart information
Reporting	Customize reports to match mandated formats (e.g., school or camp physicals or reports to school nurses)
System design	
Special privacy issues	Address adolescent privacy, genetic information, flexible guardianship data (e.g., adoption, foster care, divorce, and remarriage) and financial responsibility
Pediatric work settings	Need to function in busy pediatric practice workflows and in the presence of active children
Family member links	Maintain linkages, as appropriate, to relatives having similar social, family medical or past medical histories
Registry linkages	Share immunization, newborn screening and disease outbreak data with government registry systems to ensure timely diagnosis, notification, and follow-up
Consider policy statements	AAP policies regarding the design and use of EHR systems should be considered in the design of software systems for use in pediatric health care

Armed with this information, developers, and users can judge whether a given EHR system conforms to these standards, and therefore meets the minimum need for pediatrics providers. Likewise, the Health Level 7 (HL7) Electronic Health Record System Functional Model standard includes many of the important pediatric-specific functions identified by the AAP and the HL7 Pediatric Data Special Interest Group (HL7 PeDSSIG).[11]

32.2.2   Syntactic Standards

Standards exist to define the technical formatting of clinical data produced by EHR systems. Formatting standards, herein called syntactic standards, describe the specific method for notating the clinical data such that computer systems can properly identify and use it. Syntactic standards specify how data is packaged, including the sequence that information is encoded, the specific character codes that delimit data fields and how data are contained among the computer character codes (e.g., whether a field is between the characters '<' and '>' or '{' and '}'). Syntactic standards can be thought of as a specification for the size, shape, and color of an envelope a person may use for mailing a letter, the color and type of ink used to write the letter, and the placement of the address and the greeting line on the page, while the prose itself may be written in any language.

A commonly used syntactic standard is the eXtensible Markup Language (XML), a method designed to describe data and text.[12-14] In particular, XML specifies a method for marking up text with specific character delimiters and for describing text in a way that allows for both human- and machine-readability. In addition, XML allows for the relationships among different pieces of data to be indicated, including which data elements are more or less specific forms of other data elements (e.g., that the medication "metoclopromide" is available in the form, "oral tablets 10 mg") and attributes that modify a given data element (e.g., a medication may have attributes defining the dose, the frequency, the duration and how much should be dispensed). A sample of data describing a prescription for metoclopromide marked up using XML is presented in Fig. 32.1.

32.2.3   Semantic Standards

For clinical information to be shared among and used by different EHR systems, there must be a standardized method for describing it.[15] Semantic standards define and name the concepts that underlie clinical information and entities.[16] They ensure that the words used to describe something are consistent, regardless of where or in which EHR system it is described. For example, a patient's weight may be documented in an EHR system and called "weight." However, the same weight may be documented as "Weight," "patient weight," "dosing weight," "dry weight," "birth

```
<RXCART>
    <RXCART_ID>114068</RXCART_ID>
    <RXCART_EXTERNAL_ID></RXCART_EXTERNAL_ID>
    <RX>
        <RXID>268213</RXID>
        <MEDICATION>
            <ID>295749</ID>
            <MED_NAME>Metoclopramide (Reglan)</MED_NAME>
            <MED_DESCRIPTION>Oral Tablet 10 mg</MED_DESCRIPTION>
        </MEDICATION>
        <FREEFORM_DOSING>N</FREEFORM_DOSING>
        <SIG_ROUTE>oral</SIG_ROUTE>
        <DOSE_AMOUNT>1</DOSE_AMOUNT>
        <DOSE_UNIT>tablets</DOSE_UNIT>
        <DOSE_FREQUENCY>qid</DOSE_FREQUENCY>
        <DURATION_AMOUNT>30</DURATION_AMOUNT>
        <DURATION_UNIT>days</DURATION_UNIT>
        <SUBSTITUTION>N</SUBSTITUTION>
        <SPECIAL_INSTRUCTIONS></SPECIAL_INSTRUCTIONS>
        <COMMENTS></COMMENTS>
        <CLINICIAN_NAME></CLINICIAN_NAME>
        <DISPENSE_AMOUNT>120</DISPENSE_AMOUNT>
        <DISPENSE_UNIT>tablets</DISPENSE_UNIT>
        <SAMPLE_DISPENSE_AMOUNT>120</SAMPLE_DISPENSE_AMOUNT>
        <SAMPLE_DISPENSE_UNIT>tablets</SAMPLE_DISPENSE_UNIT>
        <REFILL_STANDARD>0</REFILL_STANDARD>
        <REFILL_EXTENDED>0</REFILL_EXTENDED>
        <RX_TYPE_STANDARD>N</RX_TYPE_STANDARD>
        <RX_TYPE_SAMPLE>Y</RX_TYPE_SAMPLE>
        <RX_TYPE_EXTENDED>N</RX_TYPE_EXTENDED>
        <STARTDATE>12/12/2006 15:46:41</STARTDATE>
    </RX>
    <ACTION>
        <TYPE>Printed</TYPE>
        <ID>0</ID>
        <NAME>local</NAME>
        <LOCATION></LOCATION>
    </ACTION>
    <FINAL_EVENT>
        <EVENT_INFO>Print Signed</EVENT_INFO>
        <COMMENTS></COMMENTS>
    </FINAL_EVENT>
</RXCART>
```

Fig. 32.1 Message encoding a medication prescription generated by a Vanderbilt University Medical Center EHR system-based prescription writer. The prescription uses XML as a syntactic standard

weight," or "weight in pounds," depending on the context or system used. In some cases, these may be considered equivalent (e.g., the first weight measured after a baby is born could reasonably be called "weight," "Weight," "birth weight," or "patient weight"). While a human may be able to look at these names and reason that they are equivalent, computer systems may not be able to do so. Using standard names to represent the same clinical information helps computer systems correctly integrate similar data and separate distinct data.

To provide semantic standards for healthcare, researchers have created numerous clinical terminologies. Terminologies are collections of standardized words and phrases, called terms, combined in a systematic fashion to represent the conceptual information that makes up a given knowledge domain, such as medical cardiology or pediatrics. For example, using either the term "streptococcal pharyngitis" or "streptococcal sore throat," a terminology can represent the disease syndrome caused by an infection of the pharynx and palatine tonsils with the bacterial microorganism *Streptococcus pyogenes*. Currently, numerous terminologies exist, and many represent given diseases and concepts using different terms from each other. To help align terminologies to a single set of semantic standards, the United States National Committee on Vital and Health Statistics (NCVHS) and the United States government's multiagency consolidated health informatics (CHI) council recommended in 2003 a core set of terminologies as standards for representing aspects of patient medical record information.[17] The recommended terminologies include the Systematized Nomenclature of Medicine Clinical Terms (SNOMED CT, for the exchange, aggregation, and analysis of patient medical information), Logical Observation Identifiers Names and Codes (LOINC, for the representation of individual laboratory tests) and several Federal Drug Terminologies such as RxNorm and the National Drug File Reference terminology (NDF-RT, for representing medications, their biological mechanisms of actions and their physiologic effects). A sample diagnosis encoded using SNOMED CT as a semantic standard is displayed in Fig. 32.2.

```
<CONCEPT>
  <CONCEPT_ID>73158014</DISEASE_ID>
  <CONCEPT_NAME>Streptococcal Pharyngitis</DISEASE_NAME>
  <PARENTS>
      <PARENT>312129004</PARENT>
      <PARENT>312118003</PARENT>
      <PARENT>312422001</PARENT>
      <PARENT>85769006</PARENT>
  </PARENTS>
  <PREFERRED_CONCEPT>73157016</PREFERRED_CONCEPT>
  <MODIFIERS>
      <HAS_COURSE>53737009</COURSE>
      <HAS_EPISODICITY></EPISODICITY>
      <HAS_ONSET></ONSET>
      <HAS_SEVERITY>24484000</SEVERITY>
  </MODIFIERS>
  <CHILDREN>
      <CHILD>76651006</CHILD>
      <CHILD>41582007</CHILD>
  </CHILDREN>
<CONCEPT>
```

Fig. 32.2 The diagnosis "severe acute streptococcal pharyngitis" encoded using XML as a syntactic standard and SNOMED CT as a semantic standard. All relationships with associated concepts, such as to parents and to modifiers, reference concepts' unique identifier numbers rather than their names

32.3 Role of the Standards Development Organization

Standards development organizations (SDOs) are the entities that consider, create, maintain, and distribute standards, often with the support or sponsorship of larger entities, such as governments or specialty groups. Standards development organizations are generally made up of individuals with expertise in the domain being standardized and in the standardization process, often working as volunteers. Domain experts may be anybody with practical, administrative, or theoretic knowledge and experience from the field being standardized. For example, when creating standards for pediatric data, the HL7 PeDSSIG assembled a group of more than 70 participants that included physicians, nurses, pharmacists, researchers, administrators and program directors, and system developers among others. Including a diverse array of participants into an SDO allows for differing views and experiences to be considered when standards are developed and evaluated. Standards development organizations may be independent groups whose primary role is to develop standards, and they may be a component of an organization meeting a special need or constituent. For example, HL7 is a standalone independent SDO having the goal of standardizing clinical and administrative data "requirements of the entire health care organization."

The process for developing standards occurs in several stages. The stages may cover the steps that take place from the conception of an idea all the way through publication and general availability. The rigor with which stages are defined and followed vary with the SDO creating the standard. The International Organization for Standardization, for example, defines six distinct stages for standards development.[18] These include the proposal stage, the preparatory stage, the committee stage, the enquiry stage, the approval stage and the publication stage, as described in Table 32.2. Other SDOs may

Table 32.2 International Organization for Standardization (ISO) stages for developing and publishing new standards[18]

Stage	Tasks and procedures
Proposal	Propose a new standard to the relevant technical committee to determine through voting whether the standard is needed and useful and to identify the project leader if the group decides to proceed
Preparatory	A working group of domain experts is convened and iteratively develops a draft set of standards, which are reviewed by the technical committee who approved developing the new standard
Committee	The draft standards are registered and then evaluated by the technical committee, which both provides feedback and votes to accept the draft. When accepted, the draft is formatted to a "draft International Standard (DIS)"
Enquiry	The DIS is reviewed for vote and comment by all organizations participating in the ISO, with approval occurring if two thirds of the organizations vote to support the standard but no more than one fourth vote against it. The approved version is called a "final draft International Standard (FDIS)"
Approval	The FDIS is circulated for vote again by organizations participating in the ISO, with approval occurring if two thirds of the organizations vote to support the standard but no more than one fourth vote against it; technical comments are not considered at this stage
Publication	The final ISO standard receives minimal copyediting and is published for use by all stakeholders

employ different methods for creating, drafting, and publishing standards; however they generally include steps in which standards are iteratively revised, consensus is generated and approval is sought from widening circles of experts.

32.4   Aligning and Certifying Standards

With multiple independent SDOs representing different stakeholders, there is the need to align their published standards. Standards are only useful if they are universally adopted and represent a broad range of needs. The Alliance for Pediatric Quality (Alliance) is a collaboration of four major national pediatric organizations formed to help align the pediatric community and bridge data standards initiatives, including the work being done by the AAP Council on Clinical Information Technology (COCIT) and the HL7 PeDSSIG. Alliance organizations include the American Academy of Pediatrics, The American Board of Pediatrics, Child Health Corporation of America and the National Association of Children's Hospitals and Related Institutions. The Alliance participates in national functional, messaging, and terminology health care data standards initiatives to ensure that they address pediatric issues, with ultimate goals of building consensus on child health care data standards and influencing adoption of these standards. Consensus-building to-date has involved the HL7 PeDSSIG and the AAP COCIT. The PeDSSIG is an active volunteer group consisting of primarily child health practitioners, chief medical information officers and informaticists. PeDSSIG participants work together to identify and to agree upon data standards important for child health care. The PeDSSIG works to ensure that the published HL7 standards include those most important in providing general child health care. COCIT is a volunteer organization made up of AAP members who have an interest in the application of information technology to clinical pediatrics. COCIT educates AAP members on health information technology, contributes to the development of AAP policy on health information technology, and provides guidance to pediatricians seeking to make decisions about the selection and use of clinical information technology in practice. In early 2007, the Alliance led an effort to combine the functional criteria identified by the PeDSSIG and COCIT into one master document that will be used to identify gaps in the HL7 standards and the Certification Commission on Health Information Technology (CCHIT) certification criteria.

Once standards have been developed, published, aligned, and accepted in the greater community, objective certification organizations can then evaluate existing products to determine whether they comply with the standards. Certification helps consumers judge whether a given product has adopted and incorporated published standards. For example, CCHIT is an independent private-sector commission that tests commercial EHR systems using an agreed-upon set of functional standards, and that certifies those systems that comply. As with SDOs, certification organizations develop certification criteria through iterative cycles of proposal, public commentary and balloting before final acceptance and publication. CCHIT originally developed as a coalition of three organizations, the American Health Information Management Association (AHIMA), the Healthcare Information and Management Systems Society (HIMSS) and The National Alliance for Health Information Technology (Alliance), which came together in 2004 to create a certification organization. In September 2005, the US Government Department of Health and Human Services awarded CCHIT a 3-year contract to develop objective criteria and a process for certifying EHR systems. In 2006, CCHIT released its first directory of certified EHR systems, and since then, the certification criteria and listing of certified vendors have evolved as SDOs have expanded lists of functional standards.

32.5 Case Study: Pediatric Growth Chart Standards

Let us explore the role of standards as they pertain to a real case. At Vanderbilt University Medical Center (VUMC), developers elected to add pediatric growth charts to the institutional EHR system in 2002. In 2002, there were no clear standards for how developers should create growth charts in EHR systems, and there were no lists of the tasks and features that they should cover. While the AAP had published in 2001 its "Special Requirements for Electronic Medical Record Systems in Pediatrics," this document only provided high-level standards for growth charts in EHR systems. In addition, at that time VUMC hosted several locally developed and commercial EHR system components, including a standalone inpatient computerized provider order entry (CPOE) system and an integrated electronic nursing intake form in which nurses could enter patient vital signs and measurements. While users could enter patient measurements, such as patient weight, in any of the systems, the values were not encoded the same way across systems and not all data were shared among systems.

To create EHR system-based growth charts, the VUMC developers needed to develop or adopt standards to allow growth data to be shared among EHR system components. The standards included content, syntactic, and semantic standards. The content standards were developed by a team that included practicing general pediatricians and pediatric subspecialists, informaticians, and software engineers. The content standards were expanded from those previously defined by the AAP, and specified that EHR system based growth charts should have the ability to record height, weight, and head circumferences; to plot these data against population-based curves such as those published by the United States Centers for Disease Control and Prevention (CDC) and its National Center for Health Statistics (NCHS); to adjust the normative curves based on patient age, gender, and possibly other demographic or diagnostic features; to calculate body mass index (BMI) and population-based percentiles; and to integrate into a busy clinical practice, among others. The complete list of growth chart specifications is in Table 32.3.

Table 32.3 Specifications for EHR system-based pediatric growth charts[19]

Workflow

Use routinely gathered growth measurements

Automatically generate growth charts

Growth charts accessible from standard EHR system components

Growth data and calculations reusable for other tasks

Growth data

Capture weight, height or length, head circumference

Calculate Body Mass Index and growth velocity

Calculate percentiles and standard deviations based on population norms

Capture data using different units of measurement (e.g., grams, kilograms, pounds)

Capture context of measurement (e.g., laying or standing, ventilated)

Support automated data capture from measurement devices (e.g., digital scales)

Presentation

Display growth data on standardized charts as the default view

Display against standard population-based normal curves

Display normal curves based on age, gender, and other demographic characteristics

Display using graphical and tabular formats

Display predictive growth curves or growth targets

Display time and date of birth for infants

Functionality

Calculate mid parental height by gender-specific parent height percentiles

Display bone age measurements with actual age measurements

Derive and display and the median age at which a given growth point is achieved

Allow addin 1 g, deleting and editing of growth points

Enable varying the scale's level of detail (i.e., zoom in or out)

Support printing and faxing

Support user preferences (i.e., connected points, superimposed values)

The specifications called for the EHR system-based growth charts automatically to generate growth charts from routinely gathered growth measurements and from multiple EHR system components. Because patient growth measures are gathered in multiple places and different EHR system components at VUMC, each with a different formatting and naming convention, they could not all be used immediately by the growth chart software. To solve this problem, developers had to create and apply syntactic standards and semantic standards to the different data sources. In this case, the developers programmed several "filters" which searched the raw data generated by the EHR system components, and then standardized any growth data it found. The filters then applied syntactic standards to normalize the data stream structure, and semantic standards to encode the data to a single common set of terms. Once the data had been standardized, the growth chart software was able automatically to display it, regardless of the source of data. An example growth chart applying content standards and containing syntactically and semantically standardized data obtained from different EHR system components, including a CPOE system and a nursing intake system, is displayed in Fig. 32.3.

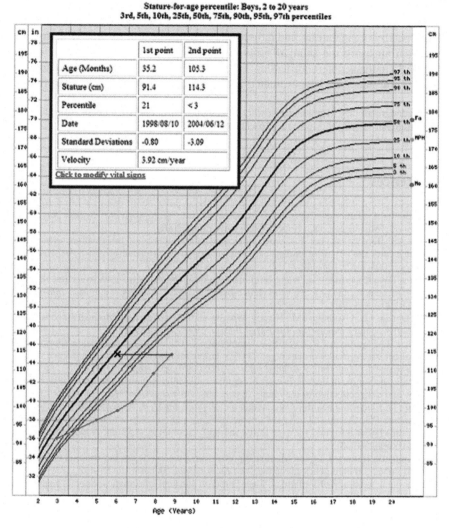

Fig. 32.3 An EHR system-based growth chart that includes features outlined by content standards and which displays data that has been normalized to syntactic and semantic standards. Content standards include use of a population-based norm, applying growth data from different EHR system components, including parental growth targets, and performing various calculations to determine Z score, growth velocity, percentiles, etc. (Adapted from Rosenbloom et al.[19])

32.6   Conclusion

Standards for Electronic Health Record (EHR) systems can improve the healthcare delivery to populations of children. Specifically, semantic and syntactic standards can improve healthcare delivery by facilitating clinical data exchange among various EHR systems, while functional standards encourage EHR systems to provide for users a consistent and expected set of functions. Standards should be developed by organizations and individuals that represent those who will ultimately benefit from using the standards and through an iterative process that allows for stages of feedback and modification. Once standards have been developed and published, compliance may be evaluated and compliant products may be certified.

Acknowledgment Dr. Rosenbloom's work was supported in part by a Grant from the United States National Library of Medicine (Rosenbloom, 5K22 LM008576-03).

References

1. Institute of Medicine. *Crossing the Quality Chasm: A New Health System for the 21st Century*. Washington, DC: National Academy Press; 2001.
2. Ash JS, Berg M, Coiera E. Some unintended consequences of information technology in health care: the nature of patient care information system-related errors. *J Am Med Inform Assoc*. 2004;11(2):104–112.
3. Bates DW, Kuperman GJ, Wang S, et al. Ten commandments for effective clinical decision support: making the practice of evidence-based medicine a reality. *J Am Med Inform Assoc*. 2003;10(6):523–530.
4. McDonald CJ, Overhage JM, Tierney WM, et al. The Regenstrief Medical Record System: a quarter century experience. *Int J Med Inform*. 1999;54(3):225–253.
5. Miller RA, Waitman LR, Chen S, Rosenbloom ST. The anatomy of decision support during inpatient care provider order entry (CPOE): empirical observations from a decade of CPOE experience at Vanderbilt. *J Biomed Inform*. 2005;38(6):469–485.
6. Apkon M, Singhaviranon P. Impact of an electronic information system on physician workflow and data collection in the intensive care unit. *Intensive Care Med*. 2001;27(1):122–130.
7. Kalra D. Electronic health record standards. *Methods Inf Med*. 2006;45(Suppl 1):136–144.
8. Biondich PG, Grannis SJ. The Indiana network for patient care: an integrated clinical information system informed by over thirty years of experience. *J Public Health Manag Pract*. 2004;Suppl:S81–S86.
9. Shapiro JS, Kannry J, Lipton M, et al. Approaches to patient health information exchange and their impact on emergency medicine. *Ann Emerg Med*. 2006;48(4):426–432.
10. American Academy of Pediatrics: Task Force on Medical Informatics. Special requirements for electronic medical record systems in pediatrics. *Pediatrics*. 2001;108(2):513–515.
11. Dolin RH, Alschuler L, Boyer S, et al. HL7 clinical document architecture, release 2. *J Am Med Inform Assoc*. 2006;13(1):30–39.
12. World Wide Web Consortium (W3C). W3C Website; 2008. Available at: http://www.w3.org/. Accessed December 21, 2008.
13. Dolin RH, Alschuler L, Behlen F, et al. HL7 document patient record architecture: an XML document architecture based on a shared information model. *Proc AMIA Symp*. 1999:52–56.
14. Dolin RH, Alschuler L, Boyer S, Beebe C. An update on HL7's XML-based document representation standards. *Proc AMIA Symp*. 2000:190–194.
15. Huff SM. Clinical data exchange standards and vocabularies for messages. *Proc AMIA Symp*. 1998:62–67.
16. Bakken S, Campbell KE, Cimino JJ, Huff SM, Hammond WE. Toward vocabulary domain specifications for health level 7-coded data elements. *J Am Med Inform Assoc*. 2000;7(4):333–342.

17. Lumpkin J, National Committee on Vital Health Statistics (NCVHS). Report to the Secretary of HHS: Uniform Data standards for Patient Medical Record Information; 2003. Available at: http://www.ncvhs.hhs.gov/hipaa000706.pdf. Accessed December 21, 2008.
18. International Organization for Standardization (ISO). Stages of Development for International Standards. ISO Website; 2008. Available at: http://www.iso.org/iso/standards_development/ processes_and_procedures/stages_description.htm. Accessed December 21, 2008.
19. Rosenbloom ST, Qi X, Riddle WR, et al. Implementing pediatric growth charts into an electronic health record system. *J Am Med Inform Assoc.* 2006;13(3):302–308.

Chapter 33
The Case for a Pediatric Terminology

George R. Kim and S. Trent Rosenbloom

Objectives

- To provide an overview of the roles and importance of terminologies in health care
- To articulate problems and challenges with current terminologies in pediatrics
- To describe current projects in pediatric terminology development

33.1 Introduction

Terminologies are structured collections of designations ("terms") that describe entities and relationships that represent the knowledge within a given domain.[1,2] Terms may consist of words, phrases, or other notations (such as numbers or symbols), and are designed to support communication, storage, retrieval, and use of knowledge and information by humans and machines. An example is the *clinical entity* of "blood pressure measured during the diastolic phase of the cardiac cycle," which is designated (in the terminology SNOMED CT) by the *preferred term* "Diastolic blood pressure" and the *concept identifier* "271650006." Terminologies can formally define and specify representation of information content, and when used with messaging standards, can support structured information exchange among different electronic patient care systems. Terminologies have been developed with differing levels of rigor, and best practices have been described.[2,8]

33.2 Terminologies in Health Care

33.2.1 Uses

There are numerous terminologies designed to support various clinical domains and operational tasks within healthcare. Examples include:

C.U. Lehmann et al. (eds.), *Pediatric Informatics: Computer Applications in Child Health,* Health Informatics,
© Springer Science+Business Media, LLC 2011

- Coding for service documentation and reimbursement:
  ○ Medical diagnosis: International Classification of Diseases (ICD9 – CM, ICD-10)
  ○ Psychiatric diagnosis: Diagnostic and Statistical Manual of Mental Disorders (DSM IV)
  ○ Evaluation, management and procedures: Common Procedural Terminology (CPT)
  ○ Documentation and study of processes and outcomes for quality improvement:
- Nursing Intervention and Outcomes Classifications (NIC, NOC)
  ○ North American Nursing Diagnosis Association (NANDA)
  ○ Ordering and tracking items used in medical work
  ○ Drug classes, specific drugs, their forms, amounts, and packaged doses (RxNorm, Multum, FirstDataBank, Micromedex)
- Laboratory and imaging test names, specifications, result units and normal ranges (Logical observations indicators names and codes (LOINC))
- Medical equipment (Food and Drug Administration Product Code Classification)
- Indexing, retrieval of and linkage to published medical knowledge
  ○ Medical Subject Headings (MeSH) for medical journal articles
  ○ CINAHL Subject Headings for nursing journal articles
  ○ Thesaurus of Psychological Index Terms for psychology journal articles
- Locating patient-specific data
  ○ Descriptive data: SNOMED CT
  ○ Health Level Seven
- Natural language processing (and applications)
  ○ The Unified Medical Language System (and MetaMap)
  ○ The Medical Entities Dictionary (and MEDLEE)
  ○ SNOMED CT (and Lingologix)
- Clinical documentation
  ○ SNOMED CT® (used in Kaiser Permanente's HealthConnect EHR,[3] among others)
  ○ Medcin® (used in the Department of Defense's Armed Forces Health Longitudinal Technology Application (AHLTA) EHR[4])
  ○ Medical Entities Dictionary (used at New York Presbyterian Hospital[5])

The central importance of terminologies in US health care was reinforced in 2005 with the development of the Federal Consolidated Health Informatics (CHI) initiative (a part of the eGovernment Business portfolio) which adopted a set of existing terminologies (and identified gaps) for use in electronic exchange of clinical information within specified health domains by the US Federal health enterprise, its clients and partner entities (see Table 33.1).[6]

33.2.2   Implementations

Technical requirements for well-constructed terminologies in biomedicine have been articulated.[8] These requirements include formal definitions, sufficient scope

Table 33.1 Consolidated health informatics terminology standards[7]

Domain	Terminology standard
Anatomy	National Cancer Institute (NCI) Metathesaurus, SNOMED CT
Diagnosis/Problem Lists	
Laboratory Results	Standardized Nomenclature of Medicine Clinical Terms (SNOMED CT)
Non-Laboratory Interventions/ Procedures	
Nursing	
Demographics	
Immunizations	
Clinical Encounters	Health Level Seven (HL7)
Text Based Reports	
Units	
Laboratory Result Names	Logical Observations Indicators Names and Codes (LOINC)
Laboratory Test Order Names	
Genes	Human Gene Nomenclature (HUGN)
	Environmental Protection Agency's (EPA)
Chemicals	Substance Registry System (SRS)
Medications:	Food and Drug Administration's (FDA)
Active Ingredients	Unique Ingredient Identifier (UNII)
Clinical Drugs	National Library of Medicine (NLM) RxNORM
Drug Classifications	National Drug File Reference Terminology (NDF-RT)
	Food and Drug Administration's (FDA)
Drug Product	National Drug Code (NDC) Product Name/Code
Manufactured Dosage Form	Food and Drug Administration (FDA)
	Center for Drug Evaluation and Research (CDER)
Package	Data Standards Manual
Special Populations	Health Level Seven Version 2.x
	Logical Observations Indicators Names and Codes (LOINC)
Structured Product Label	Clinical Structured Product Label (SPL)
HIPAA Approved Code Sets	Health Insurance Portability and Accountability Act (HIPAA) transactions and code sets
Supplies	
History & Physical	
Population Health	
Disability	No current standards
Physiology	
Proteins	
Multimedia	

and granularity of concepts to describe entities and events within a domain (to the extent and detail needed) and reusability. Different terminologies implementations include:

- *Dictionaries, catalogs*: structured collection of terms that may be related to objects, with attributes (e.g., drug formulary with generic and trade names, dose, and route information)

- *Nomenclature*: a system of objects named according to a prescribed set of rules (e.g., formal anatomic names of organs and spaces within the human body: Terminologia Anatomica[9])
- *Taxonomy*: formal classification of concepts according to hierarchical relationships (e.g., classification of viruses: ICTV[10])
- *Thesaurus*: collection of terms grouped by concept (e.g., The National Cancer Institute (NCI) Thesaurus[11])
- *Ontology*: a data model in which concepts (within a domain) are linked to each other by relationships and rules (description logic) that are used to reason and draw conclusions about the concepts within the domain (e.g., The Gene Ontology[12])

Detailed discussions on biomedical terminologies,[13] standard definitions,[14,15] natural language processing,[16] the linguistic aspects of terminology[17] are available.

33.3 Current Terminology Challenges for Pediatrics

The American Academy of Pediatrics has articulated the challenges known to representing pediatric concepts with current terminologies:

> [B]arriers that child health care providers encounter in the application of [electronic] systems relate not to functions of the system but to the inappropriate terminology used to express concepts (physical examination findings, developmental milestones, diagnoses) in the…system's user interface … [suggesting the need for advocacy for] inclusion in these systems of historical findings, psychosocial risk factors, family structural details, social history, physical examination findings, developmental problems, behavioral issues, congenital syndromes, and diagnoses of particular importance to pediatrics[18]

Examples of these challenges include:

- Inclusion of common pediatric concepts and domains that are not (yet) formalized in existing biomedical terminologies, such as developmental milestones and immunizations.
- Defining preventive and cognitive services for reimbursement as valued components of primary health care[19,20]
- Extending medication library items to meet safe pediatric practices for high-risk inpatient processes (such as continuous infusions)[21]

33.4 Current Work in Creating Pediatric Terminologies

Different approaches have been used to define and encode concepts for inclusion in pediatric terminologies:

33.4.1 Creation of a Pediatric Clinical Corpus

One approach that has been undertaken is the development of a pediatric corpus of clinical information (including text data) at the Cincinnati Children's Hospital Medical Center, including nurses and surgical notes, discharge summaries, information about symptoms, procedures, findings, and therapeutic response, genetic specimen and other data[22] for use in experiments with natural language processing tools and lexical/semantic tagging.

33.4.2 Workflow-Based Templates

Another approach to creating terminologies is to define a clinical workflow (such as a well-child visit) in terms of the data that are collected, recorded, and processed in performing the task. Representations of these data needs (descriptions of developmental stages and delays, nutrition, immunizations) are then matched to a candidate terminology (such as those in the CHI, discussed previously) proposed for use in the workflow. Evaluation of coverage and level of detail can help identify gaps within the candidate terminology in meeting the terminology needs of the clinical workflow.

The requirements of this approach are: (a) a robust terminology that is matched to the domain (such as pediatric ambulatory care); and (b) cooperation between a dedicated and representative group of clinicians (who define the data needs of the specific workflow) and informaticians (who are versed in the nuances of clinical work and terminology development). Barriers to this approach include engaging the needed expertise and its labor-intensiveness. In addition, while the structure of a terminology such as SNOMED CT may allow for the development of extensions to fill gaps in that the basic terminology does not cover, such extensions must be formally submitted for incorporation.

This approach has been studied for use in medical evaluations[23,24] and has been explored but not formally investigated for pediatric work.

33.4.3 Content Analysis of Reports

A third approach has been used to develop taxonomies for use in patient safety event reporting in general pediatrics[25] and neonatology.[26] In these cases, text reports on reported patient safety events were collected either by voluntary submission to an online database or through direct interviews with clinicians. Textual data is reviewed and classified using a constant comparative analysis method[27] in conjunction with a conceptual model of errors to develop hierarchical taxonomies of error types. Strengths of such taxonomies include structure that is both descriptive and predictive and the ability to display both the relationships between various components and the pathways from the contributing factors to the outcome.[25]

33.5 Terminology Tools

A number of tools are available for research and development of terminologies and these are summarized in Table 33.2.

Table 33.2 Terminology tools (last accessed 2 December 2008)

Tool	Terminologies	Comments
The UMLS® and MetaMap®	Many	The Unified Medical Language System (UMLS)® from the National Library of Medicine links 100 + medical terminologies by concept and semantic relationships. Contains SNOMED CT® for free use by developers (user agreement required) URL: https://kscas.nlm.nih.gov:8443/cas/login?service=http://umlsks.nlm.nih.gov/uPortal/Login
ICD codes	ICD 9, 10. International Classification of Functioning, Disability, and Health (ICF)	The International Classification of Diseases in database format f rom the National Center for Health Statistics URL: http://www.cdc.gov/nchs/icd9.htm
Relma®	LOINC®	The Regenstrief LOINC Mapping Assistant facilitates searches through the Logical Objects, Indicators, Names, and Codes database URL: http://loinc.org/relma
MeSH® browser	MeSH®	The Medical Subject Headings (MeSH)® are used to index and retrieve journal article citations from the MEDLINE/PubMed® database via the Entrez® interface URL: http://www.ncbi.nlm.nih.gov/sites/entrez?db=mesh
SNOMED CT® browsers	SNOMED CT®	SNOMED CT® is now owned by the International Health Terminology Standards Development Organisation (IHTSDO). A number of browsers exist for accessing content URL: http://www.nlm.nih.gov/research/umls/Snomed/snomed_browsers.html
Medical Entities Dictionary (MED)	MED	The Medical Entities Dictionary (MED) is a large concepts repository developed and used at the New York Presbyterian Hospital in New York URL: http://med.dmi.columbia.edu/browser.htm

33.6 Conclusion

Terminologies are an essential part of the US health care and health information technology infrastructures. There is currently a need establish an agenda to extend currently available and adopted terminologies to represent pediatric knowledge within clinical workflows to improve safety and documentation of work. This effort will require the coordination of pediatric clinicians and informaticians familiar with the terminology needs of pediatric workflows.

33.7 Additional Topics

33.7.1 Messaging Standards

In addition to terminologies, the Consolidated Health Informatics initiative specifies four messaging standards for use in eGovernment health related transactions (Table 33.3).

Messaging standards are related to but differ from terminologies in that they specify the electronic structure of health information, that is, the way it is packaged for transmission, exchange, management, and integration, including specifications for hardware, software, language, and security requirements for encoding and decoding:

- Text and numeric healthcare information (Health Level Seven)[28]
- Imaging data: Digital Imaging and Communications in Medicine (DICOM)[29]
- Electronic prescription (National Council for Prescription Drug Programs (NCPDP) SCRIPT)[30]

33.7.2 Natural Language Processing

Clinical terminologies may be used for structured entry of information by humans (such as diagnostic and procedural coding to describe clinical encounters for billing) or for automated extraction of concepts from free text (natural language processing or NLP) for summarization from pathology reports,[31] patient summaries,[32] journal

Table 33.3 Consolidated Health Informatics messaging domains and standards

Domain	Standard
Imaging	Digital Imaging and Communications in Medicine (DICOM)
Medical devices	Institute of Electrical and Electronics Engineers 1073 (IEEE 1073)
Pharmacy	National Council for Prescription Drug Programs (NCPDP) SCRIPT
Clinical	Health Level Seven (HL7)

abstracts[33] and teaching case reports.[34] An example of a clinical NLP application is GoCode (now known as Discern nCode,[35] developed at the Mayo Clinic, with adoption by several university health systems to aid in mapping of clinical text to SNOMED CT, ICD-9, and CPT for Evaluation and Management coding.

Acknowledgment Dr. Rosenbloom's work was supported in part by a Grant from the United States National Library of Medicine (Rosenbloom, 5K22 LM008576-03).

References

1. Shortliffe E, Cimino J. *Glossary. From Biomedical Informatics: Computer Applications in Health Care and Biomedicine*. 3rd ed. New York: Springer; 2006: 992.
2. Rosenbloom ST, Miller RA, Johnson KB, Elkin PL, Brown SH. Interface terminologies: facilitating direct entry of clinical data into electronic health record systems. *J Am Med Inform Assoc*. 2006;13:277–288.
3. Dolin RH, Mattison JE, Cohn S, Campbell KE, et al. Kaiser permanente's convergent medical terminology. *Medinfo*. 2004;11(Pt 1):346–350.
4. Medicomp Systems, Inc. Medcin Website; 2008. Available at: http://www.medicomp.com. Accessed December 27, 2007.
5. Columbia University Department of Biomedical Informatics. Medical Entities Dictionary Website; 2007. Available at: http://med.dmi.columbia.edu/. Accessed December 27, 2007.
6. US Department of Health and Human Services Office of the National Coordinator for Health Information Technology (ONC). Consolidated Health Informatics. Available at: http://www. hhs.gov/healthit/chi.html. Accessed December 12, 2007.
7. US Agency for Healthcare Research and Quality. Consolidated Health Informatics, United States Health Informatics Knowledgebase; 2005. Available at: http://ushik.org/chi/. Accessed December 19, 2007.
8. Cimino JJ. Desiderata for controlled medical vocabularies in the twenty-first century. *Methods Inf Med*. 1998;37(4–5):394–403.
9. Federative Committee on Anatomical Terminology. Terminologia Anatomica. Stuttgart, Germany: Thieme; 1998.
10. van Regenmortel MHV et al. eds. *Virus Taxonomy. Classification and Nomenclature of Viruses, Seventh Report of the International Committee on Taxonomy*. New York/San Diego, CA: Academic; 1999.
11. National Cancer Institute. The NCI Terminology Browser/EVS Browser Portal; 2008. Available at: http://bioportal.nci.nih.gov/ncbo/faces/index.xhtml. Accessed December 21, 2008.
12. Gene Ontology. Gene Ontology Home; 2008. Available at: http://www.geneontology.org/. Accessed December 21, 2008.
13. Hammond WH, Cimino JJ. Standards in biomedical informatics. In: Shortliffe EH et al., ed. *Biomedical Informatics: Computer Applications in Health Care and Biomedicine*. New York: Springer; 2006: 265–311.
14. International Organization for Standardization. ISO 1087-1 2000 Terminology Work – Vocabulary, Part 1 (Theory and application); 2000. Available at: http://www.iso.org/iso/iso_catalogue/catalogue_tc/catalogue_detail.htm?csnumber=20057. Accessed December 20, 2008.
15. International Organization for Standardization. ISO 1087-2 2000 Terminology Work – Vocabulary, Part 2 (Computer applications); 2000. Available at: http://www.iso.org/iso/iso_catalogue/catalogue_tc/catalogue_detail.htm?csnumber=32819. Accessed December 20, 2008.

16. Friedman C, Johnson SB. Natural language and text processing in biomedicine. In: Shortliffe EH et al., eds. *Biomedical Informatics: Computer Applications in Health Care and Biomedicine*. New York: Springer; 2006: 312–343.

17. Campbell KE, Oliver DE, Spackman KA, Shortliffe EH. Representing thoughts, words, and things in the UMLS. *J Am Med Inform Assoc*. 1998;5(5):421–431.

18. Spooner SA, Council on Clinical Information Technology, American Academy of Pediatrics. Special requirements of electronic health record systems in pediatrics. *Pediatrics*. 2007;119(3):631–637.

19. American Academy of Pediatrics Committee on Coding and Nomenclature. Application of the resource-based relative value scale system to pediatrics. *Pediatrics*. 113(5):1437–1440.

20. Goodson JD. Unintended consequences of resource-based relative value scale reimbursement. *JAMA*. 2007;298(19):2308–2310.

21. Veltri MA, Ascenzi J, Clark JS, et al. Successful Elimination of the Rule of Six in an Academic Children's Hospital Through a Medication-Use-System Redesign and Standardization of Continuous Infusions. ASHP 42nd Midyear Clinical Meeting; 2006. Available at: http://www.ashpadvantage.com/bestpractices/2006_papers/veltri.htm. Accessed December 20, 2008.

22. Pestian JP, Itert L, Duch W. Development of a pediatric text-corpus for part-of-speech tagging. In: Wierzchon ST, Trojanowski K, eds. *Intelligent information processing and web mining: Proceedings of the International IIS: IIPWM'04*; 2004 May 17–20. Zakopane, Poland/Berlin: Springer; 2004: 219–226.

23. Rosenbloom ST, Miller RA, Johnson KB, Elkin PL, Brown SH. A model for evaluating interface terminologies. *J Am Med Inform Assoc*. 2008;15(1):65–76.

24. Brown SH, Elkin PL, Bauer BA, et al. SNOMED CT: utility for a general medical evaluation template. *AMIA Annu Symp Proc*. 2006:101–105.

25. Woods DM, Johnson J, Holl JL, et al. Anatomy of a patient safety event: a pediatric patient safety taxonomy. *Qual Saf Health Care*. 2005;14(6):422–427.

26. Suresh G, Horbar JD, Plsek P, et al. Voluntary anonymous reporting of medical errors for neonatal intensive care. *Pediatrics*. 2004;113(6):1609–1618.

27. Creswell JW. *Research Design: Qualitative and Quantitative Approaches*. Thousand Oaks, CA: Sage; 1994.

28. Health Level 7. HL7 Website; 2008. Available at: http://www.hl7.org. Accessed December 21, 2008.

29. Digital Imaging and Communications in Medicine (DICOM). DICOM Website; 2008. Available at: http://medical.nema.org/. Accessed December 14, 2007.

30. US Department of Health and Human Services Centers for Medicare & Medicaid Services (CMS). Medicare program; identification of backward compatible version of adopted standard for e-prescribing and the Medicare prescription drug program (version 8.1). Interim final rule with comment period. *Fed Regist*. 2006;71(121):36020–36024.

31. Zhou L, Tao Y, Cimino JJ, et al. Terminology model discovery using natural language processing and visualization techniques. *J Biomed Inform*. 2006;39(6):626–636.

32. Friedman C, Liu H, Shagina L. A vocabulary development and visualization tool based on natural language processing and the mining of textual patient reports. *J Biomed Inform*. 2003;36(3):189–201.

33. Aronson AR. Effective mapping of biomedical text to the UMLS Metathesaurus: the MetaMap program. *Proc AMIA Symp*. 2001:17–21.

34. Kim GR, Aronson AR, Mork JG, Cohen BA, Lehmann CU. Application of a Medical Text Indexer to an online dermatology atlas. *Medinfo*. 2004;11(Pt 1):287–291.

35. Cerner Corporation. Discern nCode (formerly GoCode); 2008. Available at: http://www.cerner.com/public/Cerner_3.asp?id=31472. Accessed December 20, 2008.

Chapter 34
Pediatric Research and Informatics

Harold P. Lehmann, Paul A. Law and Allen Y. Tien

Objectives

- To articulate the types of research impacted by informatics
- To identify new types of research that can be performed only with informatics innovations
- To articulate the phases of the research cycle and how information technology supports them

34.1 Introduction: The Agenda and Scope of Pediatric Research

Pediatric research seeks to improve and optimize child health through scientific exploration and translation of the products and results of research into clinical practice. With advances in research methods and technology, scientists are progressively able to address new and persistent problems in clinical medicine, quality improvement, health services, public and population health and bioinformatics as well as in new domains. Current federal interest in speeding knowledge translation from laboratory to clinical practice to improve outcomes has led to the study of the improvement and optimization of the research process itself, and how translation and adoption of best practices occurs within the health community. As health care research and technologies to save and prolong life evolve, even more questions arise regarding the wisdom, responsibility, and the equity of their use, to protect children and their rights and the rights of their families.

The domain of pediatric research is wide: from newborns to adults, from genetics to environment, from well children to the critically ill. Units of analysis can range from individuals to families to communities and populations. Areas of study encompass all things that affect children, their growth, health, and development from in utero exposures to home, school, playground, and even society.

C.U. Lehmann et al. (eds.), *Pediatric Informatics: Computer Applications in Child Health,* Health Informatics,
© Springer Science+Business Media, LLC 2011

Information technology and informatics provide new opportunities to extend research boundaries by creating:

- Improved methods for data collection and validation
- "High-throughput" computing for processing large amounts of data quickly for complex research models
- Expanded technologies for quickly exploring very large data sets for prediction, visualization, and hypothesis generation
- New models for participation that include children and families as partners (as well as subjects)

With these new opportunities and power of data also come new responsibilities to assure the safety and rights of subjects and their families:

- To assure the protections and rights of human subjects
- To prevent the unauthorized or unintended use of personal health information
- To assure the integrity of the research process, its intent, design, validity, execution, and the representation of its findings

34.2 The Research Process and Informatics

The formalization of research has evolved to assure validity of the results of clinical studies and trials and to protect the safety and rights of human subjects.[1] Even if studies do not involve human subjects directly, they may involve protected health information (PHI) of individuals which require special procedures to assure patient/subject privacy. Formalization of research projects requires a clear statement of the plan of research (its goals, objectives, and steps), an informed review of its scientific validity and ethical base (systematic literature review, preliminary data, conflict disclosures, expected risks and benefits), determination of a budget, resources, and schedule and agreement on deliverables (a report, a product or process change) between the researcher and the research funder. A framework for research formalization in the context of informatics support is presented in Table 34.1.

34.2.1 Generating a Research Question or Hypothesis

Research begins with questions and observations not previously noted. Pasteur noted that "Chance favors only the prepared mind." With the incorporation of large data sets and data mining[2] techniques, "chance" becomes a probability of detecting previously unrecognized patterns or recurrences that can suggest hypotheses for further testing. In drug research, such an approach has been used to economize costs by suggesting likely avenues for research. In clinical medicine, physicians have shown interest in using these techniques[3] for critiquing care and forecasting needs.

Table 34.1 Seven idealized steps in performing research with idealized informatics concerns. "Organization": the context in which research is performed (inpatient or outpatient; government-sponsored pilot test or commercial multicenter trial). "Workflow": the actions taken by participants and stakeholders, at all levels. "Software": the computer programs that support the workflow within the organization to accomplish research. "Hardware": the physical infrastructure of computers and network devices within which software operates. Informatics methods and information technology should fill in each cell in this table, and where they do not is an opportunity for development or exploration.

Research Steps Informatics Concerns	Generating research question	Justifying project	Designing study	Obtaining IRB approval*	Executing protocol	Analyzing data	Publishing results
Organization							
Workflow							
Software							
Hardware							

34.2.2   Justifying a Project

The feasibility and likelihood of success of answering a research question or hypothesis definitively and safely on technical, pragmatic, and financial levels justifies investment to decision-makers and funders.

34.2.2.1   Technical

Technical justification begins with review of what is already known: a literature search of current evidence. This is done to assess: (1) what has already been done to avoid repetition, (2) if an answer to the questions or hypotheses posed already exists and (3) previous problems encountered in answering the question or confirming the hypothesis. In pediatrics, the American Academy of Pediatrics (AAP) develops pediatric clinical guidelines based on systematic reviews as a source of the strength of recommendations. AAP Guidelines[4] along with those of other organizations are assembled by the Agency for Healthcare Research and Quality (AHRQ) into the National Guideline Clearinghouse.[5] Structured evidence is also available in the form of systematic reviews (The Cochrane Collaborative[6,7] is organized into disease-related Groups and Fields (such as Child Health (although most of the pediatric reviews deal with neonatology)).[8] Because systematic reviews and guidelines are frequently out of date, it is important for the researcher to search the literature published since the last review (usually 2–3 years). The National Library of Medicine provides a resource called Clinical Queries[9] that facilitates location of published evidence on therapy, diagnosis, prognosis, etiology, and prediction rules as well as systematic reviews on a topic from PubMed citations. A medical librarian trained in evidence-based searches should also be consulted for inclusive searches of appropriate[10,11] databases, which may be a requirement for certain projects.

34.2.2.2 Pragmatic

Pragmatic justification (such as pilot studies) is needed to determine variations in data, to calculate a sample size and/or to confirm the logistical practicalities of performing a definitive study. Traditionally, an investigator performs a chart review or a small prospective study for these purposes. Electronic medical records and data-mining can facilitate this sort of data collection to guide research and may be helpful for "orphan" diseases (rare diseases where little published (or funded) research is available). Another preliminary approach is to simulate a study according to a mathematical model, using data from existing or hypothetical (virtual) patients using commercially available products.[12–13] Other pragmatic tools may provide insights as to cost-benefit or cost-effectiveness of studies. In the UK, the National Institute for Health and Clinical Excellence (NICE)[14] uses such models to justify, not only whether a research problem ought to be addressed, but also justifies the level of social financial investment.[15] Other resources include CRISP,[16] an online database of proposals funded by the NIH, and the Clinicaltrials.gov[17] databank of all ongoing clinical trials (which unfortunately lacks many pharmaceutical-company funded projects). Other trial data banks are available through online communities of interest.

34.2.2.3 Financial

Financial justification determines the level of funding needed to pay for services, salaries, and facilities. Systematic collection of data (research) requires resources beyond the operational assets typically available in the course of clinical and even administrative practice. The NIH budgets $29 billion annually for biomedical research, with $1.3 billion going to the National Institute of Child Health and Human Development.[18,19] There is a number of mechanisms of support, where the natural sequence for academic investigators starts with "K" and "F" awards (mentored research) or R21 (pilot) to R01 (investigator initiated) to P (Center grants). Other traditional sources include foundations and companies with interest in a clinical problem or particular disease, while federal agencies (such as AHRQ) fund projects in health services research and quality improvement. The World Wide Web has become the standard mechanism of announcing and locating announcements and submitting and tracking proposals. As of February 2007, all NIH research grants must be submitted electronically.

34.2.3 Designing a Study

Traditional study design is based on established methodologies and statistical models considered in the justification stage. Design is determined by the types of questions or hypotheses that are to be answered.[20,21] A central design question is "What is the unit of analysis?" or what is the entity from which data is being collected. In traditional clinical research, it is the patient (or human subject) who is the unit of analysis. In quality improvement research, it may be a clinical practice or care unit (such as a hospital). In public health research it may be a subpopulation of a community. In the evaluation of clinical information technology, it is the provider (the clinical user of IT) who is the unit of analysis (and sometimes the clinic or workplace).[22] Formalization of a study involves:

- Identification of a principal investigator and research team
- Definition of the purpose and methodology of the study
- Development of the protocol that defines subject eligibility, recruitment, enrollment, allocation, and reimbursements. Protocols also define all data, forms, and analyses that are to be collected or completed, all budgets related to the protocol and nonstandard procedures (for halting a study early, for example).

34.2.4 Obtaining Institutional Review Board Approval

The assurance of sound study design and adherence to shared principles of research ethics is the purpose of institutional review board (IRB) of a study project. The protocol submission and review process is typically complex, with multiple sources of information, participants, and steps to assure that the design and implementation of pediatric research protocols protects the population being studied. The complexity of the process has led to a number of Web-based protocol management tools to assure these steps.[23]

34.2.5 Executing the Protocol

Once IRB approval has been obtained, the processes of subject recruitment and enrollment, data collection and recording, and study management and budget tracking may be executed. Although many generic business IT and business applications that incorporate database and spreadsheet applications exist, the most important component in successful protocol execution is a competent research project manager.

34.2.5.1 Subject Recruitment and Enrollment

Subject recruitment, enrollment, registration, and group assignment depends on the number of eligible subjects. Recruitment activities may be explicitly specified, especially for children, to assure the ethical principles of autonomy, beneficence, justice, respect, non-malfeasance, and honesty. In the case of low prevalence of eligible candidates, such as children with "orphan disease," recruitment through patient communities of practice and interest, such as the Children's Oncology Group[24] may be possible and attractive to both researchers and subject populations. Such recruitment approaches may be useful in large organized communities (such as the Interactive Autism Network (IAN)[25] (see Case Study)) to raise awareness of current research trends. Enrollment, registration, and group assignments may be managed through a combination of telephone and Web site forms linked to a central database.

The Health Insurance Portability and Accountability Act of 1996[26] has impacted research in general[27] and pediatric research in particular.[28] A simulation study with eligible recruits suggests that inclusion of HIPAA-compliant language in informed consent may reduce participation by over 30% in African Americans.[29] The need for including protected health information (PHI) in informed consent has formalized recruitment and retention of research subjects.[30] The development of methods to recruit subjects without violating HIPAA conditions while creating usable datasets that are de-identified from at least the 18 defined items of PHI has been challenging.[31] Other challenges in de-identification include genomic data, which is currently not "protected," but which is specific to individuals.[32] A concise and informative examination of HIPAA, security, and research for academic institutions has been created.[33]

Pediatrics has a tradition of ambulatory-based research. Office-based, multisite research efforts have been facilitated through efforts of organizations such as the American Academy of Pediatrics Pediatric Research in Office Settings Network (PROS Net)[34,35] or the Slone Center[36,37] Large, simple randomized "studies," where patients are recruited without inclusion/exclusion or stratification criteria of traditional studies have been implemented using phone and fax, and are easier with the Internet.[38] Information technology has eased the ability of practices to join, either through facilitating registration or making data collection and participation simpler.

34.2.5.2 Data Collection and Recording

IT tools can facilitate data collection, storage, and transfer using secure wireless technology or well-designed personal digital assistant (PDA) applications. Such technologies work in locations as diverse as clinical offices, community settings and developing countries. One of the authors of this chapter (PL) has been very successful in incorporating PDA-based data collection in the Congo for the delivery of routine health information from disparate health stations to regional and then national offices. As useful as these device may be, they have their own vulnerabilities to errors: failures in uploading or downloading data and or manual entry errors.[39]

Researchers who reuse data from electronic patient records (EPR) for research studies must consider:

• Administrative privileges, including institutional review and HIPAA-related issues regarding the data collection process in the context of the study.
• The appropriateness of algorithms used to identify properly the numerators and denominators in the context of the question being asked and the population being studied.

- The appropriateness of the level of detail available and its adequacy and completeness for the research project.
- Data that is not included. In pediatrics, data fields that may not be included in adult encounter forms, such as weight or parents' names, must be considered when using electronic patient data for a protocol.
- The form of the data being collected. Photographed text records may be manually reviewable but not electronically usable. Researchers need to make allowances (including manual review and reconciliation) of a variety of data types that may be required by protocols, including photographic, biological, and genetic data.

Large collaborative efforts to collect clinical data for reuse in research include the cancer Biomedical Informatics Grid, or caBIG.[40] The NIH's recent effort in providing Clinical and Translational Science Awards[41] includes an Informatics Key Function,[42] with over ten Working groups or Taskforces, including data repositories and standards and interoperability.

34.2.5.3   Budget Management and Reporting

Decision support and scheduling tools, available through generic productivity tools for keeping track of budgets, clinical appointments and data submissions associated with research protocols are now ubiquitous and can be modified for research. Because of increasing demand for regulatory oversight of accurate and proper billing of services that are covered by clinical trials for patients who also receive medical care, continued development of tools to simplify navigation of the evolving complexities of compliance will be needed.[43]

34.2.6   Analyzing the Data

Beyond spreadsheets and programs that handle standard statistical models, specialized software that supports sophisticated modeling and data manipulation are available for data mining, factor analysis, structural equation models and belief/influence networks as well as visualization (such as geographical information systems).[44] Such tools can facilitate accurate result processing and facilitate monitoring of research for early termination of studies when a large benefit or unanticipated harm of an intervention is detected.

34.2.7   Publishing the Results

The standard model of publishing is via peer-review in recognized journals. Professional reputations are built on publications in journals according to their Impact Factor, a bibliometric measure of influence within the scientific community based on citation numbers and other factors. Publishing studies typically depends on submitting articles to journals in a standard format in which an author forfeits copyrights if the article is published.

Newer publishing models include online-only journals that allow writers to retain ownership of intellectual property. Biomed Central began in the UK as an "open access" journal. Authors pay the primary costs of publishing ranging from $195 (*Cases Journal*) to $2685 (*Genome Biology*)[45] unless their institutions are part of the BioMed Central consortium). BioMed Central hosts a number of journals, including BMC Pediatrics and Pediatric Rheumatology and BMC Public Health. The Public Library of Science (PLoS) has a similar model, provides an on-demand print options but does not have a pediatric-specific journal. As of April 7, 2008, full-text copies of all accepted final peer-reviewed manuscripts arising from NIH funds must be submitted to the NIH upon acceptance for publication[46,47] in the PubMed Central (PMC) archive, open for public access.

Yet another publishing model is making available the datasets on which studies are based into national and global[48-49] trial banks.

34.3   Information and Communication Technology and New Models for Research

Present efforts in building a national health information network (NHIN)[50,51] have shown promise for creating research opportunities on a large scale. First, regions, if not the whole country, will provide a population basis for any conclusions reached. Second, entire sets of patient data will be available, enabling high-quality outcomes. For instance, mortality and morbidity will be easier to measure, because all episodes will leave their footprints in the data set. "Population health," using data collected across medical records to provide research evidence, if only epidemiological, is a major strategic direction for the NHIN that has been outlined by the American Medical Informatics Association.[52]

34.3.1   Novel Uses of Information in Pediatric Care

Health information technology has provided novel information-based interventions. In the 1980s, the use of low-cost office-based computers to counsel adolescents about health proved successful.[53] More recently, the same approach, using Web-based applications has been part of ongoing efforts to evaluate the impact of Internet-available consumer-based information.[54] Provision of such information has been formalized as "information prescriptions,"[55] whose efficacy has already been evaluated in pediatrics.[56] One of the authors (HPL) is currently involved in a study of information prescriptions for parents of premature infants.

34.3.1.1 Analyzing Social Networks

Social network analysis (SNA) is based on theory of graphs or of how individuals are connected to each other. It is useful for studying relationships within groups of people as well as the spread through personal interaction of things as diverse as influence, infectious diseases, ideas, and adoption of technology. It is computationally-intensive, but analyses have increased with the availability of cheaper and more powerful computers and advances in computer science. SNA has been used to study pediatric phenomena such as the transmission of sexual infections,[57] bullying,[58] eating disorders[59] and tobacco use in adolescents.[60]

A key concept from the social network scientific community is that of "scale-free" networks. Scale-free means that the distribution of the number of links (to other nodes) that each node (e.g., a person, a website, a molecule) follows a power law. This means that a few nodes in a network will have a large number of links to other nodes, and hence are of central importance in the structure and operation of that network. For public health interventions, individual who are highly connected may be in a position to facilitate the dissemination of a new program to others.[61] Such individuals are often called "peer-opinion leaders."

34.3.1.2 Creating Communities of Practice

Collaborative communication and interactions, where physical distances do not pose barriers to participation, have been facilitated through the development and use of the Internet. The ability for communication among any group of people allows and empowers the development of virtual communities. In communities of practice, participants who share common interests, such as patients and families, researchers, and care providers may come together to solve common problems and to share solutions (see Case Study).

34.4 Conclusion: The Future

As research processes becomes fully represented and managed by information technology, new types of projects that were heretofore impossible or impractical can be undertaken. With widespread interoperable electronic medical and personalized health records, the NIH goal of speeding the translating of research into clinical practice can be realized by:

- Informing clinicians and patients (using decision support tools) about newly available treatments and opportunities to participate in clinical trials
- Incorporating practice into research and vice versa by IT-facilitated comparisons of the effectiveness of similar therapies using de-identified data collected from electronic records of ambulatory visits

- Integrating and warehousing data from formal and long-term studies such as the National Children's Study[62] on genetic and environment effects on children's health over time
- Providing on-demand interim analyses for pediatric safety[63]

Interoperable and connected medical records will provide a complex and rich set of observational data; all patient data will potentially provide evidence. We are only beginning to understand how to mine this new data source appropriately.

The relationship between research community and the public will change dramatically as society demands and technology provides greater transparency to the research process. With increasing availability of data from trial banks, researchers, and other readers will be able trace published results to the level of individual experiments. This level of accountability (and reproducibility) is already available in bioinformatics research as much of what is published is based on computational presentation of data,[64,65] and can be extended to novel presentations of traditional statistics[66] or "hybrid" combinations of data from heterogeneous sources.[67] As research "communities" broaden from academics to include patients and their families, new incentives and new questions for researchers and their subjects will arise, allowing knowledge translation and dissemination to feed back to sustain the research process.

34.5   Case Study: ISAAC/IAN – Informatics in Autism Research

Dr Paul Law, a pediatrician and Director of Medical Informatics at the Kennedy Krieger Institute in Baltimore, Maryland (along with Dr Allen Tien, President and Research Director at Medical Decision Logic, Inc. ("mdlogix") with IAN Research in Baltimore, Maryland), has developed information technology tools to empower research and advocacy in the area of autism.

In 1996, while working as a medical student at a reputable institution focused on developmental disabilities, I noticed inherent inefficiencies in the research process. There appeared to be little forward momentum in solving data management issues either across projects and investigators or between serial projects.

With this in mind, I began thinking about ways that technology development paths, in combination with administrative strategies, could lead to a technology platform for storing/processing data that would be more efficient and synergistic, avoiding the waste, duplication, and confusion inherent in our current way of doing things. At the same time, the Cure Autism Now Foundation was seeking a partner to develop a Web-based application to support the wide range of clinical data that would be collected as part of the Autism Genetics Resource Exchange (www.agre.org).

Keeping the future in mind, we agreed to create a system that would facilitate the efforts not only of AGRE, but of many autism researchers: the Internet System for Assessing Autistic Children (ISAAC).

34.5.1   ISAAC (Internet System for Assessing Autistic Children)

ISAAC was designed to meet an important and universal need of autism researchers: the management of data collected on paper forms. This included standard psychometric instruments with broad use as well as forms designed by single researchers for their own specific studies. After reviewing the needs of autism researchers in general and the AGRE project in particular, the following initial functions were developed:

- Form data management
- Data validation
- Automated scoring features for psychometric instruments
- User management (including role based functions)
- Data sharing features for multicenter studies or for researchers who otherwise want to share data
- Capacity to serve as a shared data warehouse
- Detailed and version specific codebooks for deciphering data
- Ability to protect proprietary content of the owners of psychometric instruments

To facilitate the integrity of this data system, all content was managed with a library of forms and questions which allowed us to repurpose content for everything from building dynamic data entry screens to automated download areas. The system was built using basic Web technology: Cold Fusion and a Microsoft SQL Server database, both hosted on a single NT server.

It is important to understand the dynamic interplay of content, functionality, and the contribution of varied projects that facilitated ISAAC's growth. Each new research project benefited from the efforts of those that had preceded it through savings in cost and effort in form design and programming. Many of the psychometric forms used in autism are already in widespread use and, once in existence, could be used at no cost, allowing time, money, and energy to be spent on research itself.

A philosophy of sharing for the greater good was essential. We were, in fact, demanding something of a paradigm shift from participants, as most researchers are accustomed to a competitive atmosphere where their work is concerned. Although early adopters experienced some anxiety about their contributions benefiting unknown colleagues and competitors, they forged ahead. It was made clear to investigators that their contributions in extending ISAAC functionality or content would be shared with other researches at no cost. Without early adopters' generosity of spirit and willingness to risk something new and untried, ISAAC would never have succeeded. The M.I.N.D. Institute of U.C. Davis, led lead by Dr. David Amaral, played a pivotal role by adopting ISAAC while it was still a very young project, contributing to it financially and promoting ISAAC's philosophy of sharing. (CAN subsidized most of ISAAC's start up cost, while the bulk of ongoing expenses was supported financially by the user-base.)

ISAAC has been a great success, ultimately used by over 60 projects, including those sponsored by four countries, the Centers for Disease Control (CDC), the National Institutes of Health (NIH), and several major universities.

34.5.2 IAN (Interactive Autism Network)

Building on experience gained through ISAAC, a revolutionary new autism research initiative was launched: the Interactive Autism Network (IAN), which includes IAN Community and IAN Research. A project of the Kennedy Krieger Institute generously funded by Autism Speaks, IAN links the autism community and researchers to accelerate the pace of autism research. IAN deals with each of the research steps discussed earlier in this chapter. The IAN Project overcomes obstacles to families' research participation while building on a philosophy of sharing. It is not a single autism research project, but a gateway to many projects.

IAN has launched IAN Exchange, an online community of practice which fosters global, interdisciplinary collaboration. Breakthroughs are often achieved when researchers depart their comfort zone, gaining exposure to ideas and theories germinating in other disciplines, in other institutions, or in other countries. IAN provides virtual meeting space, document storage and sharing capabilities, and private discussion forums to facilitate this process. It has the potential to be the virtual equivalent of an international interdisciplinary conference ... one that will go on 365 days a year. In the 3 months since its launch, IAN Exchange has engaged over 150 autism researchers working on a variety of projects.

IAN Research has two main parts: (1) for researchers, a tool for building and managing data collection forms, including detailed validation rules and also navigation rules ("skip logic"); and (2) for parents, a set of functions and interfaces that are easy to use and support parents in entering data and also seeing the results. Hence, IAN Research serves as a way for researchers to design novel surveys that can be implemented in collaboration with the IAN team. In accordance with our belief in parent collaboration, we welcome both researcher and parent feedback about the process as a whole.

IAN Research was implemented for Kennedy Krieger by mdlogix, based on the mdlogix Clinical Research Management System (CRMS), which is a suite of pure web application modules that supports and integrates a comprehensive set of health research processes, including subject recruitment, administrative management of the research, protocol execution, financial workflow, specimen tracking and banking, and data mining.

IAN is a research registry which matches researchers undertaking their own autism-focused studies and families who meet criteria for inclusion in the study. Our aim is to reduce the cost and time required to locate willing and qualified research participants while increasing sample sizes, to the benefit of all. So far, over 150 autism research projects, including the National Institutes of Health (NIH) and major universities, are recruiting subjects through IAN.

The project removes many of the obstacles to families' participation and enhances study recruitment. The parents of a child with autism face many stressors, in terms of time, freedom, and finances. They may find it impossible to overcome the demands of participating in a traditional autism study, such as having to take time off work or travel to a distant clinic or university. Through IAN, they can participate over the Internet, from home and at their convenience.

The project takes advantage of the fact that doing research on autism requires the measurement of nonbiological phenomena: behavior, communication styles and social approaches. These are usually captured by the use of psychometric tools, such as the Autism Diagnosic Interview – Revised (ADI-R), which rely on parent report. It is the people who live with a child with an autism spectrum disorder (ASD), after all, who naturally possess data on their child's behavior and way of being, over time and across settings. Using a web based interface, IAN solicits parents' knowledge and experience – information crucial to autism researchers.

IAN is designed to collect data from the parents of a child with an ASD in a secure online environment, offering a sense of privacy and other features that make data collection easier on the parent, such as being able to stop and start the process at their convenience.

We are currently collecting crucial longitudinal data on a variety of topics, from diagnosis to comorbidity, from family history to treatments and outcomes. Parents are also asked to complete the Social Communication Questionnaire (SCQ) and the Social Responsiveness Scale (SRS) – instruments measuring the core symptoms of autism over time. Content will be continually added to our online questionnaire based on the interest of families and researchers alike.

In accordance with our ongoing philosophy of sharing and dissemination, data collected is not held as proprietary, but is made available for use by the autism research community. Families are responding with enthusiasm to the opportunity to provide data and "be part of the solution." Eighteen months after the project's launch, more than 25,000 individuals are consented to participate in IAN, including over 8,000 children with ASD.

In brief, the Interactive Autism Network is utilizing a robust online shared research informatics environment, and engaging a vast array of stakeholders in every step of the research cycle, to facilitate the acceleration of autism research.

Acknowledgments Thanks to Peter Rowe for examples of scientific discovery in pediatrics.

References

1. US Food and Drug Administration. Guidances, Information Sheets, and Important Notices on Good Clinical Practice in FDA-Regulated Clinical Trials; 2008. Available at: http://www.fda.gov/oc/gcp/guidance.html. Accessed December 21, 2008.
2. Downs SM, Wallace MY. Mining association rules from a pediatric primary care decision support system. *AMIA Annu Symp*. 2000:200–204.

3. Chae YM, Kim HS, Tark KC, Park HJ, Ho SH. Analysis of healthcare quality indicator using data mining and decision support system. *Expert Syst Appl.* 2003;24(2):167–172.
4. American Academy of Pediatrics. Clinical Practice Guidelines. Available at: http://aappolicy. aappublications.org/practice_guidelines/index.dtl. Accessed December 20, 2008.
5. Agency for Healthcare Research and Quality. National Guideline Clearinghouse. Rockville, MD; 2008. Available at: http://www.guideline.gov/. Accessed December 20, 2008.
6. The Cochrane Collaboration. Cochrane Collaboration Website; 2008. Available at: http:// www.cochrane.org/. Accessed December 20, 2008.
7. Higgins JPT, Green S. Cochrane Handbook for Systematic Reviews of Interventions. Oxfordshire, UK: Wiley.
8. Cochrane Child Health Field. Cochrane Child Health Website, Edmonton, Alberta, CANADA; 2008. Available at: http://www.cochranechildhealth.ualberta.ca/index.html. Accessed December 20, 2008.
9. National Library of Medicine. PubMed Clinical Queries; 2008. Available at: http://www.ncbi. nlm.nih.gov/entrez/query/static/clinical.shtml. Accessed December 20, 2008.
10. National Library of Medicine. OLDMEDLINE; 2008. Available at: http://www.nlm.nih.gov/ databases/databases_oldmedline.html. Accessed December 20, 2008.
11. Elsevier. Embase.com; 2008. Available at: http://www.embase.com/. Accessed December 20, 2008.
12. Pharsight Corporation. Pharsight Knowledgebase Server; 2008. Available at: http://www. pharsight.com/main.php. Accessed December 20, 2008.
13. Cambridge University, MRC Biostatistics Unit. The BUGS Project; 2008. Available at: http:// www.mrc-bsu.cam.ac.uk/bugs/. Accessed December 20, 2008.
14. National Health Service's National Institute for Health and Clinical Excellence. Paediatric Guidances; 2008. Available at: http://www.nice.org.uk/search/guidancesearchresults.jsp? keywords=paediatric&searchType=guidance. Accessed December 20, 2008.
15. Claxton KP, Sculpher MJ. Using Value of Information Analysis to Prioritise Health Research: Some Lessons from Recent UK Experience. *Pharmaco Economics.* 2006;24(11):1055–1068.
16. National Institutes of Health ERA Commons. Computer Retrieval of Information on Scientific Projects (CRISP) Database; 2008. Available at: http://crisp.cit.nih.gov/. Accessed December 20, 2008.
17. National Library of Medicine. ClinicalTrials.gov; 2008. Available at: http://clinicaltrials.gov/. Accessed December 20, 2008.
18. Tauberer J. GovTrack.us: H.R. 3043–110th Congress: Departments of Labor, Health and Human Services, and Education, and Related Agencies Appropriations Act, 2008. Available at: http://govtrack.us. Accessed December 20, 2008.
19. National Institutes of Health Office of the Budget. IC Distribution of FY 2008 Enacted Level With Supplemental; 2008. Available at: http://officeofbudget.od.nih.gov/ui/fy2008elws.html. Accessed December 20, 2008.
20. Swinscow TDV. Statistics at Square One. *BMJ*; 1997. Available at: http://www.bmj.com/ statsbk. Accessed December 20, 2008.
21. Modgil S, Hammond P. Decision support tools for clinical trial design. *Artif Intell Med.* 2007;27(2):181–200.
22. Chuang JH, Hripcsak G, Heitjan DF. Design and analysis of controlled trials in naturally clustered environments: implications for medical informatics. *J Am Med Inform Assoc.* 2002;9(3):230–238.
23. Goldfarb NM. Save the planet: eIRB solutions for everyone. *J Clin Res Best Prac.* 2006;2(2). Available at: http://firstclinical.com/journal/2006/0602_eIRB.pdf. Accessed December 20, 2008.
24. CureSearch. Cancer Oncology Group. Our Research; 2005. Available at: http://www.cure-search.org/our_research/. Accessed December 20, 2008.
25. Interactive Autism Network. Research; 2006. Available at: https://www.ianresearch.org/. Accessed December 20, 2008.
26. Office for Civil Rights. HIPAA: Medical Privacy - National Standards to Protect the Privacy of Personal Health Information; 2008. Available at: http://www.hhs.gov/ocr/hipaa/consumer_ rights.pdf. Accessed December 20, 2008.

27. Shalowitz D, Wendler D. Informed consent for research and authorization under the Health Insurance Portability and Accountability Act Privacy Rule: an integrated approach. *Ann Intern Med.* 2006;144(9):685–688.

28. Barnard J, Fine D. The HIPAA Privacy Rule and its impact on pediatric research. *J Pediatr Gastroenterol Nutr.* 2003;37(5):527.

29. Dunlop AL, Graham T, Leroy Z, Glanz K, Dunlop B. The impact of HIPAA authorization on willingness to participate in clinical research. *Ann Epidemiol.* 2007;17(11):899–905.

30. Wipke-Tevis DD, Pickett MA. Impact of the Health Insurance Portability and Accountability Act on participant recruitment and retention. *West J Nurs Res.* 2008;30(1):39–53.

31. National Institutes of Health. How Can Covered Entities Use and Disclose Protected Health Information for Research and Comply with the Privacy Rule?; 2008 Available at: http://privacyruleandresearch.nih.gov/pr_08.asp. Accessed December 20, 2008.

32. Malin BA. An evaluation of the current state of genomic data privacy protection technology and a roadmap for the future. *J Am Med Inform Assoc.* 2005;12(1):28–34.

33. Masys D. Research and the HIPAA Security Rule. Association of American Medical Colleges; 2005. Available at: http://www.aamc.org/members/gir/hipaa/researchsecurityrule.pdf. Accessed July 21, 2008.

34. American Academy of Pediatrics. Pediatric Research in Office Settings (PROS); 2008. Available at: http://www.aap.org/pros/. Accessed December 20, 2008.

35. Barkin SL, Finch SA, Ip EH, Scheindlin B, Craig JA, Steffes J, et al. Is office-based counseling about media use, timeouts, and firearm storage effective? Results from a cluster-randomized, controlled trial. *Pediatr.* 2008;122(1):e15–e25.

36. Boston University Slone Epidemiology Network. Slone Center Office-based Research (SCOR) Network; 2008. Available at: http://www.bu.edu/slone/Research/Studies/SCOR/SCOR.htm. Accessed December 20, 2008.

37. Vernacchio L, Vezina RM, Mitchell AA. Management of acute otitis media by primary care physicians: trends since the release of the 2004 American Academy of Pediatrics/American Academy of Family Physicians clinical practice guideline. *Pediatr.* 2007;120(2):281–287.

38. Hilbrich L, Sleight P. Progress and problems for randomized clinical trials: from streptomycin to the era of megatrials. *Eur Heart J.* 2006;27(18):2158–2164.

39. Shelby-James TM, Abernethy AP, McAlindon A, Currow DC. Handheld computers for data entry: high tech has its problems too. *Trials.* 2007;8:5.

40. National Cancer Institute. caBIG: Cancer Biomedical Informatics Grid; 2008. Available at: https://cabig.nci.nih.gov/. Accessed December 20, 2008.

41. National Institutes of Health. Clinical and Translational Science Awards: Translating Discoveries to Medical Practice; 2008. Available at: http://www.ctsaweb.org/. Accessed December 20, 2008.

42. Clinical and Translational Science Awards. Informatics; 2008. Available at: http://www.ctsaweb.org/index.cfm?fuseaction=committee.viewCommittee&com_ID=9. Accessed December 20, 2008.

43. Boyd CE, Meade RD. Clinical trial billing compliance at academic medical centers. *Acad Med.* 2007;82(7):646–653.

44. Roberts EM, English PB, Wong M, et al. Progress in pediatric asthma surveillance II: geospatial patterns of asthma in Alameda County, California. *Prev Chronic Dis.* 2006;3(3):A92.

45. Biomed Central. Frequently asked questions about BioMed Central's article-processing charges; 2008. Available at: http://www.biomedcentral.com/info/about/apcfaq#howmuch. Accessed December 20, 2008.

46. National Institutes of Health. NIH Public Access; 2008. Available at: http://publicaccess.nih.gov/. Accessed December 20, 2008.

47. Glover SW, Webb A, Gleghorn C. Open access publishing in the biomedical sciences: could funding agencies accelerate the inevitable changes? *Health Info Libr J.* 2006;23(3):197–202.

48. American Medical Informatics Association. Global Trial Bank; 2006. Available at: http://www.amia.org/gtb/. Accessed December 20, 2008.

49. Sim I, Carini S, Olasov B, Jeng S. Trial bank publishing: phase I results. *MEDINFO.* 2004;11(Pt 2):1476–1480.

50. Thompson TG, Brailer DJ. *The Decade of Health Information Technology: Delivering Consumer-Centric and Information-Rich Health Care*. Bethesda, MD: DHHS; 2004.
51. Office of the National Coordinator. *The ONC-Coordinated Federal Health IT Strategic Plan: 2008–2012*. Bethesda, MD: National Insitutes of Health; 2008.
52. Safran C, Bloomrosen M, Hammond WE, Labkoff S, Markel-Fox S, Tang PC, et al. Toward a national framework for the secondary use of health data: an american medical informatics association white paper. *J Am Med Inform Assoc: JAMIA*. 2007;14(1):1–9.
53. Paperny DM, Aono JY, Lehman RM, Hammar SL, Risser J. Computer-assisted detection and intervention in adolescent high-risk health behaviors. *J Pediatrics*. 1990;116(3):456–462.
54. Wagner TH, Greenlick MR. When parents are given greater access to health information, does it affect pediatric utilization? *Med Care*. 2001;39(8):848–855.
55. Williams MD, Gish KW, Giuse NB, Sathe NA, Carrell DL. The Patient Informatics Consult Service (PICS): an approach for a patient-centered service. *Bull Med Libr Assoc*. 2001;89(2):185–193.
56. D'Alessandro DM, Kreiter CD, Kinzer SL, Peterson MW. A randomized controlled trial of an information prescription for pediatric patient education on the internet. *Arch Pediatr Adolesc Med*. 2004;158(9):857–862.
57. Ellen JM, Gaydos C, Chung SE, Willard N, Lloyd LV, Rietmeijer CA. Sex partner selection, social networks, and repeat sexually transmitted infections in young men: a preliminary report. *Sex Transm Dis*. 2006;33(1):18–21.
58. Bollmer JM, Milich R, Harris MJ, Maras MA. A friend in need: the role of friendship quality as a protective factor in peer victimization and bullying. *J Interpers Violence*. 2005;20(6):701–712.
59. Hutchinson DM, Rapee RM. Do friends share similar body image and eating problems? The role of social networks and peer influences in early adolescence. *Behav Res Ther*. 2007;45(7):1557–1577.
60. Hall JA, Valente TW. Adolescent smoking networks: the effects of influence and selection on future smoking. *Addict Behav*. 2007;32(12):3054–3059.
61. Valente TW, Hoffman BR, Ritt-Olson A, Lichtman K, Johnson CA. Effects of a social-network method for group assignment strategies on peer-led tobacco prevention programs in schools. *Am J Public Health*. 2003;93(11):1837–1843.
62. Landrigan PJ, Trasande L, Thorpe LE, et al. The National Children's Study: a 21-year prospective study of 100,000 American children. *Pediatrics*. 2006;118(5):2173–2186.
63. Hirtz DG, Gilbert PR, Terrill CM, Buckman SY. Clinical trials in children–How are they implemented? *Pediatr Neurol*. 2006;34(6):436–438.
64. Gentleman R. Reproducible research: a bioinformatics case study. *Stat Appl Genet Mol Biol*. 2005;4: Article 2.
65. Bova GS, Eltoum IA, Kiernan JA, Siegal GP, Frost AR, Best CJ, et al. Optimal molecular profiling of tissue and tissue components: defining the best processing and microdissection methods for biomedical applications. *Mol Biotechnol*. 2005;29(2):119–152.
66. Lehmann HP, Goodman SN. Bayesian communication: a clinically significant paradigm for electronic publication. *J Am Med Inform Assoc.: JAMIA*. 2000;7(3):254–266.
67. Cheung KH, Yip KY, Townsend JP, Scotch M. HCLS 2.0/3.0: health care and life sciences data mashup using Web 2.0/3.0. *J Biomed Inform*. 2008;41(5):694–705.

Part VII
A Vision and Current Landscape of Pediatrics

Chapter 35
The Moving Picture of Pediatric Informatics

George R. Kim and Stuart T. Weinberg

Objectives

- To envision a possible future of child health
- To outline the roles and limitations of pediatric informatics in realizing the vision
- To suggest frontiers of research, development and advocacy

35.1 Introduction

35.1.1 Case Study: A Vision of the Future of Child Health

Johnny Q is an 11-year-old boy with a history of mild intermittent asthma, who develops a slight cough and begins to wheeze while in school. He is sent to the school nurse who notes slight wheezing on auscultation. Johnny also states that his throat hurts.

The nurse measures his vital signs, pulse oximetry, and peak flow using a hand-held recording device that records the data and transmits it to her desktop computer. A computer application opens Johnny's personal health record (PHR), which opens to a problem list with records of his treatments for asthma. The encounter is time-stamped and the handheld data is entered into the new record. A text message is sent to Johnny's mother cell phone (as specified whenever Johnny's PHR is opened).

The nurse reviews Johnny's recent history. She notes his diagnosis is mild intermittent asthma, but that he has had several attacks requiring visits to the nurse and one to the emergency department of the local hospital. She asks if he has been taking his bronchodilator via metered dose inhaler (MDI) as prescribed, which he affirms, noting he has needed it several times a week, more than previously, since football season started.

The graphical results of the data collected from the handheld appear on the computer screen. Johnny's peak flow is in the "yellow" zone and his oxygen

C.U. Lehmann et al. (eds.), *Pediatric Informatics: Computer Applications in Child Health,* Health Informatics,
© Springer Science+Business Media, LLC 2011

saturation is greater than 94%. The nurse presses a "Send" button on the screen and the information is sent to Johnny's pediatric Medical Home to the practitioner in the clinic that morning. By Johnny's mother's request, a copy is also sent via text message to her.

The computer beeps. A message from the practice is returned to the nurse, which notes the pediatrician's review of the data, and that instructs her to follow an order set created for Johnny's asthma exacerbations: administration of an albuterol metered dose, with recheck of vital signs in 10 min. Johnny, who has already performed this several times, has already taken his spacer and MDI from the storage locker in the nurse's office. The nurse administers the albuterol.

The phone rings. It is Johnny's mother, who was able to excuse herself from her meeting. She asks how Johnny is doing, and the nurse reassures her and informs her of his progress. Johnny's mother asks if the doctor has called, and the nurse tells her of the assessment and order. Johnny's mother tells the nurse that she will be in a meeting, but will be reachable via cell phone. The time of the phone message is recorded, and the nurse enters a note and adds the cell phone number to the contact information in the PHR encounter.

The computer beeps again. The new vital signs return. The nurse instructs Johnny to provide a peak flow measurement and records the measurement. It is in the green zone. She sends the data to the practice office (again with a copy is sent to Johnny's mother's cell phone). The computer beeps a third time. A chat box from the practice opens. The pediatrician has reviewed the new data. The nurse sends a structured message that reviews the visit with an assessment that Johnny has improved. The pediatrician returns that Johnny should start a second protocol (that is in his PHR) with an inhaled corticosteroid dose to be given in the nurse's office, with follow up with the practice later that evening. The pediatrician also instructs the nurse to run a quick strep test, which is negative, which she enters into the encounter record. The pediatrician signs off, and the school nurse sends Johnny back to class.

The nurse completes a text message form that summarizes the visit and provides home instructions and recommends follow up care with the Medical Home physician using an appointment time provided by the pediatrician's office staff. The nurse closes the computer record, updating the medication record and vital signs in the PHR. Johnny's mother receives an e-mail alert that Johnny's PHR has been modified and a copy of the report is now available for her review (Since Johnny is still a minor, she has full access to his record according to state law). The encounter data is forwarded via a secure connection to the practice for the evening visit. The coding and billing for the visit in the nurse's office and the tele-consultation from the pediatric practice are automatically documented and forwarded to the state child health insurance program for reimbursement. The school health administrator also receives an electronic copy of the encounter for billing and to track inventory use to replace the disposable equipment used during the visit.

Later in the month, the collected clinical data from all school nurse visits in the county and the state are de-identified and sent to a regional registry created by a partnership between the school system, the pediatric practice (as a member of the local pediatric professional society) and the state child health insurance program.

The purpose of the registry is to collect data on the impact of low cost telemedicine tools in schools to extend pediatric care and reduce preventable emergency department visits for asthma exacerbations in children.

Over 1 year, there is a clinical and statistical reduction of morbidity, mortality, and emergency department utilization in the counties that used telemedicine, resulting in improved health in the pediatric asthma population and a significant savings for the insurance program. These results are presented to the state legislature, and result in expanded funding to provide telemedicine services, training for school nurses, and pediatric Medical Homes for better asthma care in all counties throughout the state. Publication of these results draws interest from researchers and health information technology vendors interested in reproducing their results in other states and in making similar health outcome improvements for other pediatric conditions.

35.1.2   Ideals and Constraints of Pediatrics

The vision and ideal of pediatrics, regardless of technology, is the attainment (and maintenance) of optimal physical, mental, and social health and well being of all infants, children, adolescents and young adults. This vision encompasses the bio-psycho-socio-cultural spectrum of children, from genetics and environmental exposures to economic, ethical and legal issues; from primary prevention to technology-based invasive procedures. This ideal includes:

- Universal and lifelong health care access and coverage
- Personalized medicine for all, coordinated through a Medical Home, with timely and ongoing translation of a patient's genomic, historical, and environmental data into effective customized care plans for maintaining health, managing emergent problems, and planning care
- Measurable and equitable improvements in health outcomes and care quality with reductions in morbidity and mortality that have heretofore been elusive
- Ongoing public health surveillance for threats to children's health with timely interventions
- Widespread and ubiquitous implementation and deployment of pediatric-specific care processes that are error-free and that provide complete transparency and accountability
- Complete partnership between patients/parents/caretakers who make informed decisions about their children's health care and a health care system that empowers patients to achieve and maintain optimum health

Current (and ongoing) constraints to realizing the pediatric vision include:

- The rising costs of health care, including technology-driven interventions
- Limitations in capital, health workforce, and pediatric expertise
- Disparities in the availability and distribution of pediatric expertise among urban and rural, academic, and community settings

- Lack of a consistent infrastructure to monitor/measure the quality and impact of health interventions and to collect data easily, accurately and in a timely fashion
- Barriers to effective communication with patients and families due to language, literacy, education, and cultural issues
- Uncertainty and complexity in medical knowledge, decision making (in domains such as pediatric oncology and rare diseases) and health care processes (such as chemotherapy and clinical trials)
- Conflicts in political and economic interests that de-prioritize the health needs of children

35.2 The Roles of Information Technology and Informatics in the Vision

35.2.1 Opportunities to Improve Pediatric Care

Information technology can help overcome these constraints by:

- Providing access to timely, appropriate pediatric expertise by remote patients and practitioners through communication and telemedicine applications
- Empowering families and physicians to control and share health care information in ways that strengthen the patient–family–pediatrician relationship, through the development and use of interoperable electronic health records and personal health records
- Assuring real-time availability, integrity and confidentiality of patient health information when and where it is needed (specialty clinics, emergency departments, disaster situations) from wherever it is (hospital/laboratory/pharmacy systems, regional health information organizations registries), coordinated and managed through interoperable Medical Home information systems
- Streamlining medical work by facilitating access to information, guiding clinical choices, providing knowledge-based alerts and reminders[1] and other forms of clinical decision support systems
- Reducing errors by automating and standardizing of health care processes (such as inpatient medication delivery) via order entry, transaction auditing, and error tracking

35.2.2 Limitations of Information Technology in the Vision

Information technology alone cannot improve outcomes. Applications may fail for many reasons, including organizational and personnel issues.[2] Fitting IT tools to clinical tasks requires understanding how health care differs from other industries:

- The central entity (and unit of analysis) in health care is the continuing patient–provider relationship, not single transactions. In pediatrics, the relationship is between the family and the health care team.
- Health care interactions go beyond simple vendor–client transactions. There are two (or more) centers of control (patient/family and providers) and disagreements in health decisions are often not solvable by a simple cancellation of transactions. In pediatrics, the responsibility of the provider to the patient may not always be aligned with the interests of the family. Transactions are only part of the ongoing interaction and relationship between patient/family and provider.
- Patient–provider relationships change over time, involving multiple decision-makers (family, patient, or guardians) and multiple providers (primary care providers and specialists) who may not be in direct communication with each other at all times. Changes in providers (care transitions that may range from inpatient "change of shifts" to the "graduation" of a teenager from a pediatric to adult Medical Home) involve transfers of information, authority, and responsibility,[3] which are often more detailed than in other industries, but which may be helped by use of tools such as standard checklists.[4] In pediatrics, an increasing number of children with special health care needs (such as those with congenital cardiac conditions[5]) are surviving to adulthood, creating new populations of vulnerable adults that need primary and speciality care for what had previously been pediatric problems.[6]
- Nuances in communications may be difficult to capture formally, but may have significant impact on outcomes. In pediatrics, these interactions may include unarticulated "hidden agendas"[7] that may be related to different segments of a child's world: family, school, social groups, etc.
- Legal requirements for confidentiality and documentation are more complex than other industries with great practice variance (such as known maternal HIV status[8] that is not formally documented). In pediatrics, such variances, which are in most cases determined by local jurisdiction, may lead to delays in appropriate care.
- Health care transactions and their documentation are subject to the same vulnerabilities to errors (misidentification, calculation errors, mistakes, slips, etc.) and deceptions (misrepresentation, counterfeiting, fraud, intentional misdiagnosis, etc.) as in other industries, but have the added impacts of the clinical consequences of those errors. Children have higher vulnerabilities to medical errors and their impacts than adults.

Information technology **cannot** replace human participation in:

- Creating policies that provide universal access to health services and information
- Designing tools that cross language and literacy barriers
- Fitting IT applications to human workflows in clinical environments
- Evaluating the impact of IT interventions on health outcomes
- Changing human behavior

Information technology **should not** replace:

- Interpersonal components of pediatric care: meeting families on the first visit (including mutual acquaintance of family and provider through comprehensive history and thorough physical examination)
- Ongoing communication and education of patients and families on anticipatory guidance and management of acute and chronic disease
- Person-to-person reassurance and guidance in patient and family decisions for care in response to the new clinical information (laboratory test results, consultations, etc.)
- Direct sharing of information (when possible) with another provider when a patient's care is transferred (either temporarily or permanently)

35.3 New Problems in Communication, Culture and Health

35.3.1 Diversity and Disparity: A New Babel?

Increasing diversity in the US population is creating an increasing need for solutions that address auditory/visual, language,[9] literacy,[10] cultural[11,12] and health literacy[13] barriers and disparities in access to health (and health information) services. Solutions to eliminate these barriers and disparities[14,15] must include information tools and services to help patients, families and providers to communicate[16,17] health information with their providers. Solutions will likely need to combine accessibility and translation tools, interpreter services and provider language training. A major challenge will include cost management of developing and maintaining resources.

35.3.2 Information Technology in Real Life: A Brave New World?

The pervasiveness information and communication technology (ICT) and media have created new needs for research into its direct effects on children's health. Biological effects associated with ICT and media have included:

- Photosensitive seizures[18,19] triggered by television, leading to technical restrictions in television programming
- Repetitive strain injury and tendonitis with computer game use and overuse[20]
- Obesity and its sequelae, associated with time-displacement, increased caloric intake and reduced metabolic rates during television viewing.[21–24] There appears to be an association with the length of time spent on ICT activities (which may be less for computers than television[25,26]), and certain computer game designs[27–29] may increase physical activity (dancing).[30]

Psychosocial and cultural effects include:

- Distraction of drivers[31] and pedestrians[32] by mobile devices may increase injury risks.
- Excessive television and computer use may have negative effects on children's sleep, learning and memory.[33] Early exposure to television may be associated with broadening knowledge, but also with attention[34,35] and school performance problems[36]
- Media use may be linked to body image and eating disorders[37]
- The portrayal of unhealthy or unsafe lifestyle practices[38–41] in television, movies, and music may be linked to promotion of such behaviors in youth.
- Social networking tools may help children and teens in health[42] and illness,[43,44] but may also pose threats to their health and safety,[45] including victimization by predators,[46] cyber-bullying,[47–49] media violence[50] and sale of unsafe products.[51] Little published evidence to date exists on the effect of Internet sites on behavior.[52]

Efforts to counter negative effects of technology for children include developing awareness of the issues[53] and education. A recent partnership between the American Academy of Pediatrics and the Microsoft Corporation has been established to help create a safe online environment[54] for children.

As society becomes progressively connected and diversified, new (and unforeseen) problems will undoubtedly emerge providing new opportunities for innovation.

35.4   Epilog: Pediatric Informatics – A Moving Picture

"Knowledge is of two kinds. We know a subject ourselves, or we know where we can find information upon it." – Samuel Johnson

Improving pediatric care and child health will require improvements in the control of information surrounding that care. However, pediatricians cannot do this alone.

- ***It requires more than just technology.*** Pediatricians must be able to share their expertise of child health, to ask appropriate questions and to understand why and how information technology can improve (or worsen) pediatric care processes. Pediatricians must be able to collaborate effectively with IT developers through clear articulation of information needs and active feedback during design, implementation and deployment of systems (such as electronic health records) to achieve health care goals.
- ***It requires political awareness and informed advocacy.*** Pediatricians must be aware of current business and regulatory issues related to health IT that affect the quality, safety and viability of pediatric care and practice. Pediatricians must be able to advocate collectively and knowledgeably as child health experts, to legislators, regulators, health care leadership and funders, on all health IT issues related to pediatrics. This may require development of alliances with other health care and information technology groups.

- *It requires multidisciplinary collaboration.* Pediatricians must establish and maintain alliances with other members of the health care team (families, specialists, nurses and pharmacists and institutional leadership) as an essential part of "systems-based practice."[55] Health care providers and developers must keep in mind that effective health information management is only part of any solution to optimize pediatric care and safety.

The development of a pediatric community of practice (CoP)[56] that includes families, physicians, nurses and other advocates can strengthen collaborations to improve child health as well as help build the infrastructure needed to improve the control of health care information. Ubiquitous tools such as e-mail, the Web, mobile computing and cellular telephones now connect practitioners to online communities of peers and experts through professional organizations (such as the American Academy of Pediatrics and the American Medical Informatics Association) for collective problem-solving in ways which would previously have been time-consuming if not impossible. In fact, it has been the shared work of such a community that created this text and forms the basis for future work in pediatric informatics.

The aim of this text is to introduce pediatric informatics (a developing area of applied clinical informatics) and its concepts, to pediatricians, other health professionals and IT developers by providing pointers to relevant literature, to online resources and to members within its growing community of practice. Unlike texts, the living community is not static, but evolves continually as the science, practice and business of pediatrics evolve. Therefore, a second aim of the book is to invite readers to explore and to participate in the community of pediatric informatics (The Appendix contains a partial list of associated organizations and resources) in your own efforts in leveraging information technology to improve child health.

References

1. Perreault L, Metzger J. A pragmatic framework for understanding clinical decision support. *J Healthcare Inf Manage.* 1999;13(2):5–21.
2. Lorenzi NM, Smith JB, Conner SR, Campion TR. The success factor profile for clinical computer innovation. *Medinfo.* 2004;11(Pt 2):1077–1080.
3. Behara R, Wears RL, Perry SJ, et al. A conceptual framework for studying the safety of transitions in emergency care. In: *Advances in Patient Safety: From Research to Implementation. Vol. 2, Concepts and Methodology.* Rockville, MD: Agency for Healthcare Research and Quality; 2005.
4. Arora V, Johnson J. National patient safety goals: a model for building a standardized hand-off protocol. *Joint Comm J Qual Patient Safety* 2006;32(11):646–655.
5. Reid GJ, Irvine MJ, McCrindle BW, et al. Prevalence and correlates of successful transfer from pediatric to adult health care among a cohort of young adults with complex congenital heart defects. *Pediatrics.* 2004;113(3 Pt 1):e197–205.
6. Barr M, Ginsburg J. *The Advanced Medical Home: A Patient-Centered, Physician-Guided Model of Health Care*, A Policy Monograph. Philadelphia, PA: American College of Physicians; 2006.

7. Menahem S. Teaching students of medicine to listen: the missed diagnosis from a hidden agenda. *J R Soc Med.* 1987;80(6):343–346.
8. Taylor AW, Ruffo N, Griffith J, et al. The missing link: documentation of recognized maternal human immunodeficiency virus infection in exposed infant birth records, 24 United States jurisdictions, 1999-2003. *Am J Obstet Gynecol.* 2007;197(3 suppl):S132–136.
9. Kuo DZ, O'Connor KG, Flores G. Minkovitz CS. Pediatricians' use of language services for families with limited English proficiency. *Pediatrics.* 2007;119(4):e920–927.
10. Sentell TL, Halpin HA. Importance of adult literacy in understanding health disparities. *J Gen Intern Med.* 2006;21(8):862–866.
11. Schyve PM. Language differences as a barrier to quality and safety in health care: the Joint Commission perspective. *J Gen Intern Med.* 2007;22(2 suppl):360–361.
12. Thibodeaux AG, Deatrick JA. Cultural influence on family management of children with cancer. *J Pediatr Oncol Nurs.* 2007;24(4):227–233.
13. Hironaka LK, Paasche-Orlow MK. The implications of health literacy on patient-provider communication. *Arch Dis Child.* 2008;93(5):428–432.
14. Partida Y. Addressing language barriers: building response capacity for a changing nation. *J Gen Intern Med.* 2007;22(2 suppl):347–349.
15. Grant R, Shapiro A, Joseph S, Goldsmith S, Rigual-Lynch L, Redlener I. The health of homeless children revisited. *Adv Pediatr.* 2007;54:173–187.
16. Ngo-Metzger Q, Sorkin DH, Phillips RS, et al. Providing high-quality care for limited English proficient patients: the importance of language concordance and interpreter use. *J Gen Intern Med.* 22(2 suppl):324–330.
17. Green AR, Ngo-Metzger Q, Legedza AT, Massagli MP, Phillips RS, Iezzoni LI. Interpreter services, language concordance, and health care quality. Experiences of Asian Americans with limited english proficiency. *J Gen Intern Med.* 2005;20(11):1050–1056.
18. Ishida S, Yamashita Y, Matsuishi T, et al. Photosensitive seizures provoked while viewing "pocket monsters," a made-for-television animation program in Japan. *Epilepsia.* 1998;39(12):1340–1344.
19. Fisher RS, Harding G, Erba G, Barkley GL, Wilkins A. Epilepsy Foundation of America Working Group. Photic- and pattern-induced seizures: a review for the Epilepsy Foundation of America Working Group. *Epilepsia.* 2005;46(9):1426–1441.
20. Zapata AL, Moraes AJ, Leone C, Doria-Filho U, Silva CA. Pain and musculoskeletal pain syndromes related to computer and video game use in adolescents. *Eur J Pediatr.* 2006;165(6):408–414.
21. Ortega FB, Ruiz JR, Sjostrom M. Physical activity, overweight and central adiposity in Swedish children and adolescents: the European Youth Heart Study. *Int J Behav Nutr Phys Act.* 2007;4(1):61.
22. Kautiainen S, Koivusilta L, Lintonen T, Virtanen SM, Rimpelä A. Use of information and communication technology and prevalence of overweight and obesity among adolescents. *Int J Obes (Lond).* 2005;29(8):925–933.
23. Robinson TN. Television viewing and childhood obesity. *Pediatr Clin North Am.* 2004;48(4):1017–1025.
24. McGavock J, Sellers E, Dean H. Physical activity for the prevention and management of youth-onset type 2 diabetes mellitus: focus on cardiovascular complications. *Diab Vasc Dis Res.* 2007;4(4):305–310.
25. Rey-Lopez JP, Vicente-Rodríguez G, Biosca M, Moreno LA. Sedentary behaviour and obesity development in children and adolescents. *Nutr Metab Cardiovasc Dis.* 2008;18(3):242–251.
26. Kautiainen S, Koivusilta L, Lintonen T, Virtanen SM, Rimpela A. Use of information and communication technology and prevalence of overweight and obesity among adolescents. *Int J Obes (Lond).* 2005;29(8):925–933.
27. Lanningham-Foster L, Jensen TB, Foster RC, et al. Energy expenditure of sedentary screen time compared with active screen time for children. *Pediatrics.* 2006;118(6):e1831–1835.

28. Maddison R, Mhurchu CN, Jull A, Jiang Y, Prapavessis H, Rodgers A. Energy expended playing video console games: an opportunity to increase children's physical activity? *Pediatr Exerc Sci.* 2007;19(3):334–343.
29. Tan B, Aziz AR, Chua K, Teh KC. Aerobic demands of the dance simulation game. *Int J Sports Med.* 2002;23(2):125–129.
30. Unnithan VB, Houser W, Fernhall B. Evaluation of the energy cost of playing a dance simulation video game in overweight and non-overweight children and adolescents. *Int J Sports Med.* 2006;27(10):804–809.
31. McCartt AT, Hellinga LA, Bratiman KA. Cell phones and driving: review of research. *Traffic Inj Prev.* 2006;7(2):89–106.
32. Hatfield J, Murphy S. The effects of mobile phone use on pedestrian crossing behaviour at signalized and unsignalized intersections. *Accid Anal Prev.* 2007;39(1):197–205.
33. Dworak M, Schierl T, Bruns T, Strüder HK. Impact of singular excessive computer game and television exposure on sleep patterns and memory performance of school-aged children. *Pediatrics.* 2007;120(5):978–985.
34. Thakkar RR, Garrison MM, Christakis DA. A systematic review for the effects of television viewing by infants and preschoolers. *Pediatrics.* 2006;118(5):2025–2031.
35. Mistry KB, Minkovitz CS, Strobino DM, Borzekowski DL. Children's television exposure and behavioral and social outcomes at 5.5 years: does timing of exposure matter? *Pediatrics.* 2007;120(4):762–769.
36. Sharif I, Sargent JD. Association between television, movie, and video game exposure and school performance. *Pediatrics.* 2006;118(4):e1061–1070.
37. Borzekowski DL, Bayer AM. Body image and media use among adolescents. *Adolesc Med Clin.* 2005;16(2):289–313.
38. Wellman RJ, Sugarman DB, DiFranza JR, Winickoff JP. The extent to which tobacco marketing and tobacco use in films contribute to children's use of tobacco: a meta-analysis. *Arch Pediatr Adolesc Med.* 2006;160(12):1285–1296.
39. Dixon HG, Scully ML, Wakefield MA, White VM, Crawford DA. The effects of television advertisements for junk food versus nutritious food on children's food attitudes and preferences. *Soc Sci Med.* 2007;65(7):1311–1323.
40. Wills TA, Sargent JD, Stoolmiller M, Gibbons FX, Worth KA, Cin SD. Movie exposure to smoking cues and adolescent smoking onset: a test for mediation through peer affiliations. *Health Psychol.* 2007;26(6):769–776.
41. Escobar-Chaves SL, Tortolero SR, Markham CM, Low BJ, Eitel P, Thickstun P. Impact of the media on adolescent sexual attitudes and behaviors. *Pediatrics.* 2005;116(1):303–326.
42. Lenhart A, Madden M, Macgill AR, Smith A. Teens and Social Media: the use of social media gains a greater foothold in teen life as they embrace the conversational nature of interactive online media. Pew Internet & American Life Project; 2007. Available at: http://www.pewinternet.org/PPF/r/230/report_display.asp. Accessed December 21, 2008.
43. Johnson KB, Ravert RD, Everton A. Hopkins teen central: assessment of an internet-based support system for children with cystic fibrosis. *Pediatrics.* 2001;107(2):e24.
44. Bers MU, Gonzalez-Heydrich J, Demaso DR. Use of a computer-based application in a pediatric hemodialysis unit: a pilot study. *J Am Acad Child Adolesc Psychiat.* 2003;42(4):493–496.
45. Committee on Communications, American Academy of Pediatrics, Strasburger VC. Children, adolescents, and advertising. *Pediatrics.* 2006;118(6):2563–2569.
46. Malesky LA Jr. Predatory online behavior: modus operandi of convicted sex offenders in identifying potential victims and contacting minors over the internet. *J Child Sex Abus.* 2007;16(2):23–32.
47. McGuinness TM. Dispelling the myth of bullying. *J Psychosoc Nurs Ment Health Serv.* 2007;45(10):19–22.
48. Kowalski RM, Limber SP. Electronic bullying among middle school students. *J Adolesc Health.* 2007;41(6 Suppl 1):S22–30.
49. Lenhert A. Cyberbullying and Online Teens. Pew Internet & American Life Project; 2007. Available at: http://www.pewinternet.org/PPF/r/216/report_display.asp. Accessed December 20, 2008.

50. American Academy of Pediatrics Committee on Public Education. Media violence. *Pediatrics*. 2001;108(5):1222–1226.
51. Brown Kirschman K, Smith GA. Resale of recalled children's products online: an examination of the world's largest yard sale. *Inj Prev* 2007;13(4):228–231.
52. Brown JD, Witherspoon EM. The mass media and American adolescents' health. *J Adolesc Health*. 2002;31(6 Suppl):153–170.
53. Villani VS, Olson CK, Jellinek MS. Media literacy for clinicians and parents. *Child Adolesc Psychiatr Clin N Am*. 2005;14(3):523–553.
54. American Academy of Pediatrics. SafetyNet; 2008. Available at: http://safetynet.aap.org/. Accessed December 21, 2008.
55. Walsh KE, Miller MR, Vinci RJ, Bauchner H. Pediatric resident education about medical errors. *Ambul Pediatr*. 2004;4(6):514–517.
56. Wenger E. Communities of Practice: A Brief Introduction; 2008. Available at: http://www.ewenger.com/theory/index.htm. Accessed November 22, 2008.

Chapter 36
Appendix: A Community of Child Health and Informatics

George R. Kim and Kevin B. Johnson

The following list of resources in informatics and child health, while far from exhaustive, provides pointers for interested learners to further resources and people.

36.1 Organizations: Pediatric-Medical Professional

The American Academy of Pediatrics (AAP): http://www.aap.org
The AAP is the professional medical organization for 60,000 pediatricians in the US and around the world. It represents the interests of children and pediatricians on many levels and publishes a number of professional journals and pediatric references, including Pediatrics and the Red Book (The Report of the Committee on Infectious Diseases). The AAP has member-driven groups that are involved in health IT include:

- The Council on Clinical Information Technology (COCIT) http://www.aapcocit.org

  COCIT provides resources on pediatric information technology, including input on policy statements on pediatric health IT, legislative updates on current bills and educational and networking tools such as the EMR Review, which is an online forum for pediatric practices to share their experiences about specific electronic health record products.

- The Section on Administration and Practice Management (SOAPM): http://www.aap.org/sections/soapm/soapm_home.cfm

  The mission of SOAPM is to "impart both basic and cutting edge administrative and practice management innovations" for its membership. It has resources for practice managers to share information on coding, compliance and employment laws and an active electronic mailing list of pediatricians in practice.

- The National Center of Medical Home Initiatives for Children with Special Needs http://www.medicalhomeinfo.org/index.html

  The Center provides leadership, information and tools to promote and develop Medical Homes. In 2008, AAP received in a federal grant to create the National

C.U. Lehmann et al. (eds.), *Pediatric Informatics: Computer Applications in Child Health,* Health Informatics,
© Springer Science+Business Media, LLC 2011

Center for Medical Home Implementation to support effective implementation of medical home among pediatric health care providers, public health professionals.

• Bright Futures http://brightfutures.aap.org/

Bright Futures is an AAP national health care promotion and disease prevention initiative funded by the Health Resources and Services Administration's (HRSA) Maternal and Child Health Bureau (MCHB) 'that "uses a developmentally based approach to address children's health needs in the context of family and community, structured in the form of the Bright Futures Toolkit, "an essential compendium of parent questionnaires, fact sheets, screening tools and other pediatric health supervision materials." '

The American Academy of Family Physicians (AAFP): http://www.centerforhit.org/

The mission of the AAFP is to improve the health of patients, families, and communities by serving the needs of its members with professionalism and creativity. The AAFP hosts a Center for Health Information Technology that is very active in promoting education and training for electronic record adoption among family practitioners.

36.2   Organizations: Medical Informatics and Information Technology

The American Medical Informatics Association (AMIA): http://www.amia.org

AMIA is a 30 year old organization that is "the professional home for biomedical and health informatics dedicated to promoting the effective organization, analysis, management, and use of information in health care in support of patient care, public health, teaching, research, administration, and related policy. AMIA members encompass an interdisciplinary and diverse group of individuals and organizations that represent over 65 countries." It publishes the Journal of the American Medical Informatics Association (JAMIA) and hosts a widely attended Annual Symposium. Its current work includes an effort to increase clinician education of informatics and to gain recognition of clinical informatics as a medical specialty.

The Healthcare Information and Management Systems Society (HIMSS) http://www.himss.org

HIMSS is "the healthcare industry's membership organization exclusively focused on providing global leadership for the optimal use of healthcare information technology (IT) and management systems for the betterment of healthcare. HIMSS represents over 300 corporate members that collectively represent organizations employing millions of people. HIMSS frames and leads healthcare public policy and industry practices through its advocacy, educational and professional development initiatives designed to promote information and management systems' contributions to ensuring quality patient care."

The American Health Information Management Association (AHIMA) http://www. ahima.org

AHIMA is a 52,000 member organization of health information management professionals. "Founded in 1928 to improve the quality of medical records, AHIMA is committed to advancing the health information management profession in an increasingly electronic and global environment through leadership in advocacy, education, certification, and lifelong learning."

The Medical Record Institute (MRI) http://www.medrecinst.com

Founded in 1983, MRI's vision is "an educational organization designed to stimulate the development of electronic medical records and electronic health records 'through health information technology.'" It hosts a number of recurring conferences, including the TEPR (Towards the Electronic Patient Record) Conference as the forum for sharing knowledge and experience about EMRs (and which presents awards for outstanding healthcare IT products for pediatric use).

The Certification Commission for Health care Information Technology (CCHIT) http://www.cchit.org

CCHIT is the "recognized certification body (RCB) for electronic health records and their networks, and an independent, voluntary, private-sector initiative. Its mission is to accelerate the adoption of health information technology by creating an efficient, credible and sustainable certification program." It currently includes pediatric certification in its list of processes.

36.3 Private Foundations

The Markle Foundation (Markle) http://www.markle.org

Markle "structures and operates projects in cooperation with our partners instead of working as a traditional grant-making organization." Connecting for Health is its public-private collaborative designed to address the barriers to development of an interconnected 'health information infrastructure "by driving" consensus on the adoption of an initial set of data standards, developing case studies on privacy and security, helping to define the electronic personal health record (PHR)" and developing an incremental Roadmap to achieve healthcare connectivity.

The eHealth Initiative http://www.ehealthinitiative.org

The eHealth Initiative and its Foundation are independent, nonprofit organizations that seek to drive improvement in the quality, safety, and efficiency of health care through information and information technology by engaging multiple stakeholders to define and then implement specific actions related to quality and safety related to information technology.

36.4 Federal Agencies Involved in Health Care and Information Management

The National Library of Medicine (NLM) http://www.nlm.nih.gov

The NLM, at the National Institutes of Health in Bethesda, Maryland, "is the world's largest medical library, with materials in all areas of biomedicine and health care, as well as works on biomedical aspects of technology, the humanities, and the physical, life, and social sciences." It produces PubMed®, MedlinePlus®, the Genetics Home Reference and a number of other medical information databases for public use. It supports medical informatics research and training on-site at the Lister Hill National Center for Biomedical Communications and through university-based training programs at many institutions throughout the US (http://www.nlm.nih.gov/ep/GrantTrainInstitute.html) that lead in clinical information technology development.

The National Cancer Institute (NCI) https://cabig.nci.nih.gov/overview

The NCI develops and hosts a number of resources for practitioners and the public on cancer. In addition to the PDQ online cancer database for adult and pediatric cancers (http://www.cancer.gov/cancertopics/pdq/pediatrictreatment), NCI is developing caBIG®, the cancer Biomedical Informatics Grid®, which is an "information network enabling all constituencies in the cancer community – researchers, physicians, and patients – to share data and knowledge."

The Centers for Disease Control and Prevention (CDC) http://www.cdc.gov

The CDC is the federal agency involved in developing an informatics and IT infrastructure relevant to public health issues, including population bio-surveillance of disease such as cancer and infectious diseases. It also hosts public health informatics training programs for health professionals.

The Agency for Healthcare Research and Quality (AHRQ) http://www.ahrq.gov

AHRQ's initiative on health information technology (health IT) is "a key element to the nation's 10-year strategy to advance the use of information technology ... It includes grants and contracts in to support and stimulate investment in health IT, especially in rural and underserved areas, to identify challenges to health IT adoption and use, solutions and best practices for making health IT work and tools that will help hospitals and clinicians successfully incorporate new IT ... As part of the initiative, AHRQ created the National Resource Center for Health Information Technology. In addition to providing technical assistance, the Center shares new knowledge and findings that have the potential to transform everyday clinical practice."

The Office of the National Coordinator for Health Information Technology (ONC) http://www.hhs.gov/healthit/onc/mission/

The ONC provides counsel to the Secretary of HHS and DHHS leadership on developing and implementing an interoperable national health information technology infrastructure to improve the quality, safety and efficiency of health care and the ability of consumers to manage their health information and health care. It also provides support for the American Health Information Community (AHIC), a federally-chartered advisory committee that advises the Secretary of HHS on digital and interoperable records to encourage market-led adoption and ensure their privacy and security (Adapted from the ONC Website).

Index